Fifth Edition

Certification Exam Review

for Pharmacy Technicians

Sarah M. Lawrence

Cheryl Aiken

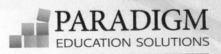

PARADIGM
EDUCATION SOLUTIONS

A DIVISION OF KENDALL HUNT

Minneapolis • Dubuque

VP of Content Strategy: Christine Hurney
Executive Acquiring Editor: Nancy Roberts
Development Editor: Brian Farrey-Latz
Director of Marketing: Keri Haas
Marketing and Communications Manager: Selena Hicks
Digital Project Manager: Tom Modl
Director of Publishing Services: Wendy S. Jochum
Publishing Specialist Supervisor: Carrie A. Maro
Supervisor of Prepress and Manufacturing: Cari M. Rieckens
Publishing Specialist: Nick Carolan
Designer: Jack Ross

Care has been taken to verify the accuracy of information presented in this book. However, the authors, editors, and publisher cannot accept responsibility for web, email, newsgroup, or chat room subject matter or content, or for consequences from the application of the information in this book, and make no warranty, expressed or implied, with respect to its content.

Trademarks: Some of the product names and company names included in this book have been used for identification purposes only and may be trademarks or registered trade names of their respective manufacturers and sellers. The authors, editors, and publisher disclaim any affiliation, association, or connection with, or sponsorship or endorsement by, such owners.

Photo Credits: Following the index

We have made every effort to trace the ownership of all copyrighted material and to secure permission from copyright holders. In the event of any question arising as to the use of any material, we will be pleased to make the necessary corrections in future printings. Thanks are due to the authors, publishers, and agents listed in the Photo Credits for permission to use the materials therein indicated.

Cover image © Shutterstock.com

© 2021 Paradigm Education Solutions, a division of Kendall Hunt
7900 Xerxes Avenue S STE 310
Minneapolis, MN 55431-1118
Email: CustomerService@ParadigmEducation.com
Website: ParadigmEducation.com

ISBN: 978-0-7638-9305-7

Published in the United States of America

Brief Contents

* Study Supplements that can be accessed through the eBook/Cirrus include: Top 200 Drugs, Top Hospital Drugs, Vulnerable Populations Resources and Drugs to Avoid, Common Palliative Care and Hospice Drugs, HIPAA Regulations Pertaining to Pharmacy Medical Terminology, and Tips for Multicultural Healthcare Service.

Table of Contents

Chapter 7
Sterile and Hazardous
Compounding 209

Chapter 8
Pharmacy Inventory Management . . . 239

Certification Exam Review for Pharmacy Technicians
What Makes This New Edition Exciting?

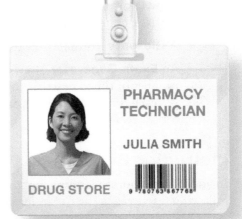

As a pharmacy technician, you want to build knowledge and establish a skills base for exceptional, safe service to patients. With certification, you will be able to continually advance in your career. *Certification Exam Review for Pharmacy Technicians,* Fifth Edition, has been updated to help you accomplish these goals. The Fifth edition features include:

- Alignment with PTCE domains and ExCPT topical areas, covering the subjects in a logical order and clear language
- Convenient eBook with study and assessment materials that are easily accessed through eBook links for the self-study course and through the Cirrus learning platform for the instructor-guided course
- Numerous information tables and appendixes for organized studying and memorization
- Leading pharmacy topics covered in the rigorous certification exams
- Extensive instructor input in every aspect of the new edition
- Web links for additional online pharmacy resources.
- Helpful margin features:

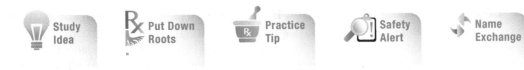

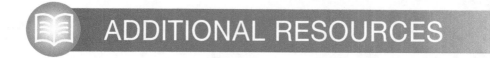

The following student resources can be accessed through eBook links. The only exception is that students enrolled in an instructor-guided course may only access their chapter tests through the Cirrus learning management system.

- **Supplemental Resources** include lists of Top 200 Drugs, Most Common Hospital Drugs, Common Palliative Care and Hospice Drugs, Vulnerable Populations Resources and Drugs to Avoid, HIPAA Regulations, and other useful study resources based on the most recommended pharmaceutical and medical websites.

- **New Digital Flash Card Sets** on pharmacy laws, generic/brand drug names, drug suffixes, controlled substances, and other information make studying these topics easy.

- A **Glossary** compiles key terms and definitions in one easy-to-access document.

- An **Exam Generator** draws from a test bank of +1,000 questions and offers an infinite number of timed practice exams that simulate the PTCE with similar amounts of questions per each domain. Students can take a new exam as often as they like to judge their readiness for the real exam.

Instructor Resources

In addition to course planning materials, instructors receive the following resources in the Cirrus learning management system:

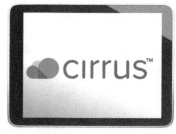

- **PowerPoint Slides** highlight key points of chapter content and can be downloaded and customized to meet your course needs.

- **Prebuilt Chapter Tests and Final Answer Keys** may be edited and instructors may add to these prebuilt tests directly in Cirrus or by importing the provided RTF files into your own learning management system.

About the Authors

Sarah M. Lawrence

Sarah M. Lawrence, PharmD, MA, BCGP has over 15 years of experience in the profession of pharmacy, as a technician, intern, and pharmacist. Her pharmacy experience includes community pharmacy, corporate long-term care, medical education, and academia. She is board certified in Geriatrics. Dr. Lawrence served as program director of an ASHP-accredited pharmacy technician program and in 2019 was awarded the Roy Kemp Award, which recognizes the national pharmacy technician educator of the year. She has taught students at all levels of higher education, including undergraduate, masters, and doctoral students. Dr. Lawrence works as a medical grant writer and pharmacy technician educational consultant for Knowfully Learning Group, a leading provider of continuing education. Dr. Lawrence served as national president of the Pharmacy Technician Educators Council from 2019 - 2020.

Cheryl Aiken

Cheryl Aiken, BS, PharmD, RPh, is an assistant manager and pharmacy informatics specialist at the Brattleboro Retreat, a private psychiatric hospital in Brattleboro, Vermont. In addition to her work in the psychiatric field, she has served as a community pharmacist for independent and chain pharmacies, and as a staff pharmacist at the Brattleboro Memorial Hospital. She serves as the preceptor for IPPE and APPE Pharmacy Interns from Albany College of Pharmacy, Western New England College of Pharmacy and Husson University. In 2002, she helped establish an associate's degree and the Pharmacy Technician Training Program certificate at Vermont Technical College.

Acknowledgements

The quality of this body of work is a testament to the many contributors and reviewers who participated in the creation of *Certification Exam Review for Pharmacy Technicians,* Fifth Edition. We offer a heartfelt thank-you for your commitment to producing high-quality instructional materials for pharmacy technician students.

Textbook Consultants and Reviewer

Sara Byars, BS, CPhT, Ph, TR is the Lead Faculty and Clinical Liaison for the Pharmacy Technician department of San Jacinto Community College's North Campus in Houston, TX, and also holds the role of primary advisor of the Phi Theta Kappa Honors Organization's Alpha Alpha Omega Chapter. She graduated with honors and holds a bachelor's degree in Analytical Chemistry from Sam Houston State University in Huntsville, TX. She has been a certified and registered pharmacy technician for 14 years, and teaching in this discipline for eight. Her specialties lie in retail, long-term care, and compounding pharmacy, and she is very active in the Pharmacy Technician Educators Council (PTEC).

Nicole Barriera, CPhT, became a pharmacy technician in 2001 and PTCB-certified in 2003. In 2007, Nicole became the department chair and program coordinator for the ASHP/ACPE-accredited pharmacy technician program at Pikes Peak Community College in Colorado Springs, Colorado. She became certified in extemporaneous compounding, credentialed in online pedagogy, and trained in providing IV certification and education. Her program was recognized with the Outstanding CTE Program award by the state of Colorado in 2009. It was the first accredited program to offer an Advanced Pharmacy Practice Certificate in the state and it remains the only Associate of Applied Science (AAS) degree in Pharmacy Technology available in Colorado.

Test Bank Reviewers

Melissa Burgess, CPhT—LVT Program Coordinator of the Pharmacy Technology and Health Science Technology Programs at West Kentucky Community and Technical College in Paducah, KY

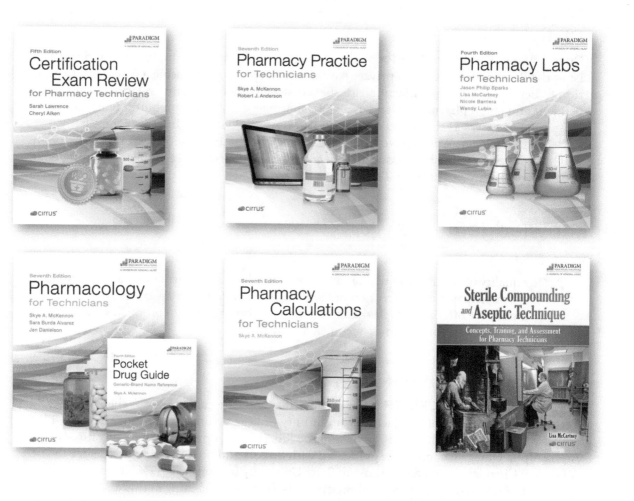

Paradigm's Comprehensive Pharmacy Technician Series

In addition to *Certification Exam Review for Pharmacy Technicians*, Fifth Edition, Paradigm Education Solutions.
offers other titles designed specifically for the pharmacy technician curriculum.

- *Pharmacy Practice for Technicians*, Seventh Edition
- *Pharmacy Labs for Technicians*, Fourth Edition
- *Pharmacology for Technicians*, Seventh Edition
- *Pocket Drug Guide: Generic Brand Name Reference*, Fourth Edition
- *Pharmacy Calculations for Technicians*, Seventh Edition
- *Sterile Compounding and Aseptic Technique* Second Edition
- *Career Readiness & Externships: Soft Skills for Pharmacy Technicians* to the list.

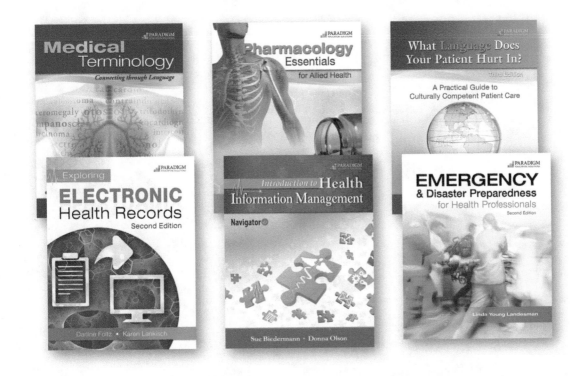

Additional Health Careers Courseware

The following learning solutions are particularly useful for pharmacy technicians:

- *Medical Terminology: Connecting through Language*
- *Emergency & Disaster Preparedness for Health Professionals*, Second Edition
- *Pharmacology Essentials for Allied Health*
- *What Language Does Your Patient Hurt In?: A Practical Guide to Culturally Competent Care*, Third Edition
- *Exploring Electronic Health Records*
- *Introduction to Health Information Management*

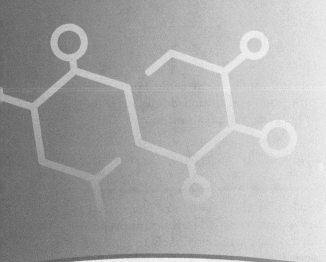

INTRODUCTION
Preparing for a High-Stakes Exam

Learning Objectives

1 Discuss the importance of certification for a pharmacy technician.

2 Explain the elements of certification, registration, and licensure.

3 Describe the major testing components of the PTCE and ExCPT examinations.

4 Make a study plan for the examination.

5 Use techniques for successfully taking a multichoice examination.

A certification exam is a nationally recognized test used to measure competency in a professional area of practice. The exam's purpose is to protect the public interest by evaluating candidates' knowledge in a specific area. In this case, it is the knowledge necessary to perform the duties of a pharmacy technician. A nongovernmental agency develops the exam and implements the rules and policies related to certification based on criteria for the profession.

Certification Exam Review for Pharmacy Technicians, Fifth Edition, is intended to help you study for and pass a pharmacy technician certification exam. Two national exams are offered: the **Pharmacy Technician Certification Exam (PTCE)** and the **Exam for the Certification of Pharmacy Technicians (ExCPT)**. Individual states may recognize just the PTCE or both exams. Check your state's requirements before deciding which exam to take.

Certification recognizes that an individual has met predetermined qualifications in a specific area of study. A technician who successfully passes the exam may use the designation Certified Pharmacy Technician (CPhT) after his or her name. The Pharmacy Technician Certification Board's (PTCB's) associate director, William Schimmel, explained to an interviewer for *Pharmacy Times* that "national certification becomes a portable credential that can travel from state to state and job to job." Employers place a considerable value on certification because it demonstrates your knowledge as a technician and your commitment to your role in pharmacy. As we see things change in the profession and advanced roles for technicians open up, certification will open a number of new opportunities.

Why Become Certified?

Pharm Facts

According to the National Pharmacy Technician Association, there are more than 39,000 jobs for technicians available every year!

In a 2016 survey by the Pharmacy Workforce Center, three-fourths of pharmacy customers said that they would choose a pharmacy with certified technicians over one that does not have them. Parents with children were particularly likely to state this. These customers, and their employers, understand fully how the effective and safe delivery of pharmaceuticals depends on competent and knowledgeable technicians. Through certification, pharmacy technicians have demonstrated the ability, knowledge, and skills necessary to function effectively in a pharmacy team.

With certification, you become a marketable sales asset to any pharmacy, assisting in the care of patients and the success of the business or healthcare institution. You are open to increased responsibilities, job opportunities, and promotions, along with increased respect from your peers. In addition, certification offers a sense of accomplishment and the potential for greater job satisfaction.

As the profession of pharmacy advances, providing ever more medication therapy management and healthcare services, the possible career advancement opportunities multiply. There is an increasing need for qualified pharmacy technicians of many different experiences and skill sets ready to take on duties in pharmacy management, tech-check-tech roles, medication history profiles, medication reconciliation, insurance and billing, inventory, pharmacy informatics, patient assistance, hazardous drug handling, and nonsterile, sterile, and hazardous compounding.

State Practice Requirements

State pharmacy boards determine whether pharmacy technicians need to be registered, licensed, and/or certified. State requirements for pharmacy technicians may include one or all of these components. Many states stipulate a maximum ratio of technicians (including pharmacy interns) to pharmacists, which varies from 2:1 to 4:1. The ratio may be dependent on the number of certified pharmacy technicians employed at a site. Some states may use a higher technician-to-pharmacist ratio if at least one technician is certified. Only four states did not have laws regulating pharmacy technicians as of mid-2020: Wisconsin, Pennsylvania, New York, and Hawaii, but likely it is only a matter of time until they do.

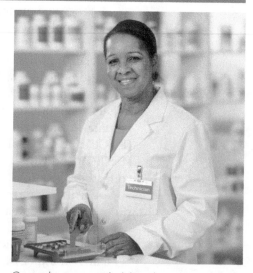

Once pharmacy technicians have passed their certification exam, they can proudly where the designation of CPhT.

Registration

In the majority of states, pharmacy technicians are required to be "registered," or listed on the state board of pharmacy's official list of pharmacy technicians before starting to practice in any licensed pharmacy. This is a way to control access to the restricted area of the pharmacy and track who is permitted to assist the pharmacist. Pharmacy technicians who are not registered, or have allowed their registration to lapse, cannot legally work in the restricted pharmacy area in these states.

Another of the main reasons for registration is to report and monitor any serious disciplinary action (such as stealing drugs or money) before the disciplined technician applies for another pharmacy technician job or is hired at another pharmacy within or outside the state. If a technician changes employment within the state, he or she must notify the board of pharmacy. Registration cannot be reciprocated or transferred to another state. States have varying continuing education requirements for annual re-registration.

There is no test required for registration, but the process generally includes an application to the state board of pharmacy and payment of appropriate fees. The application process may include a background check. Registration may be denied if the applicant has a history of criminal activity or charges related to drugs or alcohol use. Registration will be denied or revoked for actions that compromise the lawful activities of a pharmacy, and the state may levy fines against pharmacies that allow unregistered individuals in restricted areas. A majority of states also have training requirements, but these are not yet standardized across the states.

Licensure

Some states require pharmacy technicians to be licensed. Licensure is a more rigorous application process than registration. The process varies by state. Passing a licensure exam is often a key component. The license exam may be on state pharmacy laws or on the state laws plus practice in general. In addition, the license applicants may need to be certified and/or a graduate (associate degree or higher) of an accredited college program specializing in pharmacy technology. Individual states also have continuing education requirements for license renewal.

Visit your state board of pharmacy website for information on individual state requirements. To learn more about state licensure requirements, visit the National Association of Boards of Pharmacy website at http://CertExam5e.ParadigmEducation.com/napb/pharmacyboards and click on Boards of Pharmacy.

Certification

By seeking to pass a certification exam, you are ahead of the game. More than half the states have made national certification either mandatory or preferred for licensure or practice, and the number of states making this a requirement is continuing to grow. In states with fewer requirements, employers often make certification a requirement to promote medication safety and efficiency.

There are strong financial reasons to become certified. Community pharmacies increasingly expect their technicians to be certified; it may be a requirement for initial employment (especially in large hospitals) or strongly encouraged within the first year of employment. Sometimes the cost of the exam and even training are covered for a valued employee.

Most hospital pharmacies require certification and will often expect prior experience or advanced training, especially if the technician will be working with sterile IV products and chemotherapy. Hospital accreditation depends on trained staffing. Some hospitals offer their own training or a monetary incentive for certification.

Successful completion of a national certification exam qualifies you to work in a variety of pharmacy settings including retail, institutional, mail order, administration, and educational. Employer-specific examinations, such as those offered by some chain pharmacies may test an individual's ability to work in one specific pharmacy environment, but those exams are generally not comprehensive enough to demonstrate the skills needed to work in many different pharmacy environments. If certification is required, the state board of pharmacy determines which certification exam(s) will be accepted.

Choose the Right Exam

A certification exam for pharmacy technicians is a high-stakes, professional exam. The exam is similar to other high-level prerequisite tests, such as those for college or graduate school. To successfully complete the PTCE or ExCPT, you must become proficient in the knowledge and skills necessary to be a pharmacy technician and practice good test-taking strategies.

Certification Exam Review for Pharmacy Technicians, Fifth Edition, is designed to prepare you for either test you choose. It includes 8 chapters that review the content of the PTCE and the ExCPT. Overviews of the PTCE and ExCPT test plans and their domains are shown in Tables 0.1 and 0.2 on the next pages.

Pharm Facts

The PTCE is the more long-standing and recognized of the two tests. It has been offered since 1995.

Pharmacy Technician Certification Exam

The longstanding recognized national certification is the Pharmacy Technician Certification Exam (PTCE), sponsored by the Pharmacy Technician Certification Board. The examination grew out of efforts by two states (Michigan and Illinois), the American Society of Health-System Pharmacists, and the American Pharmacy Association to develop technician standards. The board developed the PTCE based on task analyses of the actual work of pharmacy technicians in both the retail and hospital pharmacy settings. In 2001, the National Association of Boards of Pharmacy joined this coalition to offer a certification program for pharmacy technicians.

The PTCE for pharmacy technician certification is accepted by all 50 states and the District of Columbia as a legitimate certification for the profession, and in almost half of the states it is the only test mentioned as a practice standard. Since 1995, the PTCB has granted over 700,000 certifications.

Exam for the Certification of Pharmacy Technicians

An additional test evolved out of the efforts of the National Community Pharmacists Association and the National Association of Chain Drug Stores. The Exam for the Certification of Pharmacy Technicians (ExCPT) is offered through the NHA, which offers other health career certification exams as well. The ExCPT is similar in content to the PTCE and is accepted by the majority of states.

Test and Certification Eligibility

The PTCE and ExCPT have different eligibility requirements. Candidates should consult the official requirements for each exam to confirm eligibility.

TABLE 0.1 PTCE Testing Content—90 Questions (80 Scored)

Chapter	Domain	Description	Weight
Chapter 1	Medications	**1.1** Generic names, brand names, and classifications of medications	40%
		1.2 Therapeutic equivalence	
		1.3 Common and life-threatening drug interactions and contraindications (e.g., drug-disease, drug-drug, drug-dietary supplement, drug-laboratory, drug-nutrient)	
		1.4* Strengths/dose, dosage forms, routes of administration, special handling and administration instructions, and duration of drug therapy	
		1.5 Common and severe medication side effects, adverse effects, and allergies	
		1.6 Indications of medications and dietary supplements	
		1.7 Drug stability (e.g. oral suspensions, insulin, reconstitutables, injectables, vaccinations)	
		1.8 Narrow therapeutic index (NTI) medications	
		1.9 Physical and chemical incompatibilities related to non-sterile compounding and reconstitution	
		1.10 Proper storage of medications (e.g. temperature ranges, light sensitivity, restricted access)	
Chapter 2	Federal Requirements	**2.1** Federal requirements for handling and disposal of non-hazardous, hazardous, and pharmaceutical substances and waste	12.5%
		2.2* Federal requirements for controlled substance prescriptions (i.e., new, refill, transfer) and DEA controlled substances schedules	
		2.3 Federal requirements (e.g., DEA, FDA) for controlled substances (i.e., receiving, storing, ordering, labeling, dispensing, reverse distribution, take-back programs, and loss or theft of)	
		2.4* Federal requirements for restricted drug programs and related medication processing (e.g., pseudoephedrine, Risk Evaluation and Mitigation Strategies [REMS])	
		2.5 FDA recall requirements (e.g. medications, devices, supplies, supplements, classifications)	
Chapter 3	Patient Safety and Quality Assurance	**3.1** High-alert/risk medications and look alike/sound-alike [LASA] medications	26.25%
		3.2 Error prevention strategies (e.g., prescription or medication order to correct patient, Tall Man lettering, separating inventory, leading and trailing zeros, bar code usage, limit use of error-prone abbreviations)	
		3.3* Issues that require pharmacist intervention (e.g., drug utilization review [DUR], adverse drug event [ADE], OTC recommendation, therapeutic substitution, misuse, adherence, post-immunization follow-up, allergies, drug interactions)	
		3.4 Event reporting procedures, (e.g., medication errors, adverse effects, and product integrity, MedWatch, near miss, root-cause analysis [RCA])	
		3.5* Types of prescription errors (e.g. abnormal doses, early refill, incorrect quantity, incorrect patient, incorrect drug)	
		3.6 Hygiene and cleaning standards (e.g., handwashing, personal protective equipment [PPE], cleaning counting trays, countertop, and equipment)	

continues

TABLE 0.1 PTCE Testing Content—90 Questions (80 Scored)—Continued

Chapter	Domain	Description	Weight
Chapter 4	Order Entry and Processing	4.1* Procedures to compound non-sterile products (e.g., ointments, mixtures, liquids, emulsions, suppositories, enemas) 4.2* Formulas, calculations, ratios, proportions, alligations, conversions, Sig codes (e.g., bid, tid, Roman numerals), abbreviations, medical terminology, and symbols for days supply, quantity, dose, concentration, dilutions 4.3* Equipment/supplies required for drug administration (e.g., package size, unit dose, diabetic supplies, spacers, oral and injectable syringes) 4.4* Lot numbers, expiration dates, and National Drug Code (NDC) numbers 4.5 Procedures for identifying and returning dispensable, non-dispensable, and expired medications and supplies (e.g., credit return, return to stock, reverse distribution)	21.25%

*Domain may require calculation knowledge (addressed in Chapter 5).

TABLE 0.2 ExCPT Testing Plan—100 questions (and 20 Pretest Questions)

Chapter	Domain	Description	Weight
Chapter 2 Chapter 8	Overview and Laws	• Role, Scope of Practice, and General Duties of the Pharmacy Technician • Laws and Regulations • Controlled Substances	25%
Chapter 1	Drugs and Drug Therapy	• Drug Classification • Frequently Prescribed Medications	15%
Chapter 4 Chapter 5 Chapter 6 Chapter 7	Dispensing Process	• Prescription and Medication Order Intake and Entry • Preparing and Dispensing Prescriptions • Calculations • Sterile and Nonsterile Products, Compounding, Unit Dose, and Repackaging	45%
Chapter 3	Medication Safety and Quality Assurance		15%

PTCE Eligibility and Scheduling

To be eligible to apply for PTCB CPhT Certification, candidates must complete one of two pathways. Applicants can complete a PTCB-recognized education/training program or demonstrate equivalent work as a pharmacy technician (minimum 500 hours). In addition, candidates must disclose all criminal and State Board of Pharmacy registration or licensure actions and comply with all applicable PTCB certification policies.

The PTCE is a computer-based test offered at Pearson Professional testing centers. Each certification exam testing site has a secure, comfortable, properly lit, temperature-controlled environment. You will be given one hour and fifty minutes to complete the 90-question examination.

The PTCE is organized into four domains or sections, each of which is weighted differently. Skills and knowledge from both the community and institutional settings are required to pass this examination, including basic compounding knowledge and skills. Out of the 90 multiple choice questions, only 80 are scored. Each question comes with four possible choices. Only one answer is correct. *You should answer every question whether you are sure of the answer or not*, because the final score is based on the total number of questions answered correctly rather than the percentage of correct answers. Educated guesses are encouraged. After the exam, in the final 10 minutes, you will take a post-exam survey and receive your unofficial results onsite.

ExCPT Eligibility and Scheduling

Pharm Facts

ExCPT candidates must have a high school diploma or GED/high school equivalency, or be within 60 days of earning either.

In addition to the secondary education requirement, all ExCPT candidates must have completed a pharmacy technician training program from a state-recognized institution within the past five years. In lieu of this, you can have passed an employer-based academic training program that has been approved by the state board of pharmacy or have 1,200 hours of employer-supervised, pharmacy-related experience within any one year of the past three years. Those with pharmacy-related training in the military are also eligible. The student must prepare a "candidate profile" and agree to an attestation statement before sitting for the exam.

The ExCPT is generally offered as a computer-based examination. Test takers are given two hours and ten minutes to complete the 100 multiple-choice questions (and 20 pretest questions) from a large test bank.

The ExCPT is organized into four domains, each of which is weighted differently. Skills and knowledge from both the institutional and community settings are required to pass this examination, including basic calculation knowledge. Out of 120 questions, only 100 are scored. As with the PTCE, you should answer every question and educated guesses are encouraged.

Test Preparation Strategies

Preparation is an important part of taking a high-stakes exam. There are three areas of preparation: study, preparation for thorough knowledge of the subjects, and test-taking skills. This section discusses important exam preparation skills and strategies. The main chapters review the pharmacy knowledge and skills needed by technicians interwoven with study ideas.

Practice exams can help to determine where to focus your study efforts. That is why *Certification Exam Review for Pharmacy Technicians*, Fifth Edition, offers end-of-chapter and final test with exam-like questions and an end-of-course test generator that provides a nearly infinite number of timed mock exams with the same proportion of questions per domain, depending on which exam is being taken.

How and When to Study

Study Idea

Do not cram at the last minute—set up a study schedule over the course of a few weeks to prepare for the exam.

Do not wait to study until just before the exam. Talk to graduates from your program and other certified pharmacy technicians about their experiences studying for and taking the exam and get their tips. Cramming raises test anxiety and harms the memory. Start studying now to become familiar with the skills and concepts on the exam.

Budget Time to Study

Make a timeline and plan, schedule in a few hours each day to study uninterrupted by family or friends. Spread your review over a period of weeks. Focused reviews conducted over time are more effective than cramming at the last minute. As a certified pharmacy technician, you will use this information for years to come, not just on the exam. By developing your skills and knowledge slowly over time, you will retain more information and improve your recall in the future.

Study Idea

Carry your flash cards with you wherever you go, and any time you have a few minutes, review the drug brand and generic names.

Study Resources

Study well all the tables in each chapter and the appendices, memorizing some. This course also includes other key supplements, such as "Top 200 Drugs, "HIPAA Regulations," Common Drugs to Avoid for Vulnerable Populations," and others. These can be accessed through eBook links. Additional resources include digital flashcards and a full book glossary. Then at the end of the course, take the final and generate timed exams to simulate the actual exam experience. The Paradigm Health Careers *Drugs & Terms* smartphone app can help you study generic and brand drug names and medical terms.

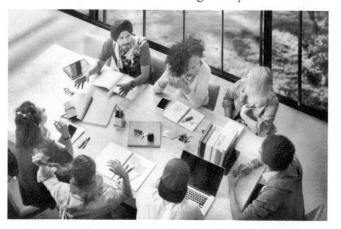

Study groups help provide associates for encouragement and to hold each other accountable for set times to study.

Study Groups

Study groups can also be an effective way to review and discuss information. If you work in a pharmacy, ask your colleagues for help. If you do not work in a pharmacy, ask a local pharmacy if you may shadow one of their technicians. (You may do this through your program or have to register with the state board of pharmacy to be behind the pharmacy counter.) Getting hands-on experience to observe and assist in the work of practicing pharmacists and pharmacy technicians is an excellent way to study for the exam.

Ask your instructors to identify areas where you need to focus your attention. If you know a pharmacist well or work with one, ask for help in areas like pharmacology and pharmacy calculations.

Practice Tip

Remember, the name on your identification must be identical to the name provided to the testing center when you registered.

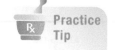

Study Idea

Form a study group with others studying to work out problems together, share tips, and quiz each other with flash cards.

Develop Relaxation Techniques

Taking a high-stakes professional exam can be stressful. Cheer yourself on like an athlete, and practice relaxation techniques if you start feeling anxious to keep your mind clear. Deep breathing, positive thinking, and visualization exercises can help prepare the body and mind for the challenge and allow you to focus on studying and the exam questions. It may be helpful to drive by the test site before the exam to become familiar with the area so you know where it is.

Prepare in Advance for Test Day

Think of preparing for the exam as you would for a trip. Get the proper directions and know where you will park if you are driving there. The night before the exam, pack all the items needed for the test. Depending on which exam you take, you will need a government-issued photo identification, such as a valid passport, driver's license, US

Armed Forces identification card, or nondriver identification issued by your state Department of Motor Vehicles. (The Take Note on page 12 lists approved IDs.)

Pack only the necessary items. You will not need pencils, paper, calculator, phone, or anything else. Anything needed to take the exam will be provided at the test site. You will be supplied with a secure locker to store items not permitted in the exam area. No electronic devices such as cell phones, tablets, or calculators are allowed in the testing room. Calculators will be provided online or will be available upon request from the testing monitor.

Pharm Facts

Tissues, earplugs, and noise-canceling headphones must be provided by the testing center for the PTCE, if needed.

Follow Good Sleeping and Eating Habits

The night before the exam, do not pull an all-nighter cramming for the exam. Get a good night's sleep. Set the alarm and wake up on time, refreshed and ready. Eat a nutritious meal or snack before the test to help maintain energy. Avoid eating high-fat foods or excessive sugar before the exam, as these foods can make you groggy or sleepy in the middle of the test.

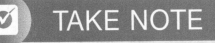

TAKE NOTE

Be sure to bring valid identification, which is defined as an unexpired, government-issued ID that has a photograph and signature. If the identification does not include a signature, a secondary ID will be required. This could be a social security card, credit/debit/ATM card, or employee/school ID. The testing center may also require biometric identification, such as a fingerprint scan or a palm vein scan.

The Day of the Exam

Don't be afraid of the exam or that feeling of pretest jitters. They show instead that your body and mind are recognizing a challenge and are preparing to meet it, like an athlete before a race. So don't fear it; lean into it and use the energy. Use the sense of stress to motivate yourself to study ahead of time, and understand that stress is a natural part of the process and should be used as an asset to help you focus.

Breathe, breathe, breathe, and stretch before you sit down, just like an athlete. Be on the top of your game, and go for it! Your mind, which has been trained and prepared, will run for you and do that exam.

Study Idea

Allow plenty of time to get there, even if you have to wait. It is better to not have the stress of cutting it close, and you can study while you wait, stretching your mind like an athlete stretches the body before going into a race.

Arrive Early

On the day of the scheduled exam, you should arrive 30 minutes early (having made sure ahead of time that you have the directions and know where to park). Getting lost and/or missing the starting time will result in the cancellation of your appointment and loss of your exam fee.

Table 0.3 provides a list of key things to do on the day of the exam.

TABLE 0.3 The Day of the Exam

Get enough sleep the night before the test. Also, make sure to get adequate sleep the week before the test.

Dress casually and comfortably. Take extra time to plan what to wear.

Check the directions to the site and bring the proper ID(s) and anything else necessary.

Arrive at the testing center early, and choose a comfortable work area.

Before the test, go the bathroom.

Pump yourself up and tell yourself you can do it! Breathe deep to fill your brain with oxygen, and do this any time you feel stressed while taking the test.

The Testing Environment

Study Idea

Test stress can be good! It can help you rise to the challenge. Become your own cheerleader for this event. You can do it!

At the exam site, you will be provided with an erasable board to serve as a scratch pad. A calculator will be available on the exam computer. Practice with and become proficient using your computer's calculator so this does not slow you down during the exam. You are not allowed to ask the exam site staff questions concerning the test content. There are no scheduled breaks. If you must leave the testing area to use the restroom, you will not be given additional time to complete the test. You must present identification to re-enter the test area. Remember, cell phones, calculators, recording devices, and photography equipment are not allowed in the test area.

You will be given time to view a tutorial before the exam. You must agree to all PTCB or NHA testing policies prior to starting the appropriate exam. You may download the tutorial in advance from the Pearson VUE website: http://CertExam5e. ParadigmEducation.com/Pearson-tutorial. This may help to reduce test anxiety.

Tips for Taking Multiple-Choice Tests

Study Idea

Slow down and read the entire question to make sure you know what the question is asking before answering. You can guess on an answer and flag it; then after you have finished them all, go back for second thoughts.

One of the advantages of taking a multiple-choice test is that the correct answer is provided in the list of possible answers. There is no penalty for guessing. Pace yourself so you can answer every question. If you are unsure of the correct answer, follow some standard test-taking tips to choose a best-guess response.

- Plan your time. You will have two hours to answer 90 multiple-choice questions for the PTCE, or 2 hours and 10 minutes for 100 multiple choice questions and 20 pretest questions for the ExCPT. Do not get stuck on a troublesome question. If you are not sure of an answer that doesn't require calculations, answer the question in 30 to 60 seconds, select an answer, flag the question, and move on. Return to the question later.

- Read the whole question before answering. Make sure you understand what the question is, and take the question at face value. Do not waste time looking for trick questions.

- *Answer the question in your head before reviewing the choices.* This will prevent you from being influenced by the answers provided.

- Remember there is *only one best answer listed*, although more than one answer may appear to be correct. So look for the most complete answer. When writing multiple-choice questions, one correct answer and three distractors are provided. The distractors are usually terms you know but are not fully correct.

- *If you do not know the answer, use a process of elimination.* Eliminate the most obviously wrong answer first, then the second, and make your best decision from the remaining two choices. This tactic gives you a 50% chance of selecting the correct answer.

- In calculation questions, the distractors may use the correct numbers in incorrect ways and often include answers you might get if you are unsure how to do the calculation or make a mistake with the decimal point. Solving the problem before you look at the choices provided helps eliminate distractors.

- Do not look for patterns in the answers. Computerized tests are written without concern for answer placement.

- If you are still unsure of the correct answer, select the longer or more descriptive answer of the remaining choices, although a good test writer will make all of the answers approximately the same length.

- If the answer set presents a range of numbers and you are not sure of the correct answer, it often works to eliminate the highest and lowest choices and select from the middle range of numbers.

- Watch out for negative words in a question. Be alert for words such as *not* or *except* or *only*. These questions ask you to identify the false statement instead of the true statement. Read the question carefully and make sure you understand what is asked.

- Beware of questions and answers that contain absolutes, such as *always*, *never*, *must*, *all*, and *none*, which severely limit the meaning of the item. Answers that contain absolutes are often incorrect except in terms of safety, aseptic procedures, and identifying the strictest laws.

- Become familiar with the computerized timed testing process and take simulated practice tests with the eBook's exam generator. It is there to help you get comfortable with the exam process.

- If you feel a question is ambiguous, misleading, or deficient in accuracy or content, fill out the comment section at the end of exam. This may help your grade if the question is found to be faulty.

Table 0.4 summarizes some key tips to consider while taking the certification exam.

TABLE 0.4 During the Exam

Listen, read, and follow directions carefully.
Read each question carefully. Do not skim or you can miss key words, especially negatives! Make sure to follow the computer screen prompts.
Answer easy questions first, and come back to the more difficult questions.
Never leave a question unanswered. Use the process of elimination! There is no penalty for guessing.
Manage your time.
Change your answer only if you are certain you made a mistake. Your first answer is usually correct.
Do not leave the testing area unless you must.

After the Exam

After completing the exam, you will receive your results immediately as pass or fail. Your numerical score will be sent to you or made available online at a later date. Each exam has its own scoring system.

If you do not pass the exam on the first attempt, identify why you think you did not pass. Work on those areas for more study, and practice for the next attempt.

- Check the requirements for practice in your state and what possible changes to these requirements are coming down the pipeline.

- As you study, imagine the vast number of career opportunities that certification opens up, which would be unattainable without the CPhT certification.

- Strategize on which national certification exam suits your current and future career plans—the PTCE or the ExCPT—and schedule your appointment.

- Make a realistic study plan that spaces out the chapters, with sufficient time for studying each and testing by chapter section.

- With each chapter, study the tables, appendices, and supplements, and take the end-of-chapter tests.

- Leave a few weeks to take a number of mock timed exams for yourself with the exam generating program, which provides tests with questions in similar proportions to the actual exams. These will help build your confidence.

- Remember the tips for succeeding at multiple-choice questions and the power of the process of elimination. If you don't know the answer for sure, knock out all the options that you know are wrong and choose from what is left.

- Don't be afraid of test-taking stress. Like an athlete, use that adrenaline to do better than you would have done without it.

- Be confident. If you have practiced, you will do well.

- Pack for the test the night before, prepare early, eat a good breakfast, and arrive a half hour ahead of time with the proper ID(s) and registration materials.

- Take the test and succeed!

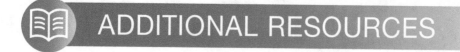

ADDITIONAL RESOURCES

To see how much you remember, take the Study Skills test that can be accessed the the ebook link for the self-study course and through Cirrus for individuals enrolled in the instructor-guided course.

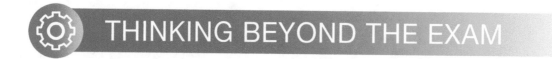

THINKING BEYOND THE EXAM

1. Many state boards of pharmacy are considering adopting new rules and regulations concerning the certification, registration, or licensure of pharmacy technicians. Find out what your state board of pharmacy is considering. Write a brief paragraph or essay explaining your choice to seek certification or your thoughts your state's qualifications for practice.

2. Why is a chain store's technician exam not adequate to earn the national designation of CPhT? Write a brief paragraph.

1

Medications

Learning Objectives

1. Define pharmacology and related terminology pertaining to medications. (Section 1.1)

2. Identify strengths, doses, dosage forms, and routes of administration of commonly used medications. (Section 1.2)

3. Classify drugs into therapeutic classes. (Sections 1.3–1.13)

4. List common drug interactions, adverse reactions, and contraindications. (Sections 1.3–1.13)

5. Match brand and generic names of commonly used medications and vaccines. (Sections 1.3–1.13)

6. Match common prescription and over-the-counter medications with their indications. (Sections 1.3–1.13)

7. Identify biotechnology and other miscellaneous medications. (Sections 1.14 and 1.15)

8. Match common prescription and over-the-counter medications with their indications. (Section 1.16)

9. Identify common alternative medicines and dietary supplements. (Section 1.17)

10. Describe proper storage of medications and vaccines. (Section 1.18)

11. Identify principles of drug stability, including physical and chemical incompatibilities related to compounding and reconstitution. (Section 1.19)

12. Identify principles of drug stability, including physical and chemical incompatibilities related to compounding and reconstitution. (Section 1.19)

13. Identify common drug suffixes and prefixes. (Section 1.20)

14. Identify common auxiliary labels and the common drugs that require these labels. (Section 1.20)

Access eBook links for resources and an exam generator, with 1,000+ questions.

There are numerous drugs on the market for many indications. This chapter reviews and discusses the basic pharmacology of commonly dispensed drugs in community and hospital pharmacies. Pharmacy technicians should have a clear understanding of generic and brand names of the most common medications, their primary indications, and common side effects. Technicians also need to know the common auxiliary warning labels that accompany these drugs and which commonly prescribed drugs are controlled substances or are on lists of high-risk drugs. It is important for technicians to have this knowledge to function effectively in the pharmacy and it is also covered on certification exams. Essential pharmacological information is necessary to help technicians better understand Drug Utilization Review alerts and enhance patient education and compliance with prescribed medications.

1.1 Essential Pharmacology Knowledge for Technicians

Pharm Fact

The PTCE domain 1 on medications will be 40% of that certification exam. The ExCPT domain 2 on drugs and drug therapy will be 15% of that certification exam.

Pharmacology is defined as the scientific study of drugs and how they work (their mechanisms of action) along with side effects, adverse reactions, and drug interactions. In its broadest sense, pharmacology encompasses specialized scientific disciplines about drugs, including:

- **therapeutics**—appropriate uses of drugs for targeted medicinal purposes
- **pharmacodynamics**—mechanisms of drugs and their biochemical and physiological effects
- **toxicology**—symptoms, mechanisms, detection, and treatment of poisonous effects and side effects of drugs
- **pharmaceutics**—various dosage forms and routes of administration of drugs, and their drug-releasing capabilities
- **pharmacokinetics**—movement of drugs within the body: absorption, distribution, metabolism, and elimination (ADME) of drugs from the body, and harmful drug interactions
- **pharmacognosy**—natural sources of drugs and herbs.

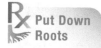

Put Down Roots

Pharmacology comes from the Greek word *pharmakon*, or "drug," and the Latin suffix *-logia*, or "study of."

It takes pharmacists many years of studying these basic and applied elements of pharmacology for thousands of drugs before they begin to practice, which is why patient questions about drugs must always be directed to the pharmacist.

Most prescriptions are written for brand-name drugs, though a generic drug that is bioequivalent is often dispensed. To be bioequivalent, a generic drug must be both pharmaceutically and therapeutically equivalent to the brand-name drug. To be pharmaceutically equivalent, the generic drug must have the same amount of active ingredient in the same dosage form. For two drugs to have therapeutic equivalence, they must have the same clinical effect and safety profile. Pharmacy technicians must be aware of the correct substitutions and situations when generic drugs can be legally substituted for brand-name drugs and when they cannot. (A more detailed discussion of this issue can be found in Chapter 4.)

Pharm Fact

Brand-name drugs are always listed as a proper name with the first letter capitalized. Generic drugs will usually not be capitalized.

Technicians also need to know each drug's **primary indications**, or the common intended uses to treat specific diseases, and each drug's **contraindications**, or the specific situations in which the drug should not be used because it will be harmful to a patient. For instance, the primary indication of atorvastatin (Lipitor) is treatment of high cholesterol, and the drug is contraindicated in pregnancy.

For every intended drug action, there are related unintended reactions, or **side effects**, that must always be considered. They can be mild or severe, such as varying intensities of nausea, constipation, diarrhea, itchiness and other skin reactions, drowsiness, pain, muscle aches, headaches, shakiness, and numbness.

Drug interactions occur when a drug affects the intended indication of another agent or reacts poorly with it. Interactions can happen between a prescribed drug and another prescribed or nonprescribed, or **over-the-counter (OTC)** drug, food, or multiple drugs. The mechanism, or primary means by which the interaction occurs, varies widely depending on the interacting agents. Drugs in combination with other agents can cause many difficulties as they react with each other, and their side effects build up.

Even vitamins, nutrients, or herbal and other dietary supplements can enhance or interfere with a drug's potency or cause intense reactions; so, the vitamins and supplements a patient is taking must be added to the patient profile and also considered. Finally, a drug intended to treat one disease might make another disease or condition the patient is experiencing worse. Types of drug interactions are listed in Table 1.1.

TABLE 1.1 Drug Interactions

Interaction	Mechanism	Examples
drug-drug	occurs when a drug interferes with or reacts with another drug; may result in reduced efficacy or toxicity	warfarin and nonsteroidal anti-inflammatory drugs (NSAIDs): additive risk of bleeding selective serotonin reuptake inhibitors (SSRIs) and Triptans: risk of serotonin syndrome
		nitrates and phosphodiesterase-5 (PDE-5) inhibitors (nitroglycerin and Viagra): risk of fatal hypotension
		angiotensin-converting enzyme (ACE) inhibitors and potassium-sparing diuretics: risk of hyperkalemia
drug-disease	occurs when a drug interferes with a patient's existing medical condition(s)	antihistamines: may cause difficult urination due to enlarged prostate
		decongestants: may worsen heart disease or high blood pressure
		NSAIDs: may cause fluid retention and increase blood pressure
drug-dietary supplement	occurs when a drug interacts with a dietary supplement that the patient is taking	warfarin and ginkgo: may increase bleeding St. John's wort and SSRIs: may increase drowsiness and risk of serotonin syndrome
drug-laboratory	occurs when a drug causes an abnormality in laboratory testing	antibiotics: may cause falsely elevated glucose test results
		psychiatric medications: may cause false positives on drug screens
drug-nutrient	occurs when food and beverages alter the effects of a patient's drug(s)	grapefruit juice: may alter the effects of statins and calcium channel blockers.
		cranberry juice and green leafy vegetables: may decrease the effects of warfarin

An **adverse drug reaction (ADR)** is an injury or severe harmful response caused by a single dose or an extended use of a drug. ADRs can arise from side effects, contraindications, allergic reactions, and incorrect use, or they may result from combining a drug with one or more other medications, vitamins, or herbal supplements. These events can range in severity from relatively mild symptoms, like shaking, vomiting, or hives, to other, more serious occurrences, like paralysis, blindness, or death. That is why technicians must look carefully at the patient profiles containing medications, allergies, history of use, and software alerts, which often update information on drugs. The technician serves as the first line of inquiry and defense against prescription errors, while the pharmacist counsels and makes the final decisions.

According to the Food and Drug Administration (FDA), **narrow therapeutic index (NTI)** medications are drugs for which small differences in dose or blood concentration may lead to serious therapeutic failures or ADRs. This means that, for NTI medications, the effective dose is very close to the toxic dose. NTI medications require regular monitoring to make sure that the patient's blood levels of the drug stay within the therapeutic range. A list of commonly used NTI medications can be found in Table 1.2.

TABLE 1.2 Narrow Therapeutic Index Medications

NTI Medication	Major Indication
carbamazepine	antiepileptic agent used in the management of seizures
cyclosporine	immunosuppressant used in management of organ transplant and inflammatory conditions such as rheumatoid arthritis and ulcerative colitis
digoxin	cardiac glycoside used in treatment and management of heart failure
levothyroxine	synthetic hormone used to treat hypothyroidism
lithium carbonate	treatment of manic episodes of bipolar disorder
phenytoin	anticonvulsant drug used in the management of seizures
theophylline	xanthine used to manage symptoms of asthma and COPD
warfarin	vitamin K antagonist used to treat various clotting and related disorders

Safety Alert

Technicians should read all boxed warnings as they become familiar with the drugs they will be working with.

The Institute for Safe Medication Practices (ISMP) has created lists of high-alert medications for community and ambulatory healthcare settings, long-term care settings, and acute care settings. These can be found at the ISMP website at CertExam5e.ParadigmEducation.com/ISMPrecommendations. There are also lists designed to address medication concerns for vulnerable populations, such as older adults (Beers Criteria) and pregnant individuals. A study supplement on these lists for vulnerable populations and other drug lists can be accessed through eBook links.

Formerly known as black box warnings, **boxed warnings** are mandated by the FDA for drugs that have serious, life threatening risks. Boxed warnings highlight dangerous side effects, interactions, and cautions for use.

1.2 Dosage Forms, Routes of Administration, and Drug Delivery

It is important for technicians to understand the different dosage forms and routes of administration for the medications they dispense. The **dosage form** is the physical form of the dose that is intended for administration to the patient. Common dosage forms include tablet, capsule, and oral liquid. The **route of administration (ROA)** is the path by which the drug enters the body. (See an extended list of drug forms and ROAs in Table 1.3.)

Common routes of administration include oral, parenteral, and inhalation. Some oral dosage forms are designed to deliver their dose to the body over an extended period of time. See Table 1.4 for examples.

To ensure patient safety, technicians must have extensive knowledge of all dosage forms, routes of administration, and drug delivery types. Patients may be harmed if the technicians prepare medications incorrectly, and the pharmacist does not notice. That is why an exam may include questions on common dosage forms, ROA, and drug delivery abbreviations. Study Tables 1.3 and 1.4 to review.

TABLE 1.3 Common Dosage Forms, Routes of Administration, and Dispensing

Dosage Form(s)	Route of Administration (ROA)	Dispensing Description and Tips
oral tablet	oral (PO [*per os*], or by mouth)	available as compression, multiple compression, chewable, oral disintegrating, and caplet with possible coatings: sugar coated, film coated, enteric coated, and buffered for different purposes and release delivery modes; modified-release tablets should not be crushed for administration
capsule	oral (PO [*per os*], or by mouth)	available in hard and soft gelatin; transparent, semi-transparent, or opaque; hard gelatin capsules may sometimes be opened and mixed with food or liquid
oral liquid	oral (PO [*per os*], or by mouth)	available as solution, syrup, suspension, elixir, emulsion, magma, colloid, aromatic water, fluid extract, solid extract, tincture, or spirit; dispense with dosing cups or oral syringes according to the appropriate patient age; include "By mouth" auxiliary label for liquids; include "Shake well" auxiliary label for suspensions, emulsions, and colloids
powders for reconstitution; effervescent tablets; other powders	oral (PO [*per os*], or by mouth)	Due to short expiration dates for some drugs, the active ingredient is supplied as a powder or effervescent tablet with instructions on how much water or other liquid is to be mixed with the drug for a given concentration. Check manufacturer label for the beyond-use date (BUD) for the reconstituted product. Include "Shake well" auxiliary label for oral liquids. Dispense with appropriate measuring spoon/cup or oral syringe
buccal products	oral (PO [*per os*], or by mouth); transmucosal (delivered via a mucous membrane, such as the eyes, ears, or nose) for gum, tablet, lozenge (troche), and lollipop	instructions should include, "Place between gum and inner lining of cheek..."; include "Keep out of reach of children" auxiliary label; dispense in child-resistant packaging, since these dosage forms may look like candy to a child; nicotine gum should be dispensed with directions for how to chew it to prevent nicotine overdose
sublingual (SL) tablets, sprays, and solutions	oral (PO [*per os*], or by mouth)	usually available as tablets and sprays, though compounding pharmacies and homeopathic practitioners may have solutions in which a given number of drops are placed under the tongue; nitroglycerin sublingual tablets must be dispensed in their original glass bottles and be replaced every six months
ophthalmic solutions, suspensions, ointments, and inserts	transmucosal (delivered via a mucous membrane, such as the eyes, ears, or nose)	Solutions and suspensions are not interchangeable. Label in which eye or both eyes the drop is to be placed. Include "Shake well" auxiliary label for suspensions. Ophthalmic drops may be used in the ears

continues

TABLE 1.3 Common Dosage Forms and Routes of Administration—*Continued*

Dosage Form(s)	Route of Administration (ROA)	Dispensing Description and Tips
otic solutions and suspensions	transmucosal (delivered via a mucous membrane, such as the eyes, ears, or nose)	Solutions and suspensions are not interchangeable. Instructions should include, "With affected ear facing up, place X drops in ear canal, keep head tilted for 2–5 min. May insert cotton plug to prevent leakage. Repeat…". Include "Shake well" auxiliary label for suspensions. Never use otic drops in the eye
nasal/intranasal solutions and suspensions	transmucosal (delivered via a mucous membrane, such as the eyes, ears, or nose)	available as a liquid solution or as a suspension in an atomizer that is sprayed up the nose; include "Shake well" auxiliary label for suspensions
rectal suppositories, enemas, creams, and ointments	transmucosal (delivered via a mucous membrane, such as the eyes, ears, or nose)	available as suppositories, enemas, creams, and ointments; suppositories may be for systemic or local indications; instructions for suppositories should include, "Remove wrap, insert into rectum small tapered end first."; most suppositories are stored at room temperature, but some should have the auxiliary label "Keep refrigerated" and be stored accordingly until pickup; enemas should include instructions telling patient to lie on side with knees bent, insert nozzle in rectum, squeeze bottle to release enema into rectum, remain in position for as long as directed; creams and ointments may come with an applicator, which is inserted rectally, and the tube is squeezed to administer the topical preparation
vaginal/intravaginal creams, ointments, tablets, foams, films, gels, and inserts	transmucosal (delivered via a mucous membrane, such as the eyes, ears, or nose)	Hormone replacement therapy is for systemic indication. Anti-infectives and antifungals are for local infection. Instructions should include, "Insert 1 applicatorful (or tablet) into vagina…"
dermal ointments, creams, lotions, pastes, plasters, gels, collodions, jellies, and irrigation solutions	topical (delivered externally via the skin)	usually for local indication; instructions should include, "Apply sparingly to affected area…"; apply "For external use only" auxiliary label
transdermal adhesives	topical (delivered externally via the skin)	includes patches and discs that consist of adhesive fabric with a drug reservoir and a rate-controlling membrane; provides slow, controlled release of drug to be absorbed systemically through the skin; instructions should include, "Apply topically to hair-free, scar-free skin…", "Rotate sites to prevent skin irritation…", and "Discard used patches safely…"; apply "For external use only" auxiliary label
transdermal gel, lotion, or spray	topical (delivered externally via the skin)	includes gels, lotions, and sprays in which the drug is used for a systemic indication; potent active ingredients are absorbed through the skin; patients should be directed to wear gloves for application; specific dose is premeasured or a tool to measure doses must be provided; product should be allowed to dry after application; apply "For external use only" auxiliary label

continues

TABLE 1.3 Common Dosage Forms and Routes of Administration—*Continued*

Dosage Form(s)	Route of Administration (ROA)	Dispensing Description and Tips
aerosols and metered-dose inhalers (MDIs)	inhalation (inhaled through the mouth into the lungs)	Aerosol devices dispense a measured dose per puff. If the patient has difficulty coordinating the device, a spacer may be used to facilitate administration. Instructions should include, "Inhale X puffs by mouth…"; label each container with a "Shake well" auxiliary label. Patients should be advised to rinse their mouth after use and to clean plastic dispensers regularly
micronized powders and non-aerosolized inhalers	inhalation (inhaled through the mouth into the lungs)	Common inhalers include Accuhaler, Turbohaler, Diskhaler, Diskus, and HandiHaler. Patient labeling must instruct the patient to activate dose and to breathe in deeply and strongly to pull the powder into the lungs. Instructions should include, "Use X vial(s) via nebulizer. Rinse mouth after use…"
inhalation solutions and nebulizers	inhalation (inhaled through the mouth into the lungs)	liquid drug solution that must be administered using a nebulizer; solutions may be premixed and ready to use or in a concentrated solution that must be mixed with sterile saline; multiple drugs may be mixed together in one treatment for patient convenience; instructions should include, "Inhale X mL (or packets) with nebulizer…"
volatiles	inhalation (inhaled through the mouth into the lungs)	Volatile medications are liquids that can be used with a vaporizer to help relieve breathing problems. Instructions should clearly direct the patient not to take internally or apply externally
solutions for intravenous (IV) injection	parenteral (delivered via injection)	allows for sterile solutions to be administered into a vein; usually for systemic use; must be particulate-free and administered by a healthcare professional; may be a small-volume parenteral (SVP) solution for an intravenous piggyback (IVPB) or bolus dose, or a large-volume parenteral (LVP) solution for continuous intravenous infusion
solutions for intramuscular (IM) injection	parenteral (delivered via injection)	allows for sterile solutions or suspensions to be injected into the muscle; depending on drug salt and diluent, IM dosage form can provide immediate or delated effect; effects of depot injection drugs are designed to last for weeks to months; usually administered by a healthcare professional
solutions for subcutaneous (SubQ) injection	parenteral (delivered via injection)	allows for sterile solutions or suspensions to be injected through the skin into the subcutaneous tissue for systemic effect; includes many vaccinations and insulin; patients should be instructed on how to store and administer the drug
solutions for intradermal (ID) injection	parenteral (delivered via injection)	allows a small volume of sterile solution to be injected between layers of skin for diagnostic purposes or vaccination; administered by a healthcare professional

continues

TABLE 1.3 **Common Dosage Forms and Routes of Administration—***Continued*

Dosage Form(s)	Route of Administration (ROA)	Dispensing Description and Tips
vaginal rings	inserts and implants (delivered via an existing opening or placed by a physician or surgeon)	flexible drug-treated plastic rings; inserted vaginally every month as a contraceptive; should be stored in the refrigerator; some new inserts have microbials and chemotherapy drugs
intrauterine devices	inserts and implants (delivered via an existing opening or placed by a physician or surgeon)	*T*-shaped plastic devices; fitted into the uterus through the vagina by a healthcare professional as a contraceptive
surgical implants	inserts and implants (delivered via an existing opening or placed by a physician or surgeon)	catheters, drug pumps, radioactive seeds, or hormonal pellets that deliver medication either systemically or locally

TABLE 1.4 **Drug Delivery Abbreviations**

Abbreviation	Meaning
DR	delayed release
CR	controlled release
CD	controlled delivery
LA	long acting
TR	timed release
SR	sustained release
XR	extended release
XL	extended length/release

1.3 Anatomical Classification of Drugs

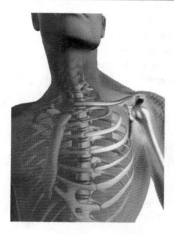

To study and remember common generic and brand-name drugs, it is often easiest to consider them according to their classification by anatomical system or organ and by their pharmaceutical action. For example, metoprolol succinate (Toprol XL) and lisinopril (Prinivil, Zestril) are found in the cardiovascular (heart-blood system) category; both are used to treat high blood pressure, but each lowers the blood pressure in a different way. The generic names of certain classes of drugs for specific indications often share the same suffix at the end of their generic names. (Notice the suffix *-pril* at the end of lisinopril and related drugs enalapril and ramipril.)

As technicians memorize generic drug names, it will be easier to learn them in their class or category (see Table 1.5). A resource list of generic drug name prefixes and suffixes can be found at the end of this chapter.

TABLE 1.5 Sample of Common Generic Name Suffixes with Drug Class/Category

Suffix	Generic Examples	Class/Category
-sone	dexamethasone, methylprednisolone, prednisone	corticosteroid, anti-inflammatory
-cillin	amoxicillin, ampicillin, nafcillin	penicillin-derivative, antibiotics
-dipine	amlodipine, nicardipine, nifedipine	calcium channel blockers, cardiovascular

Drug Facts and Comparisons® (F&C) is a primary reference for doing brand-name to generic drug substitutions, organized by bodily systems and indications. It provides factual, up-to-date information on drug product availability, indications, administration and doses, pharmacological actions, contraindications, warnings, precautions, adverse reactions, overdoses, and patient instructions. F&C is available as a hard-copy publication and as an online subscription.

For the hospital setting, the American Hospital Formulary Service (AHFS) serves as a primary reference for drug information. Although community and hospital pharmacies dispense some of the same drugs, drugs used in hospital settings also include injectable antibiotic and biotechnology drugs.

1.4 Central Nervous System Agents

The central nervous system (CNS) consists of specialized nerve cells called neurons, which are located in the brain and spinal cord. Neurons within the CNS communicate with other neurons primarily through chemicals known as *neurotransmitters*, including serotonin, norepinephrine, dopamine, acetylcholine, and histamine. Prescribed drugs often alter the neurotransmitter activity at the neuron level to produce medicinal effects, which also produce side effects that must be considered.

CNS Medications to Treat Anxiety and Insomnia

Most medicines that work on the CNS are considered to be **psychoactive drugs**, or medications that modify brain functions to influence mood, perception, and consciousness. **Hypnotic** drugs are drugs that induce sleep. The commonly dispensed antianxiety and sleep medications listed in Table 1.6 are CNS depressants, so they can interact with psychiatric medications, OTC sleeping medications, or alcohol.

The psychoactive drugs in the **benzodiazepine (BZD)** family (the *benzos*) are used to treat anxiety, panic attacks, seizures, and insomnia. (Notice the common suffix *-pam* or *-lam* in the generic drugs in Table 1.6.) Drugs in the BZD family can cause physical or psychological dependence if used long term.

Drugs in the BZD family and other CNS depressants should not be taken with opioids. Combining them can lead to unresponsiveness, extreme dizziness, and slowed, labored breathing.

Study Idea

Names of drugs in the BZD family generally end in *-lam* or *-pam*.

The hypnotics zolpidem (Ambien) and eszopiclone (Lunesta) are used for insomnia and are similar in action to benzodiazepines. Because of their potential to cause dependence, the listed hypnotics and benzodiazepines have been classified by the US Drug Enforcement Administration (DEA) as Schedule IV (C-IV) controlled substances (see Chapter 2 for more information on controlled substances schedules). Refills of C-IV drugs must occur within six months of the original prescription date and are limited to five refills. Prescriptions must be monitored for early refills and abuse. Most of these medications are recommended for short-term, as needed, or nightly use. In practice, though, many are used on a long-term, routine basis for anxiety or insomnia. The FDA has recommended dosage reductions in certain individuals for zolpidem and eszopiclone because of next-day drug hangovers that adversely impact safe driving.

Buspirone (BuSpar) is a non-benzodiazepine medication indicated to treat anxiety. Buspirone is not a controlled substance and is not habit-forming. Buspirone is non-sedating and can be administered with or without food. See Table 1.6 for a list of CNS agents to treat anxiety and insomnia.

TABLE 1.6 CNS Agents to Treat Anxiety and Insomnia

Generic Name	Brand Name	Route(s) of Administration	Dosage Form(s)	Common Dosage Amounts
Benzodiazepines (BZD)				
alprazolam	Xanax	oral	liquid, tablet, extended-release tablet	0.25 mg, 0.5 mg, 1 mg, 2 mg, 3 mg, 1 mg/mL
clonazepam	Klonopin	oral	tablet, disintegrating tablet	0.125 mg, 0.25 mg, 0.5 mg, 1 mg, 2 mg
diazepam	Valium	oral, parenteral	tablet, oral liquid, solution for injection	2 mg, 5 mg, 10 mg, 5 mg/mL
lorazepam	Ativan	oral, parenteral	oral liquid, tablet, solution for injection	0.5 mg, 1 mg, 2 mg, 2 mg/mL
temazepam	Restoril	oral	capsule	7.5 mg, 15 mg, 22.5 mg, 30 mg
Hypnotics				
eszopiclone	Lunesta	oral	tablet	1 mg, 2 mg, 3 mg
zolpidem	Ambien	oral	tablet, extended-release tablet	5 mg, 6.25 mg, 10 mg, 12.5 mg
Antianxiety Agent				
buspirone	BuSpar	oral	tablet	5 mg, 7.5 mg, 10 mg, 15 mg, 30 mg

Antidepressant and Antipsychotic CNS Medications

Antidepressant and antipsychotic CNS agents generally act directly on the neurotransmitters, such as serotonin, norepinephrine, and dopamine, to achieve a therapeutic effect.

These drugs can work for a period of time and then lose their effectiveness as the body develops a tolerance. Some of these drugs can **bioaccumulate**, or collect in the fat cells of the body, resulting in the development of side effects after taking a drug for a period of time. Patient education and compliance are important while taking antipsychotics and antidepressants; a patient may experience **withdrawal symptoms**, which may include anxiety, sweating, nausea, and shaking, if the drug is stopped abruptly. These drugs should always be tapered off.

Antidepressants

Safety Alert

The antidepressant Celexa is often confused with the arthritis treatment celecoxib (Celebrex). Watch every letter!

Antidepressants are used to treat depression. Antidepressant CNS agents work through different mechanisms, and the specific type and dose must be tailored to each patient to achieve the desired therapeutic response. Antidepressants carry boxed warnings because of the increased risk of suicidal ideation and behavior in children, adolescents, and young adults.

Several analgesic and muscle relaxant prescription (and some OTC) drugs, such as tramadol (Ultram) and cyclobenzaprine (Flexeril), can cause unsafe levels of serotonin when used with certain antidepressants, such as fluoxetine (Prozac), sertraline (Zoloft), and paroxetine (Paxil), causing confusion and agitation, among other symptoms. They should not be taken together. Alcohol should not be used with these drugs.

Some antidepressants block the reabsorption of serotonin so that more of the secreted serotonin circulates for positive effects. Several antidepressants, including fluoxetine (Prozac), work in this way. These drugs are known as **selective serotonin reuptake inhibitors (SSRIs)**. SSRIs are used to treat depression, anxiety, and obsessive-compulsive disorder. Side effects include nervousness, weight loss, and decreased libido. Patients should be cautioned that SSRIs take longer to work, and up to three weeks may be required for therapeutic effects to be experienced.

Amitriptyline (Elavil), a **tricyclic antidepressant (TCA)**, is an older antidepressant drug that offers a mild tranquilizing, soothing action. It is still used for depression, to enhance the effect of pain medications, and to prevent migraine headaches. This drug commonly causes drowsiness and is sometimes prescribed as a sleep medication for insomnia. Amitriptyline can cause dry mouth and blurry vision.

Other antidepressants block the reuptake of both serotonin and norepinephrine. Known as **serotonin-norepinephrine reuptake inhibitors (SNRIs)**, these drugs include venlafaxine (Effexor) and duloxetine (Cymbalta). They can cause insomnia if given at bedtime and should be used cautiously in patients with high blood pressure as they can raise blood pressure levels. Cymbalta is also often given to help patients with neuropathy.

Monoamine-oxidase inhibitors (MAOIs) are older medications for depression and not used as frequently as other classes. This class includes phenelzine (Nardil) and tranylcypromine (Parnate). Patients taking MAOIs must avoid specific foods, including aged cheeses and certain wines, because of a dangerous drug-food interaction with a chemical in the foods called *tyramine*. MAOIs can also cause dry mouth, urinary retention, and blurred vision.

Trazodone (Desyrel) has a different mechanism from some of the other drugs but is also used as an antidepressant. The side effects of trazadone are similar to other antidepressants, including dry mouth, vision changes, and drug hangover. Because it can cause drowsiness, it is sometimes prescribed for insomnia. Patients taking trazodone should avoid sun exposure, and patients with penises should be warned about the risk of priapism, or a prolonged painful erection. Trazodone can cause cramps in ankles and feet and some loss of fine motor function after prolonged use in some patients.

Bupropion (Wellbutrin) is another antidepressant agent that works in a slightly different way. Bupropion blocks the reuptake of dopamine and norepinephrine. It is indicated to treat depression and for smoking cessation. In contrast to other antidepressants, bupropion does not cause as much sexual dysfunction or sleepiness and may result in weight loss. For a list of antidepressant CNS agents discussed in this section, see Table 1.7.

TABLE 1.7 Antidepressant CNS Medications

Generic Name	Brand Name	Route(s) of Administration	Dosage Form(s)	Common Dosage Amount(s)
Selective Serotonin Reuptake Inhibitors (SSRIs)				
citalopram	Celexa	oral	solution, tablet	10 mg, 20 mg, 40 mg, 10 mg/5 mL
escitalopram	Lexapro	oral	solution, tablet	5 mg, 10 mg, 20 mg, 5 mg/mL
fluoxetine	Prozac	oral	capsule, solution, tablet	10 mg, 20 mg, 40 mg, 20 mg/5 mL
paroxetine	Paxil	oral	suspension, tablet, extended-release tablet	10 mg, 12.5 mg, 20 mg, 25 mg, 30 mg, 37.5 mg, 40 mg, 10 mg/5 mL
sertraline	Zoloft	oral	solution, tablet	25 mg, 50 mg, 100 mg, 20 mg/mL
vilazodone	Viibryd	oral	tablet	10 mg, 20 mg, 40 mg
vortioxetine	Trintellix	oral	tablet	5 mg, 10 mg, 20 mg
Tricyclic Antidepressants (TCAs)				
amitriptyline	Elavil	oral	tablet	10 mg, 25 mg, 50 mg, 75 mg, 100 mg, 150 mg
desipramine	Norpramin	oral	tablet	25 mg, 50 mg, 75 mg, 100 mg, 150 mg
doxepin	Silenort, Sinequan	oral	capsule, liquid	10 mg, 25 mg, 50 mg, 75 mg, 100 mg, 150 mg, 10 mg/mL
imipramine	Tofranil	oral	capsule, tablet	10 mg, 25 mg, 50 mg, 75 mg, 100 mg, 125 mg, 150 mg
nortriptyline	Pamelor	oral	capsule, solution	10 mg, 25 mg, 50 mg, 75 mg
Serotonin–Norepinephrine Reuptake Inhibitors (SNRIs)				
duloxetine	Cymbalta	oral	capsule	20 mg, 30 mg, 40 mg, 60 mg

continues

TABLE 1.7 Antidepressant CNS Agents—*Continued*

Generic Name	Brand Name	Route(s) of Administration	Dosage Form(s)	Common Dosage Amount(s)
Serotonin–Norepinephrine Reuptake Inhibitors (SNRIs)				
venlafaxine	Effexor	oral	tablet, extended-release tablet, extended-release capsule	25 mg, 37.5 mg, 50 mg, 75 mg, 100 mg, 150 mg
Monoamine Oxidase Inhibitors (MAOIs)				
phenelzine	Nardil	oral	tablet	15 mg
tranylcypromine	Parnate	oral	tablet	10 mg
Tetracyclic Antidepressant				
mirtazapine	Remeron	oral	tablet, disintegrating tablet	15 mg, 30 mg, 45 mg
Miscellaneous Antidepressants				
bupropion	Wellbutrin	oral	tablet, extended-release tablet	75 mg, 100 mg, 150 mg, 200 mg, 300 mg
trazodone	Desyrel	oral	tablet	50 mg, 100 mg, 150 mg, 300 mg

Antipsychotics

Antipsychotic drugs are medications used to manage disordered thought and behavior.

The first generation of antipsychotic drugs developed, including chlorpromazine (Thorazine) and thioridazine (Mellaril), were used to treat schizophrenia (mental and emotional fragmentation and faulty reality perception). These drugs are rarely prescribed today because of the high incidence of side effects, including blurred vision, dry mouth and related dental problems, and dementia-like symptoms. Other drugs and formulations have a higher level of success with fewer difficult side effects due to the blockage of certain brain functions.

Newer antipsychotic medications are referred to as *atypical* antipsychotics. Aripiprazole (Abilify), olanzapine (Zyprexa), quetiapine (Seroquel), and risperidone (Risperdal) are considered atypical antipsychotic drugs because they target specific neurotransmitters. These drugs are often used to enhance the antidepressant effects of traditional antidepressants. In addition to modulating the mood swings of bipolar depression (excessively low mood, energy, and activity) and mania (excessively high mood, energy, and activity), these drugs are used in adults to treat schizophrenia and severe agitation.

Atypical antipsychotic drugs may cause or aggravate metabolic syndrome, characterized by obesity, hypertension, type 2 diabetes, and hyperlipidemia. These agents should be used cautiously in older adult patients due to potential cardiovascular adverse reactions. If a patient experiences any rigidity, tremor, or involuntary muscle twitching, their physician should be notified immediately. Alcohol should not be used while taking these drugs. For a list of common antipsychotic CNS agents discussed in this section, see Table 1.8.

TABLE 1.8 Antipsychotic CNS Agents

Generic Name	Brand Name(s)	Route(s) of Administration	Dosage Form(s)	Common Dosage Amounts
First Generation				
chlorpromazine	Thorazine	oral, parenteral (IM, IV)	tablet, solution for injection	10 mg, 25 mg, 50 mg, 100 mg, 200 mg, 25 mg/mL
fluphenazine	Prolixin	oral, parenteral (IM)	tablet, oral liquid, solution for injection	1 mg, 2.5 mg, 5 mg, 10 mg, 25 mg/mL
haloperidol	Haldol	oral, parenteral (IM)	tablet, oral liquid, solution for injection	0.5 mg, 1 mg, 2 mg, 5 mg, 10 mg, 20 mg, 2 mg/mL, 5 mg/mL
loxapine	Loxitane	oral	capsule	5 mg, 10 mg, 25 mg, 50 mg
thioridazine	Mellaril	oral	tablet	10 mg, 25 mg, 50 mg, 100 mg
thiothixene	Navane	oral	capsule	1 mg, 2 mg, 5 mg, 10 mg, 20 mg
trifluoperazine	Stelazine	oral	tablet	1 mg, 2 mg, 5 mg, 10 mg
Atypical				
aripiprazole	Abilify	oral, parenteral (IM)	tablet, oral solution, oral disintegrating tablet, solution for long-acting injection	2 mg, 5 mg, 10 mg, 15 mg, 20 mg, 30 mg, 300 mg, 400 mg, 1 mg/mL
brexpiprazole	Rexulti	oral	tablet	0.25 mg, 0.5 mg, 1 mg, 2 mg, 3 mg, 4 mg
clozapine	Clozaril	oral	tablet, disintegrating tablet	12.5 mg, 25 mg, 50 mg, 100 mg, 150 mg, 200 mg
iloperidone	Fanapt	oral	tablet	1 mg, 2 mg, 4 mg, 6 mg, 8 mg, 10 mg, 12 mg
lurasidone	Latuda	oral	tablet	20 mg, 40 mg, 60 mg, 80 mg, 120 mg
olanzapine	Zyprexa	oral, parenteral (IM)	tablet, disintegrating tablet, solution for injection, solution for long-acting injection	2.5 mg, 5 mg, 7.5 mg, 10 mg, 15 mg, 20 mg, 210 mg, 300 mg, 405 mg
paliperidone	Invega	oral, parenteral (IM)	extended-release tablet, solution for long-acting injection	1.5 mg, 3 mg, 6 mg, 9 mg

continues

TABLE 1.8 Antipsychotic CNS Agents—*Continued*

Generic Name	Brand Name(s)	Route(s) of Administration	Dosage Form(s)	Common Dosage Amounts
Atypical				
quetiapine	Seroquel, Seroquel XR	oral	tablet, extended-release tablet	25 mg, 50 mg, 100 mg, 150 mg, 200 mg, 300 mg, 400 mg
risperidone	Risperdal	oral, parenteral (IM)	tablet, oral disintegrating tablet, oral solution, solution for long-acting injection	0.25 mg, 0.5 mg, 1 mg, 2 mg, 3 mg, 4 mg, 1 mg/mL, 12.5 mg, 25 mg, 37.5 mg, 50 mg
ziprasidone	Geodon	oral, parenteral (IM)	capsule, solution for injection	20 mg, 40 mg, 60 mg, 80 mg

Study Idea

There are many drugs in the serotonin agonist class to treat migraines, and all have the suffix -triptan.

Medications for Other CNS Conditions

Additional CNS agents include drugs for many different indications and conditions of the nervous system.

The diagnosis of attention deficit hyperactivity disorder (ADHD) is on the rise in pediatric and adult patients. ADHD manifests in difficulty focusing or concentrating, overactivity, and difficulty with impulse control. Commonly prescribed ADHD medications, such as methylphenidate (Concerta, Ritalin, others) and amphetamines, stimulate rather than depress the CNS, and this helps support the brain in focusing attention and behavior. Common side effects are insomnia and loss of appetite. These drugs should be taken in the morning or early afternoon.

Methylphenidate is available as both an immediate-release drug (Ritalin, others) and as a extended-release drug (Concerta, others). Adderall and Mydayis (short- and long-acting formulations) are combinations of amphetamine salts (dextroamphetamine and amphetamine). Lisdexamfetamine (Vyvanse) is also prescribed for ADHD. Agents for ADHD are classified as Schedule II (C-II) controlled substances—no refills are authorized without a new prescription.

To slow the progression of moderate to severe Alzheimer's disease, other CNS agents, such as memantine (Namenda, Namenda XR) and donepezil (Aricept, Aricept ODT are used. Memantine is sometimes used in combination with donepezil, but drowsiness is a common side effect. Donepezil is metabolized in the liver, so it is susceptible to drug interactions. The main side effects of these drugs are gastrointestinal, such as diarrhea, nausea, and vomiting.

Parkinson's disease (PD) is a neurological disorder. Patients with PD develop progressively worsening problems with movement. Medications to treat PD focus mainly on increasing the amount of dopamine in the body by different mechanisms. These medications include levodopa / carbidopa (Duopa, Rytary, Sinemet) and pramipexole (Mirapex, Mirapex ER). Ropinirole (Requip, Requip XL) is a medication for PD that is also commonly prescribed at bedtime to treat restless legs syndrome (involuntary twitching of the legs). Side effects of these agents may include nausea and orthostatic hypotension.

Epilepsy is a disease in which a patient suffers from seizures, which are spasms caused by an overfiring the neurons in the brain and nervous system. Patients are given anticonvulsant (antiseizure) medications that try to calm the nervous system by inhibiting the overly rapid and excessive firing of neurons. Some common drugs for treating epilepsy are phenytoin (Dilantin), divalproex sodium (Depakote , Depakote ER, Depakote Sprinkle), and lamotrigine (Lamictal, Lamictal CD, Lamictal ODT, Lamictal XR). Anticonvulsants are also used for other indications. For instance, topiramate (Qudexy XR, Topamax, Trokendi XR) is often used for migraine headache and to promote weight loss.

Gabapentin (Neurontin) and pregabalin (Lyrica, Lyrica CR) were initially used to control seizures. Today, though, these drugs are primarily used to reduce nerve pain associated with diabetes, chronic pain, shingles, and spinal cord injuries. Pregabalin is sometimes prescribed for fibromyalgia, or severe chronic muscle fatigue. (Pregabalin is a Schedule V (C-V) controlled substance.) The most common side effects of these anticonvulsant drugs are drowsiness, dizziness, and swelling of the ankles.

Lithium (Lithobid) is a medication used to treat bipolar disorder. Lithium helps reduce the frequency and severity of manic episodes. In addition to having a narrow therapeutic index, lithium can affect kidney and thyroid function, so patients taking it must have periodic blood tests to monitor their lithium levels. Side effects can include hand tremor, increased thirst and urination, and gastrointestinal effects.

Sumatriptan (Imitrex), which is a serotonin receptor agonist, is used as an abortive treatment for migraine headaches. It is available in various dosage formulations and must be used with caution in patients with heart disease and individuals who can become pregnant. There are many serotonin receptor agonists in this class used to treat migraines, and all have the suffix -triptan. For a list of CNS agents to treat the conditions listed in this section, see Table 1.9.

TABLE 1.9 Medications for Other CNS Conditions

Generic Name	Brand Name(s)	Route(s) of Administration	Dosage Form(s)	Common Dosage Amount(s)
Attention Deficit Hyperactivity Disorder (ADHD)				
atomoxetine*	Strattera	oral	capsule	10 mg, 18 mg, 25 mg, 40 mg, 60 mg, 80 mg, 100 mg
dexmethylphenidate	Focalin, Focalin XR	oral	capsule, tablet	2.5 mg, 5 mg, 10 mg, 15 mg, 20 mg, 25 mg, 30 mg, 35 mg, 40 mg
dextroamphetamine / amphetamine	Adderall, Mydayis	oral	capsule, tablet	5 mg, 7.5 mg, 10 mg, 12.5 mg, 15 mg, 20 mg, 30 mg
lisdexamfetamine	Vyvanse	oral	capsule, chewable tablet	10 mg, 20 mg, 30 mg, 40 mg, 50 mg, 60 mg, 70 mg
methylphenidate	Concerta, Ritalin, others	oral, topical (transdermal)	tablet, extended-release tablet, chewable tablet, extended-release oral suspension, transdermal patch	5 mg, 10 mg, 15 mg, 20 mg, 30 mg, 40 mg, 50 mg, 60 mg, 25 mg/ 5 mL, 10 mg/9 hr, 15 mg/9 hr, 20 mg/9 hr, 30 mg/9 hr

continues

TABLE 1.9 **Medications for Other CNS Conditions**—*Continued*

Generic Name	Brand Name(s)	Route(s) of Administration	Dosage Form(s)	Common Dosage Amount(s)
Alzheimer's Disease				
donepezil	Aricept, Aricept ODT	oral	tablet, disintegrating tablet	5 mg, 10 mg, 23 mg
galantamine	Razadyne, Razadyne ER	oral	capsule, tablet, liquid	4 mg, 8 mg, 12 mg, 16 mg, 24 mg
memantine	Namenda, Namenda XR	oral	extended-release capsule, solution, tablet	5 mg, 7 mg, 10 mg, 14 mg, 21 mg, 28 mg, 10 mg/5 mL
rivastigmine	Exelon	oral, topical (transdermal)	capsule, oral liquid, transdermal patch	1.5 mg, 2.5 mg, 3 mg, 6 mg, 4.6 mg/24 hr, 9.5 mg/24 hr
Parkinson's Disease				
benztropine	Cogentin	oral, parenteral (IV)	tablet, solution for injection	0.5 mg, 1 mg, 2 mg, 1 mg/mL
entacapone	Comtan	oral	tablet	200 mg
levodopa / carbidopa	Duopa, Rytary, Sinemet	oral	capsule, suspension, tablet	10 mg/100 mg, 25 mg/100 mg, 25 mg/250 mg, 50 mg/200 mg
pramipexole	Mirapex, Mirapex ER	oral	tablet, extended-release tablet	0.125 mg, 0.25 mg, 0.375 mg, 0.5 mg, 0.75 mg, 1 mg, 1.5 mg, 2.25 mg, 3.75 mg, 4.5 mg
ropinirole	Requip, Requip XL	oral	tablet	0.25 mg, 0.5 mg, 1 mg, 2 mg, 3 mg, 4 mg, 5 mg, 6 mg, 8 mg, 12 mg
rotigotine	Neupro	topical (transdermal)	transdermal patch	1 mg/24 hr, 2 mg/24 hr, 3 mg/24 hr, 4 mg/24 hr, 6 mg/24 hr, 8 mg/24 hr
Anticonvulsants				
carbamazepine	Carbatrol, Epitol, Equetro, Tegretol	oral	capsule, suspension, tablet	100 mg, 200 mg, 300 mg, 400 mg, 100 mg/5 mL
divalproex sodium	Depakote, Depakote ER, Depakote Sprinkle	oral, parenteral (IV)	capsule, delayed-release tablet, extended-release tablet, oral solution, solution for injection	125 mg, 250 mg, 500 mg, 100 mg/mL, 250 mg/5 mL

continues

TABLE 1.9 Medications for Other CNS Conditions—*Continued*

Generic Name	Brand Name(s)	Route(s) of Administration	Dosage Form(s)	Common Dosage Amount(s)
Anticonvulsants				
ethosuximide	Zarontin	oral	capsule, suspension	250 mg, 250 mg/mL
gabapentin	Neurontin	oral	capsule, solution, tablet	250 mg, 250 mg/mL
lamotrigine	Lamictal, Lamictal CD, Lamictal ODT, Lamictal XR	oral	tablet, extended-release tablet	2 mg, 5 mg, 25 mg, 100 mg, 150 mg, 200 mg
levetiracetam	Elepsia XR, Keppra, Keppra XR, Roweepra, Spritam	oral, parenteral	oral solution, tablet, solution for injection	250 mg, 500 mg, 750 mg, 1,000 mg, 100 mg/mL, 500 mg/100 mL, 1,000 mg/100 mL, 500 mg/5 mL
phenytoin	Dilantin	oral, parenteral (IV)	capsule, oral suspension, chewable tablet, solution for injection	50 mg, 100 mg, 200 mg, 300 mg, 50 mg/ mL, 125 mg/5 mL
pregabalin	Lyrica, Lyrica CR	oral	capsule, solution, extended-release tablet	25 mg, 50 mg, 75 mg, 82.5 mg, 100 mg, 150 mg, 165 mg, 200 mg, 225 mg, 300 mg, 330 mg, 20 mg/mL
topiramate	Qudexy XR, Topamax, Trokendi XR	oral	capsule, extended-release capsule, tablet	15 mg, 25 mg, 50 mg, 100 mg, 200 mg
zonisamide	Zonegran	oral	capsule	25 mg, 50 mg, 100 mg
Bipolar Disorder				
lithium	Lithobid	oral	capsule, oral solution, tablet, extended-release tablet	150 mg, 300 mg, 600 mg, 300 mg ER, 450 mg, 8 mEq/5 mL
Migraine Headache				
almotriptan	Axert	oral	tablet	6.25 mg, 12.5 mg
eletriptan	Replax	oral	tablet	20 mg, 40 mg
frovatriptan	Frova	oral	tablet	2.5 mg
rizatriptan	Maxalt	oral	tablet, oral disintegrating tablet	5 mg, 10 mg
sumatriptan	Imitrex	oral, transmucosal (intranasal), parenteral (SubQ)	tablet, nasal spray, solution for injection	5 mg, 20 mg, 25 mg, 50 mg, 100 mg, 6 mg/0.5 mL, 12 mg/mL

continues

TABLE 1.9 Medications for Other CNS Conditions—*Continued*

Generic Name	Brand Name(s)	Route(s) of Administration	Dosage Form(s)	Common Dosage Amount(s)
Migraine Headache				
zolmitriptan	Zomig	oral, transmucosal (intranasal)	tablet, oral disintegrating tablet, nasal spray	2.5 mg, 5 mg

*Atomoxetine is the only non-stimulant ADHD drug; it is not classified as a C-II controlled substance.

1.5 Cardiovascular Medications

Cardiovascular disease is a major health threat in the United States and includes conditions like coronary artery disease, heart failure, and hypertension. The complications of untreated or undertreated high blood pressure include kidney failure, stroke, and heart attack. The risk of cardiovascular disease may be partly genetic, but hypertension is often the result of lifestyle choices as well, such as smoking, unhealthy food choices, being overweight, and lack of exercise. Elevated cholesterol is an important risk factor for hypertension and general heart disease.

Medications to Treat High Blood Pressure

There are many **antihypertensive agents** (see Table 1.10) that work to lower blood pressure by dilating blood vessels, slowing heart rate, and increasing the elimination of salt and fluid from the body. Often, more than one drug is needed to reach the desired blood pressure range, usually below 120/80 mm Hg.

Angiotensin-converting enzyme (ACE) inhibitor medications reduce blood pressure and prevent heart failure by blocking or reducing the liver's production of a hormone that constricts the blood vessels. Their first cousins, **angiotensin II receptor blocker (ARB) medications**, block the reception and action of the same constrictive hormone. These drugs help dilate blood vessels, supporting increased blood flow and lowering blood pressure. These drugs also protect the kidneys from the damage caused by diabetes and hypertension. However, ACE inhibitors and ARBs can cause the body to retain potassium and must be used with caution by patients also taking potassium supplements or potassium-sparing diuretics and by patients with declining kidney function. Because of the risk of birth defects, ACE inhibitors and ARBs should not be given to pregnant patients.

The most common side effect of the ACE inhibitors is a drug-induced dry cough caused by the buildup of bradykinin, which promotes inflammation and histamine release. If the cough continues, the patient is usually switched from and ACE inhibitor to an ARB. The most serious adverse effect of ACE inhibitors is angioedema, a swelling under the skin that can be a life-threatening allergic reaction when it manifests as a swelling of the tongue, lips, or eyes. If these symptoms occur, the drug must be discontinued immediately, and the patient should be referred to emergency care.

Study Idea

The names of many ACE inhibitors end in *-pril*, whereas the names of many ARBs end in *-sartan*.

Study Idea

Note that names of some calcium channel blockers end in *-dipine*. Also, watch for the *-olol* ending for the beta blocker drugs.

Name Exchange

Epinephrine is also known by the British term "adrenaline" or as the "stress hormone" (for fight or flight). Norepinephrine, another stress hormone, is "noradrenaline."

Calcium channel blocker (CCB) medications stop calcium from entering the cells of the heart and blood vessels, making them more flexible and able to relax and widen, reducing blood pressure. The most often prescribed CCB is amlodipine (Norvasc), which can cause side effects including headaches, dizziness, and sometimes ankle swelling. CCBs can increase risk of heart failure and should generally be avoided in patients with both hypertension and heart failure.

Beta-adrenergic blocker (beta blocker) medications are drugs that stop the blood pressure-raising effects of the hormone epinephrine (also known as *adrenaline*), which makes your heart beat faster. Beta blockers can make the heart beat slower with less force, and they include atenolol (Tenormin) and the newest agent, nebivolol (Bystolic). Notice the suffix *-olol* in every generic drug name mentioned here. Beta blockers are commonly used to treat heart failure. Some beta blockers are also used for glaucoma and migraines.

Metoprolol succinate (Toprol XL) is available in an extended-release dosage form; metoprolol tartrate (Lopressor) is in an immediate-release dosage form. These different salts cannot be interchanged. They are generally well tolerated, but patients must not run out of these medications—if the drug is withdrawn for 48 to 72 hours, blood pressure can rebound to unsafe levels, leading to severe chest pain or even a heart attack.

Some beta blockers are selective and exert most of their effects on the heart. Others are nonselective and affect beta receptors elsewhere in the body. Non-selective beta blockers should be avoided in patients with asthma and COPD because they can cause bronchoconstriction. Cardio-selective beta blockers include acebutolol (Sectral), atenolol (Tenormin), bisoprolol (Zebeta), metoprolol succinate (Toprol XL), metoprolol tartrate (Lopressor) and nebivolol (Bystolic).

Patients with diabetes who are prone to low blood sugar (hypoglycemia) must use beta blockers with caution because the drugs can mask symptoms of low blood sugar. For a list of antihypertensive agents discussed in this section, see Table 1.10.

TABLE 1.10 Antihypertensive Agents

Generic Name	Brand Name(s)	Route(s) of Administration	Dosage Form(s)	Common Dosage Amount(s)
Angiotensin-Converting Enzyme (ACE) Inhibitors				
benazepril	Lotensin	oral	tablet	5 mg, 10 mg, 20 mg, 40 mg
captopril	Capoten	oral	tablet	12.5 mg, 25 mg, 50 mg, 100 mg
enlapril	Vasotec	oral	solution, tablet	2.5 mg, 5 mg, 10 mg, 20 mg, 1 mg/mL
fosinopril	Monopril	oral	tablet	10 mg, 20 mg, 40 mg
lisinopril	Prinivil, Zestril	oral	tablet	2.5 mg, 5 mg, 10 mg, 20 mg, 30 mg, 40 mg
moexipril	Univasc	oral	tablet	7.5 mg, 15 mg
perindopril	Aceon	oral	tablet	2 mg, 4 mg, 8 mg
quinapril	Accupril	oral	tablet	5 mg, 10 mg, 20 mg, 40 mg

continues

TABLE 1.10 Antihypertensive Agents—*Continued*

Generic Name	Brand Name(s)	Route(s) of Administration	Dosage Form(s)	Common Dosage Amount(s)
Angiotensin-Converting Enzyme (ACE) Inhibitors				
ramipril	Altace	oral	capsule	1.25 mg, 2.5 mg, 5 mg, 10 mg
trandolapril	Mavik	oral	tablet	1 mg, 2 mg, 4 mg
Angiotensin II Receptor Blockers (ARBs)				
azilsartan	Edarbi	oral	tablet	40 mg, 80 mg
candesartan	Atacand	oral	tablet	4 mg, 8 mg, 16 mg, 32 mg
eprosartan	Teveten	oral	tablet	400 mg, 600 mg
irbesartan	Avapro	oral	tablet	75 mg, 150 mg, 300 mg
losartan	Cozaar	oral	tablet	50 mg, 75 mg, 100 mg
olmesartan	Benicar	oral	tablet	5 mg, 20 mg, 40 mg
telmisartan	Micardis	oral	tablet	20 mg, 40 mg, 80 mg
valsartan	Diovan	oral	tablet	40 mg, 80 mg, 160 mg, 320 mg
Calcium Channel Blockers (CCBs)				
amlodipine	Norvasc	oral	tablet	2.5 mg, 5 mg, 10 mg
diltiazem	Cardizem, Cardizem CD, others	oral, parenteral (IV)	extended-release capsule, tablet, extended-release tablet, solution for injection	30 mg, 60 mg, 90 mg, 120 mg, 180 mg, 240 mg, 300 mg, 360 mg, 420 mg, 5 mg/mL
felodipine	Plendil	oral	tablet	2.5 mg, 5 mg, 10 mg
nicardipine	Cardene	oral, parenteral (IV)	capsule, solution for injection	20 mg, 30 mg, 2.5 mg/mL
nifedipine	Procardia, Procardia XL, others	oral	capsule, extended-release tablet	10 mg, 20 mg, 30 mg, 60 mg, 90 mg
verapamil	Calan, Verelan, others	oral, parenteral (IV)	extended-release capsule, extended-release tablet, solution for injection	40 mg, 80 mg, 100 mg, 120 mg, 180 mg, 200 mg, 240 mg, 300 mg, 360 mg
Beta-Adrenergic Blockers (Beta Blockers)				
acebutolol	Sectral	oral	capsule	200 mg, 400 mg
atenolol	Tenormin	oral	tablet	25 mg, 50 mg, 100 mg

continues

TABLE 1.10 Antihypertensive Agents—*Continued*

Generic Name	Brand Name(s)	Route(s) of Administration	Dosage Form(s)	Common Dosage Amount(s)
Beta-Adrenergic Blockers (Beta Blockers)				
bisoprolol	Zebeta	oral	tablet	5 mg, 10 mg
carvedilol	Coreg, Coreg CR	oral	tablet, extended-release capsule	3.125 mg, 6.25 mg, 10 mg, 12.5 mg, 10 mg, 25 mg, 40 mg, 80 mg
labetalol	Trandate	oral, parenteral (IV)	tablet, solution for injection	100 mg, 200 mg, 300 mg, 5 mg/mL
metoprolol succinate	Toprol XL	oral	extended-release tablet	25 mg, 50 mg 100 mg, 200 mg
metoprolol tartrate	Lopressor	oral, parenteral (IV)	tablet, solution for injection	25 mg, 37.5 mg, 50 mg, 75 mg, 100 mg, 5 mg/5 mL
nadolol	Corgard	oral	tablet	20 mg, 40 mg, 80 mg
nebivolol	Bystolic	oral, parenteral (IV)	tablet	2.5 mg, 5 mg, 10 mg, 20 mg
propranolol	Inderal, Inderal LA	oral, parenteral (IV)	extended-release capsule, tablet, solution for injection	10 mg, 20 mg, 40 mg, 60 mg, 80 mg, 120 mg, 160 mg, 1 mg/mL

Diuretics, which reduce water retention, are also prescribed for high blood pressure. Diuretics are often available in combination dosage forms with other antihypertensive agents, such as ACE inhibitors and ARBs. Diuretics are addressed in the Section 1.11 on renal and genitourinary medications.

Medications to Lower Cholesterol

Study Idea

It is easy to remember that the antihyperlipidemic drugs, or "statins," end in -*statin*.

Antihyperlipidemic agents are cardiovascular drugs that fight the buildup of **lipids** by lowering a patient's level of dangerous **cholesterol** (fatty acids) and **triglycerides** (three fatty acids combined with glycerol). Cholesterol consists of two main types of fatty acids: **low-density lipoprotein (LDL)**—bad cholesterol—and **high-density lipoprotein (HDL)**—good cholesterol.

Antihyperlipidemic agents that work to prevent the production of LDL cholesterol are commonly referred to as **statins**. Statins are also called **HMG-CoA redutase inhibitors**. They can lower LDL cholesterol up to 50% or more. Statins should not be taken with grapefruit juice as this may decrease metabolism of statins and increase the risk of side effects. Muscle fatigue is a common side effect, especially when these drugs are combined with other agents, such as gemfibrozil, verapamil, diltiazem, macrolide antibiotics, and amiodarone. See Table 1.11 for examples of HMG Co-A Reductase Inhibitors or statins.

TABLE 1.11 HMG-CoA Reductase Inhibitors (Statins)

Generic Name	Brand Name(s)	Route(s) of Administration	Dosage Form(s)	Common Dosage Amount(s)
atorvastatin	Lipitor	oral	tablet	10 mg, 20 mg, 40 mg, 80 mg
fluvastatin	Lescol, Lescol XL	oral	capsule, extended-release tablet	20 mg, 40 mg, 80 mg
lovastatin	Mevacor	oral	tablet	10 mg, 20 mg, 40 mg, 60 mg
pitavastatin	Livalo	oral	tablet	1 mg, 2 mg, 4 mg
pravastatin	Pravachol	oral	tablet	10 mg, 20 mg, 40 mg, 80 mg
rosuvastatin	Crestor	oral	tablet	5 mg, 10 mg, 20 mg, 40 mg, 80 mg
simvastatin	Zocor	oral	tablet	5 mg, 10 mg, 20 mg, 40 mg, 80 mg

Ezetimibe (Zetia) is another antihyperlipidemic medication. Ezetimibe blocks the absorption of cholesterol from the diet. It is available in a combination product with simvastatin (Vytorin). Nicotinic acid (Niaspan) is a B_3 vitamin with a broad spectrum of activity. In large doses, it lowers the amounts of LDL and triglycerides in the body and improves HDL cholesterol. Nicotinic acid is available as a prescription and OTC drug, but patients should be made aware that liver function should be tested periodically while using this drug. The dose must be slowly increased over several weeks to avoid flushing (warmth, redness, itching, tingling of skin) and headaches. Flushing can be prevented by predosing with aspirin 30 minutes prior to taking nicotinic acid. The dose is usually taken at bedtime with a snack.

Fenofibrate (TriCor) lowers triglycerides rather than cholesterol and is usually well tolerated. However, it must be used with caution in patients who take statins, warfarin, and other blood thinners. Another agent that lowers triglycerides is gemifibrozil (Lopid).

Omega-3 fatty acids are also effective for lowering triglycerides. Salmon is high in omega-3 fatty acids and can help naturally lower triglycerides. Natural fish oil, or a fish oil supplement, is effective for lowering triglycerides. For patients who are allergic or intolerant to seafood, Lovaza is a prescription omega-3 fatty acid. Vascepa is another prescription omega-3 fatty acid product indicated to reduce cardiovascular risk in patients with elevated triglycerides.

Alirocumab (Praluent) and evolocumab (Repatha) are proprotein convertase subtilisin/kexin type 9 (PCSK9) inhibitors, antihyperlipidemic treatments that can be considered for patients who do not meet their cholesterol treatment goals with dietary modification and other lipid-lowering therapies. Both are monoclonal antibodies administered by subcutaneous injection that work to lower LDL levels. See Table 1.12 for examples of antihyperlipidemic agents that either work in a different way than statins or that work in combination with a statin.

TABLE 1.12 Other Antihyperlipidemic Agents

Generic Name	Brand Name(s)	Route(s) of Administration	Dosage Form(s)	Common Dosage Amount(s)
Blocks Cholesterol Absorption				
ezetimibe	Zetia	oral	tablet	10 mg
simvastatin / ezetimibe	Vytorin	oral	tablet	10 mg/10 mg, 10 mg/20 mg, 10 mg/40 mg, 10 mg/80 mg
Decreases LDL and Triglycerides				
nicotinic acid	Niaspan	oral	extended-release tablet	250 mg, 500 mg, 750 mg, 1,000 mg
Decreases Triglycerides				
fenofibrate	TriCor	oral	tablet	40 mg, 48 mg, 54 mg, 120 mg, 145 mg, 160 mg
gemfibrozil	Lopid	oral	tablet	600 mg
omega-3 fatty acids	Lovaza, Vascepa	oral	capsule	0.5 g, 1 g
PCSK9 Inhibitors (Decreases LDL)				
alirocumab	Praluent	parenteral (SubQ)	solution for injection	75 mg/mL, 150 mg/mL
evolocumab	Repatha	parenteral (SubQ)	solution for injection	140 mg/mL

Miscellaneous Cardiovascular Agents

In addition to drugs to fight high blood pressure and cholesterol, other cardiovascular agents are used to treat arrhythmia (abnormal heartbeat), heart failure, and angina pectoris (severe chest pain). The agents for heart failure all work differently and are sometimes used in combination with each other or with that ACE inhibitors or ARBs.

Digoxin (Lanoxin) is an older drug that helps a weak heart beat stronger. While in use, patients' serum blood levels should be monitored to prevent toxic levels and side effects, including abnormal heart rhythms (arrhythmias). Digoxin can slow heart rate and cause nausea and vomiting when toxic levels are reached, especially if blood potassium levels are low.

Isosorbide mononitrate (Imdur) and isosorbide dinitrate (Isordil) belong to the nitrate family. The **nitrates** all work similarly—they dilate the blood vessels, particularly those of the heart, to increase oxygen and blood flow, to relieve chest pain, and reduce the workload on the heart. Nitrates can all cause headaches and a dangerous drop in blood pressure when combined with erectile dysfunction drugs, including the well-known brands Viagra, Levitra, and Cialis. Isosorbide dinitrate is often prescribed with hydralazine (Apresoline) for treatment of heart failure.

Nitroglycerin is often taken at the first sign of chest pain, with repeated doses every five minutes for three doses. If chest pain continues, the patient is advised to take a crushed aspirin tablet and get to the emergency room as quickly as possible.

Nitroglycerin sublingual (under the tongue) tablets are sensitive to air and light and should be replaced every three to six months. Because of its use in emergencies, nitroglycerin should be dispensed in the original container and never in a child-resistant container.

Sacubitril / valsartan (Entresto) is a combination medication approved for treatment of heart failure. Sacubitril is a neprilysin inhibitor that promotes vasodilation, and valsartan is an ARB. Entresto should not be taken with ACE inhibitors, and, if switching to Entresto from an ACE inhibitor, a 36-hour washout period is required. For a list of the miscellaneous cardiovascular agents discussed in this section, see Table 1.13.

TABLE 1.13 Miscellaneous Cardiovascular Agents

Generic Name	Brand Name(s)	Route(s) of Administration	Dosage Form(s)	Common Dosage Amount(s)
Cardiac Glycoside				
digoxin	Lanoxin	oral, parenteral (IV)	oral solution, tablet, solution for injection	125 mcg, 250 mcg, 0.05 mg/mL, 0.25 mg/mL
Vasodilator				
hydralazine	Apresoline	oral, parenteral (IV, IM)	tablet, solution for injection	10 mg, 25 mg, 50 mg, 100 mg, 20 mg/mL
Nitrates				
isosorbide dinitrate	Isordil	oral	extended-release capsule, tablet	5 mg, 10 mg, 20 mg, 30 mg, 40 mg
isosorbide mononitrate	Imdur	oral	tablet, extended-release tablet	10 mg, 20 mg, 30 mg, 40 mg
nitroglycerin	Nitrostat, Nitrolingual, others	oral, topical, parenteral (IV)	sublingual (SL) tablet, SL spray, transdermal patch, solution for injection	0.3 mg, 0.4 mg, 0.6 mg, 0.4 mg/spray, 0.1 mg/hr, 0.2 mg/hr, 0.6 mg/hr
Neprilysin Inhibitor/Angiotensin Receptor Blocker (ARB)				
sacubitril / valsartan	Entresto	oral	tablet	24 mg/26 mg, 49 mg/51 mg, 97 mg/103 mg

1.6 Medications to Treat Infections

Anti-infective agents include antibiotics, antifungals, and antivirals. Anti-infective agents are indicated to treat infections from a variety of pathogens, including bacteria, fungi, and viruses. Antiretrovirals are a specific type of antiviral that treats infection with human immunodeficiency virus (HIV). Anti-infective agents are available in a variety of dosage forms.

Antibiotics

Safety Alert

It is important for the technician to double-check the allergy history in the patient profile prior to dispensing any antibiotic prescription—looking especially for penicillin allergies.

Antibiotics treat bacterial infections by killing or weakening the bacteria. Most antibiotics work by slowing down the growth of bacteria, or by disrupting the integrity of the bacterial cell. There is no one type of antibiotic that cures every infection. Antibiotics are divided into classes based on their structure and function.

Penicillins

Among the most common antibiotics is penicillin (Veetids, Pen VK) and its derivatives: amoxicillin (Amoxil) and amoxicillin / clavulanate (Augmentin). These are commonly used to treat upper respiratory, sinus, and ear infections in children and adults. Ampicillin / sulbactam (Unasyn) and nafcillin (Unipen) are used primarily in the hospital to treat infections resistant to traditional penicillins. Common side effects of penicillins include stomach upset, diarrhea, rash, and allergic reaction. It is important to check patient profiles for penicillin allergies. For a list of penicillins, see Table 1.14.

TABLE 1.14 Penicillins

Generic Name	Brand Name(s)	Route(s) of Administration	Dosage Form(s)	Common Dosage Amount(s)
amoxicillin	Amoxil	oral	capsule, suspension, tablet, chewable tablet	250 mg, 500 mg, 875 mg, 125 mg/5 mL, 200 mg/5 mL, 250 mg/5 mL, 400 mg/5 mL
amoxicillin / clavulanate	Augmentin	oral	suspension, tablet, chewable tablet, extended-release tablet	200 mg/28.5 mg, 250 mg/125 mg, 500 mg/125 mg, 875 mg/125 mg, 1,000 mg/62.5 mg, 200 mg/28.5 mg/5 mL, 250 mg/62.5 mg/5 mL, 400 mg/57 mg/5 mL, 600 mg/42.9 mg/5 mL
ampicillin	Omnipen	oral, parenteral (IV)	capsule, solution for injection	125 mg, 250 mg, 1 g, 2 g, 10 g
ampicillin / sulbactam	Unasyn	parenteral (IV, IM)	solution for injection	1.5 g, 3 g, 10 g
nafcillin	Unipen	parenteral (IV)	solution for injection	1 g, 2 g, 10 g
penicillin V potassium	Pen VK, Veetids	oral	solution, tablet	250 mg, 500 mg, 125 mg/5 mL, 250 mg/5 mL
piperacillin / tazobactam	Zosyn	parenteral (IV)	solution for injection	2.25 g, 3.375 g, 4.5 g

Cephalosporins

Cephalosporins are a class of antibiotics that are related to penicillin. They are commonly used in both the community and hospital setting to treat respiratory infections, pneumonia, and infections related to dental work. Common cephalosporins include cefazolin (Ancef), ceftazidime (Fortaz, Tazicef), ceftriaxone (Rocephin), and cephalexin (Keflex). Common adverse reactions to cephalosporins include diarrhea, rash, upset stomach, and allergic reaction. While cephalosporins are similar to penicillin, fewer than 5% of those allergic to penicillins are also allergic to cephalosporins. However, if a patient has an anaphylactic reaction (severe allergy) to penicillins, cephalosporins should be avoided. For a list of cephalosporins, see Table 1.15.

TABLE 1.15 Cephalosporins

Generic Name	Brand Name(s)	Route(s) of Administration	Dosage Form(s)	Common Dosage Amount(s)
cefazolin	Ancef	parenteral (IV)	solution for injection	500 mg, 1 g, 2 g, 10 g, 20 g
cefdinir	Omnicef	oral	capsule, suspension	300 mg, 125 mg/ 5 mL, 250 mg/5 mL
cefepime	Maxipime	parenteral (IV)	solution for injection	1 g, 2 g
cefixime	Suprax	oral	powder for suspension, tablet	400 mg, 100 mg/ 5 mL, 200 mg/5 mL, 500 mg/5 mL
ceftazidime	Fortaz, Tazicef	parenteral (IV)	solution for injection	1 g, 2 g, 6 g
ceftriaxone	Rocephin	parenteral (IV, IM)	solution for injection	150 mg, 500 mg, 1 g, 2 g, 6 g
cephalexin	Keflex	oral	capsule, suspension, tablet	250 mg, 500 mg, 750 mg, 125 mg/ 5 mL, 350 mg/5 mL

 TAKE NOTE

When a patient does not complete an antibiotic therapy to kill all microorganisms, those that survive will reproduce, creating more resistant bacteria by natural selection, and decreasing the effectiveness of the antibiotic.

Consequently, stronger doses of the antibiotic or additional drugs need to be prescribed, which, in turn, creates a higher risk of side effects. Due to drug resistance, the required dose of amoxicillin to treat ear infections in children has doubled in the past 30 years. A more serious example in the hospital environment is the development of methicillin-resistant *Staphylococcus aureus* (MRSA), which can be so unresponsive to antibiotics that it can cause death.

Pharmacy technicians should stress the importance of completing the entire course of antibiotic therapy to reduce the incidence of antibiotic resistance and recurring infections.

Macrolides

Macrolides are a class of antibiotics that include azithromycin (Zithromax, Z-Pak). Azithromycin works by stopping bacteria from making their own proteins. It is commonly prescribed as a tablet (Z-Pak) or suspension for the treatment of upper respiratory infections in children and adults. Azithromycin has the advantage of a five-day course of therapy (instead of a two-week or longer regimen), which may improve patient compliance. Azithromycin should be taken with a meal or snack to lessen gastrointestinal side effects. Unlike some antibiotic suspensions, which should be refrigerated, azithromycin suspensions can be kept at room temperature. Azithromycin commonly interacts with other drugs, so the patient's medication profile and medication use must be assessed by the pharmacist. For a list of macrolides, see Table 1.16.

TABLE 1.16 Macrolides

Generic Name	Brand Name(s)	Route(s) of Administration	Dosage Form(s)	Common Dosage Amount(s)
azithromycin	Zithromax, Z-Pak	oral, parenteral (IV)	oral suspension, tablet, solution for injection	250 mg, 500 mg, 125 mg/5 mL, 250 mg/5 mL
clarithromycin	Biaxin	oral	suspension, tablet, extended-release tablet	250 mg, 500 mg, 125 mg/5 mL, 250 mg/5 mL
erythromycin	Ery-Tab	oral	delayed-release capsule, delayed-release tablet	250 mg, 333 mg, 500 mg

Fluoroquinolones

Fluoroquinolones are a class of potent antibiotics that include ciprofloxacin (Cipro) and levofloxacin (Levaquin). They are indicated to treat pneumonia, respiratory infections, and urinary tract infections. They should not be taken with milk, dairy products, or antacids. In rare but serious cases, these drugs can cause ruptured tendons or severe tendonitis with strenuous exercise, as described in the required Medication Guide. Fluoroquinolones come in many routes of administration and dosage forms, including oral, injection, otic (ear drops), and ophthalmic (eye drops). Ciprofloxacin and levofloxacin may interact with diabetes medications for lowering blood sugar, which can lower blood sugar to dangerous levels. For a list of Fluoroquinolones, see Table 1.17.

TABLE 1.17 Fluoroquinolones

Generic Name	Brand Name(s)	Route(s) of Administration	Dosage Form(s)	Common Dosage Amount(s)
ciprofloxacin	Cipro	oral, parenteral (IV)	oral suspension, tablet, solution for injection	250 mg, 500 mg, 750 mg, 250 mg/ 5 mL, 500 mg/5 mL

continues

TABLE 1.17 Fluoroquinolones—*Continued*

Generic Name	Brand Name(s)	Route(s) of Administration	Dosage Form(s)	Common Dosage Amount(s)
levofloxacin	Levaquin	oral, parenteral (IV), transmucosal (ophthalmic)	oral solution, tablet, solution for injection, eye drops	250 mg, 500 mg, 750 mg, 25 mg/mL, 250 mg/50 mL, 0.5%
moxifloxacin	Avelox, Vigamox	oral, transmucosal (ophthalmic)	tablet, eye drops	400 mg, 0.5%
ofloxacin	Floxin	oral, transmucosal (ophthalmic, otic)	tablet, eye drops, ear drops	300 mg, 400 mg, 0.3%

Tetracyclines

Tetracyclines are a class of antibiotics that include minocycline (Minocin) and doxycycline (Vibramycin). Doxycycline is an all-purpose antibiotic commonly used to treat various bacterial infections, including acne and chronic bronchitis. Tetracyclines must not be taken by pregnant or nursing patients or children under 12 years of age. In addition, they must not be taken at the same time as dairy, antacids, iron, or calcium supplements. Patients taking tetracyclines should avoid sun exposure as they may increase risk of sunburn. For a list of tetracyclines, see Table 1.18.

TABLE 1.18 Tetracyclines

Generic Name	Brand Name	Route(s) of Administration	Dosage Form(s)	Common Dosage Amount(s)
doxycycline	Vibramycin	oral, parenteral (IV)	capsule, oral suspension, tablet, solution for injection	50 mg, 75 mg, 100 mg, 150 mg, 25 mg/5 mL
minocycline	Minocin	oral, parenteral (IV)	capsule, solution for injection	50 mg, 75 mg, 100 mg
tetracycline	Sumycin	oral	capsule	250 mg, 500 mg

Other Common Antibiotics

Other common antibiotics treat specific conditions and provide alternatives for people with allergies to other antibiotics. Clindamycin (Cleocin) is an alternative antibiotic for use in patients who are allergic to penicillin; it can cause severe diarrhea. Clindamycin is commonly prescribed for dental infections, because it can treat anaerobic bacteria, which is common in oral cavities. If patients develop bloody diarrhea, they should contact their physician immediately, because they may have developed colitis from the antibiotic or a *Clostridioides difficile* infection. In the hospital, clindamycin and metronidazole (Flagyl) are used to treat or prevent severe post-surgical anaerobic infections. They are also used topically to treat acne in adolescents and adults.

Metronidazole is also frequently prescribed for five to seven days to treat vaginal infections. The use of alcohol with this drug can cause severe nausea, elevated heart rate, vomiting, and warmth/redness under skin, and death. All forms of alcohol must be avoided for 72 hours after last use.

Vancomycin (Vancocin) is a common antibiotic used to treat methicillin-resistant *Staphylococcus aureus* (MRSA), the bacterium responsible for many hard-to-treat infections in the hospital. Gentamicin (Garamycin, Gentak) is an intravenous aminoglycoside antibiotic that is frequently used in combination with other antibiotics to treat serious infections. Kidney function and levels of drug in the blood must be carefully monitored with both vancomycin (Vancocin) and gentamicin to adjust dosing. At toxic levels, these drugs can cause hearing loss; care must be taken to ensure accurate dosing levels.

Sulfamethoxazole / trimethoprim (Bactrim, Septra) is a sulfonamide antibiotic used to treat urinary tract infections, skin and soft tissue infections, and ear infections. Sulfonamides should be taken with adequate amounts of water and must be used cautiously with blood thinners like warfarin and other drugs. Sunscreen precautions should be recommended as sulfonamides cause photosensitivity.

Meropenem (Merrem) and ertapenem (Invanz) are intravenous antibiotics used in hospital settings for serious infections. They are indicated to treat community-acquired pneumonia, complicated urinary tract infections, and intra-abdominal infections. Linezolid (Zyvox) is indicated for the treatment of multi-drug-resistant bacteria, including MRSA. Side effects include thrush and abdominal discomfort.

Since antibiotics kill or weaken bacteria, they also kill good bacteria and commonly cause side effects such as diarrhea, yeast infections, and so on. Yogurt or probiotics often offset diarrhea, but yeast infections may require treatment with OTC or prescription drugs. Also, with many antibiotics, the patient should take precautions in the sun because these agents can cause sun sensitivity. Some kinds of antibiotics may lower the effectiveness of birth control, so patients on birth control medications must be made aware of this. See Table 1.19 for examples of other common antibiotics.

TABLE 1.19 Other Common Antibiotics

Generic Name	Brand Name(s)	Route(s) of Administration	Dosage Form(s)	Common Dosage Amount(s)
clindamycin	Cleocin	oral, parenteral (IV)	capsule, solution for injection	75 mg, 150 mg, 300 mg
ertapenem	Invanz	parenteral (IV, IM)	solution for injection	1 g
gentamicin	Garamycin, Gentak	parenteral (IV)	solution for injection	10 mg/mL, 40 mg/mL
linezolid	Zyvox	oral, parenteral (IV)	oral suspension, tablet, solution for injection	600 mg, 600 mg/ 300 mL, 100 mg/ 5 mL
meropenem	Merrem	parenteral (IV)	solution for injection	1 g
metronidazole	Flagyl	oral, parenteral (IV)	capsule, tablet, solution for injection	250 mg, 375 mg, 500 mg
vancomycin	Vancocin	oral, parenteral (IV)	capsule, oral solution, solution for injection	125 mg, 250 mg, 250 mg/5 mL, 5 g, 10 g
sulfamethoxazole / trimethoprim	Bacrtim, Septra	oral, parenteral (IV)	oral suspension, tablet, solution for injection	800 mg/160 mg, 400 mg/80 mg, 200 mg/40 mg/ 5 mL

Antifungals

Antifungals fight fungal infections like athlete's foot and thrush. The antifungal drug fluconazole (Diflucan) is commonly prescribed as a one-time or short-term oral treatment for fungal yeast infections. Amphotericin B (Ambisome) is an intravenous antifungal used in hospitals to treat systemic fungal infections. It must be infused slowly over six hours. Some antifungal drugs are available OTC such as miconazole (Monistat) and clotrimazole (Lotrimin). For a list of commonly prescribed antifungals, see Table 1.20.

TABLE 1.20 Antifungals

Generic Name	Brand Name(s)	Route(s) of Administration	Dosage Form(s)	Common Dosage Amount(s)
amphotericin B	Ambisome	parenteral (IV)	IV suspension	50 mg
caspofungin	Cancidas	parenteral (IV)	solution for injection	50 mg, 70 mg
clotrimazole*	Lotrimin	oral, topical, trans-mucosal (vaginal)	cream, lozenge, troche	10 mg, 1%
fluconazole	Diflucan	oral, parenteral (IV)	oral suspension, tablet, solution for injection	50 mg, 100 mg, 150 mg, 200 mg, 10 mg/mL, 40 mg/mL
ketoconazole	Nizoral	oral, topical	tablet, cream, shampoo	200 mg, 1%, 2%
miconazole*	Monistat	transmucosal (vaginal)	cream, suppository	100 mg, 200 mg, 2%
nystatin	Mycostatin	oral, topical	oral suspension, cream, powder	250 mg, 1%
terbinafine*	Lamisil	oral, topical	tablet, cream, spray	

*some strengths and dosage forms available over-the-counter (OTC)

Antivirals and Antiretrovirals

Antivirals work to fight or control infections caused by viruses. For viral herpes infections, acyclovir (Zovirax) and valacyclovir (Valtrex) are used topically (Zovirax ointment), orally, and intravenously. Oseltamivir (Tamiflu) is an antiviral drug used for flu outbreaks in both children and adults in a five-day therapy.

Antiretrovirals are a type of antiviral agent commonly prescribed to treat HIV. Some examples of the most commonly prescribed antiretroviral drug classifications are the nucleoside/nucleotide reverse transcriptase inhibitors (NRTIs), non-nucleoside reverse transcriptase inhibitors (NNRTIs), and protease inhibitors. These drugs make it difficult for the virus to replicate itself. Many HIV treatments come as combination products with three to four drugs in one tablet. Patients should follow labeled instructions and not miss a dose.

See Tables 1.21 and 1.22 for commonly prescribed antiviral and antiretroviral agents.

TABLE 1.21 Antivirals

Generic Name	Brand Name(s)	Route(s) of Administration	Dosage Form(s)	Common Dosage Amount(s)
acyclovir	Zovirax	oral, topical	capsule, oral suspension, tablet, ointment	200 mg, 400 mg, 800 mg, 200 mg/5 mL, 5%
baloxavir marboxil	Xofluza	oral	tablet	40 mg, 80 mg
oseltamivir	Tamiflu	oral	capsule, suspension	30 mg, 45 mg, 75 mg, 6 mg/mL
valacylovir	Valtrex	oral	tablet	500 mg, 1,000 mg

TABLE 1.22 Antiretrovirals

Generic Name	Brand Name(s)	Route(s) of Administration	Dosage Form(s)	Common Dosage Amount(s)
abacavir	Ziagen	oral	solution, tablet	300 mg, 20 mg/mL
atazanavir	Reyataz	oral	capsule	50 mg, 150 mg, 200 mg, 300 mg
darunavir	Prezista	oral	tablet	150 mg, 400 mg, 600 mg, 800 mg
efavirenz	Sustiva	oral	capsule, tablet	50 mg, 200 mg, 600 mg
emtricitabine	Emtriva	oral	capsule, solution	200 mg, 10 mg/mL
emtricitabine / tenofovir disoproxil	Truvada	oral	tablet	100 mg/150 mg, 133 mg/200 mg, 167 mg/250 mg, 200 mg/300 mg
ritonavir	Norvir	oral	solution, tablet	100 mg, 80 mg/mL
tenofovir disoproxil	Viread	oral	tablet	300 mg

1.7 Endocrine Medications

The **endocrine** system is the network of glands that secrete hormones into the circulatory system to regulate bodily functions, including metabolism, or the processes of producing energy from nutrients. Various endocrine agents are frequently dispensed in the community pharmacy. The most common types of these medications are used to treat diabetes and thyroid conditions.

Medications to Treat Diabetes

Diabetes is one of the fastest growing chronic diseases in the world, especially in the United States. Diabetes drugs all lower blood sugar but by different mechanisms of action. With type I diabetes (previously known as *juvenile diabetes*), the body stops producing insulin, and patients need daily doses of insulin for replacement. Type 2 diabetes, also called *adult onset diabetes*, is a type of diabetes in which the body does not use insulin properly, so blood sugar levels go up and down. Blood sugar levels must be modulated with oral medications or adjusted with injections of insulin. Most patients with diabetes have type 2 diabetes. To treat diabetes, patients need nutrition and life-style changes, oral medications, and/or insulin injections.

Non-Insulin Medications

All drugs for type 2 diabetes work to lower blood glucose, but by different mechanisms of action. Patients often need more than one drug to attain target levels. **Metformin (Glucophage, Fortamet, Glumetza, Riomet)** is the most frequently prescribed medication for type 2 diabetes and is considered first-line therapy. It is available in both an immediate-release and extended-release tablet, and as an oral liquid. Metformin should be taken with food, and patients may need to take a vitamin B12 supplement while taking long-term metformin. Metformin is often prescribed with other medications for diabetes, especially sulfonylureas, DPP-4 inhibitors, GLP-1 agonists, and SGLT2 inhibitors.

The **sulfonylureas** are another class of drugs for diabetes. Sulfonylureas stimulate the cells of the pancreas to produce more insulin. Drugs in this class include glipizide (Glucotrol, Glucotrol XL) and glyburide (Micronase, DiaBeta). When taking sulfonylureas, patients must carefully monitor their blood glucose to prevent hypoglycemia (low blood sugar) caused by an overabundance of insulin. In addition to hypoglycemia, sulfonylureas can also cause sensitivity to the sun.

DPP-4 inhibitors like sitagliptin (Januvia) and linagliptin (Tradjenta) help control blood glucose by causing the pancreas to release insulin after glucose is consumed in the diet. They have a lower risk of hypoglycemia than sulfonylureas, and this makes them a safer choice to treat diabetes in the older adult population. Like DPP-4 inhibitors, the **GLP-1 agonists** also signal the pancreas to release insulin after the patient has consumed glucose in the diet. GLP-1 agonists like exenatide (Byetta) and liraglutide (Victoza) are injectable in either daily or weekly formulas. Their main side effects are nausea, vomiting, and irritation at the site of injection.

Thiazolidinediones (TZDs) include pioglitazone (Actos) and rosiglitazone (Avandia). TZDs lower blood glucose by increasing the sensitivity of cells to insulin without increasing insulin secretion. TZDs can cause fluid retention, weight gain, and adverse gastrointestinal effects. They can worsen heart failure and are not recommended for patients who have symptomatic heart failure.

The **SGLT2 inhibitors** are a newer class of medications that treat diabetes by preventing the kidneys from reabsorbing glucose back into the blood. This allows glucose to be excreted in the urine and lowers blood glucose levels. Canagliflozin (Invokana) and dapagliflozin (Farxiga) are both SGLT2 inhibitors. Because SGLT2 inhibitors cause glucose to concentrate in the urine, they increase the risk of urinary tract and yeast infections.

Other medications to treat diabetes include pramlintide (Symlin), which is a synthetic analog of a human amylin and helps reduce mealtime glucose by several mechanisms. Pramlintide is administered by subcutaneous injection and is indicated in type 1 and type 2 diabetes. Other classes include alpha-glucosidase inhibitors, meglitinides, and combination products. For a list of diabetes medications described in this section, see Table 1.23.

TABLE 1.23 Non-Insulin Medications to Treat Diabetes

Generic Name	Brand Name(s)	Route(s) of Administration	Dosage Form(s)	Common Dosage Amount(s)
Biguanide				
metformin	Glucophage, Fortamet, Glumetza, Riomet	oral	liquid, tablet, extended-release tablet	500 mg, 750 mg, 850 mg, 1,000 mg, 500 mg/5 mL
Sulfonylureas				
glimepiride	Amaryl	oral	tablet	1 mg, 2 mg, 4 mg
glipizide	Glucotrol, Glucotrol XL	oral	tablet, extended-release tablet	2.5 mg, 5 mg, 10 mg
glyburide	Micronase, DiaBeta	oral	tablet	1.25 mg, 1.5 mg, 2.5 mg, 3 mg, 5 mg, 6 mg
DPP-4 Inhibitors				
alogliptin	Nesina	oral	tablet	25 mg
linagliptin	Tradjenta	oral	tablet	5 mg
saxagliptin	Onglyza	oral	tablet	2.5 mg, 5 mg
sitagliptin	Januvia	oral	tablet	25 mg, 50 mg, 100 mg
GLP-1 Agonists				
dulaglutide	Trulicity	parenteral (SubQ)	solution for injection	0.75 mg, 1.5 mg
exenatide	Byetta	parenteral (SubQ)	solution for injection	5 mcg, 10 mcg
liraglutide	Victoza	parenteral (SubQ)	solution for injection	0.6 mg, 1.2 mg, 1.8 mg
lixisenatide	Adlyxin	parenteral (SubQ)	solution for injection	10 mcg, 20 mcg
semaglutide	Ozempic, Rybelsus	oral, parenteral (SubQ)	tablet, solution for injection	0.25 mg, 0.5 mg, 1 mg, 3 mg, 7 mg, 14 mg
Thiazolidinediones (TZDs)				
pioglitazone	Actos	oral	tablet	15 mg, 30 mg, 45 mg
rosiglitazone	Avandia	oral	tablet	2 mg, 4 mg, 8 mg
SGLT2 Inhibitors				
canagliflozin	Invokana	oral	tablet	100 mg, 300 mg
dapagliflozin	Farxiga	oral	tablet	5 mg, 10 mg
empagliflozin	Jardiance	oral	tablet	10 mg, 25 mg

continues

TABLE 1.23 Non-insulin Medications to Treat Diabetes—*Continued*

Generic Name	Brand Name(s)	Route(s) of Administration	Dosage Form(s)	Common Dosage Amount(s)
SGLT2 Inhibitors				
ertugliflozin	Steglatro	oral	tablet	5 mg, 15 mg
Amylin Analog				
pramlintide	Symlin	parenteral (SubQ)	solution for injection	60 mcg
Alpha-Glucosidase Inhibitors				
acarbose	Precose	oral	tablet	25 mg, 50 mg, 100 mg
miglitol	Glyset	oral	tablet	25 mg, 50 mg, 100 mg
Meglitinides				
nateglinide	Starlix	oral	tablet	60 mg, 120 mg
repaglinide	Prandin	oral	tablet	0.5 mg, 1 mg, 2 mg
Combination Products				
alogliptin / metformin	Kazano	oral	tablet	12.5 mg/500 mg, 12.5 mg/1,000 mg
alogliptin / pioglitazone	Oseni	oral	tablet	12.5 mg/15 mg, 12.5 mg/30 mg, 12.5 mg/45 mg, 25 mg/15 mg, 25 mg/30 mg, 25 mg/45 mg
canagliflozin / metformin	Invokamet, Invokamet XR	oral	tablet, extended-release tablet	50 mg/500 mg, 150 mg/500 mg, 50 mg/1,000 mg, 150 mg/1,000 mg
dapagliflozin / metformin	Xigduo XR	oral	extended-release tablet	2.5 mg/1,000 mg, 5 mg/500 mg, 5 mg/1,000 mg, 10 mg/500 mg, 10 mg/1,000 mg
dapagliflozin / saxagliptin	Qtern	oral	tablet	5 mg/5 mg, 10 mg/5 mg
empagliflozin / linagliptin	Glyxambi	oral	tablet	10 mg/5 mg, 25 mg/5 mg
empagliflozin / linagliptin / metformin	Trijardy XR	oral	extended-release tablet	5 mg/2.5 mg/ 1,000 mg, 10 mg/5 mg/ 1,000 mg, 25 mg/5 mg/ 1,000 mg

continues

TABLE 1.23 Non-Insulin Medications to Treat Diabetes—*Continued*

Generic Name	Brand Name(s)	Route(s) of Administration	Dosage Form(s)	Common Dosage Amount(s)
Combination Products				
ertugliflozin / metformin	Segluromet	oral	tablet	2.5 mg/500 mg, 2.5 mg/1,000 mg, 7.5 mg/1,000 mg
ertugliflozin / sitagliptin	Steglujan	oral	tablet	5 mg/100 mg, 15 mg/100 mg
glipizide / metformin	Metaglip	oral	tablet	2.5 mg/250 mg, 2.5 mg/500 mg, 5 mg/500 mg
pioglitazone / glimepiride	Duetact	oral	tablet	30 mg/2 mg, 20 mg/4 mg
pioglitazone / metformin	Actoplus MET	oral	tablet	15 mg/500 mg, 15 mg/850 mg
repaglinide / metformin	PrandiMet	oral	tablet	1 mg/500 mg, 2 mg/500 mg
saxagliptin / metformin	Kombiglyze XR	oral	tablet	2.5 mg/1,000 mg, 5 mg/500 mg, 5 mg/1,000 mg
sitagliptin / metformin	Janumet, Janumet XR	oral	tablet, extended-release tablet	50 mg/500 mg, 50 mg/1,000 mg, 100 mg/1,000 mg

Safety Alert

Insulin mix-ups and misspellings are the most common source of medication errors.

Insulins

Many types of insulin are available on the market today. A **basal insulin** is an insulin that controls blood sugar between meals and during sleep. Insulin glargine (Lantus) is one of the most commonly prescribed basal insulins; it is often taken at bedtime. It does not peak or trough but simply provides a level reduction of blood sugar over a 24-hour period.

A **bolus insulin** is an insulin that controls mealtime blood sugar. Bolus insulins should be taken 15 to 30 minutes prior to a meal,

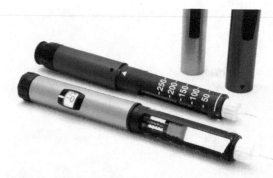

Many patients find using an insulin pen, such as the ones pictured above, more convenient than using an insulin vial and syringe.

depending on the type of insulin. Some mealtime insulins such as Novolin R and Humulin R can be sold without a prescription. Bolus insulins include insulin glulisine (Apidra) and insulin lispro (Ademlog, Humalog).

Many insulins now come in a pen form. For patient convenience, the dose of insulin is dialed into the pen and administered, eliminating the need for syringes. Technicians should make sure pen needles are dispensed to the patient to administer insulin with their insulin pen.

Frequently, insulins are prescribed separately or as mixtures of a rapid-release and slower-release insulin to be administered with syringes or pens. Be aware that Novolin and Humulin insulins are different from Novolog and Humalog insulins, and they should not be substituted for each other. Humalog and Novolog are rapid-acting, shorter-lasting insulins that should be used with meals.

Insulin must be refrigerated prior to use, and an open vial or pen must be used within a certain period once out of the refrigerator. Helping patients locate the manufacturer-recommended beyond-use date (BUD) instructions will prevent them using sub-potent insulin. For a list of insulins described in this section, see Table 1.24

TABLE 1.24 Insulins

Generic Name	Brand Name(s)
Rapid Acting	
insulin aspart	Fiasp, Novolog
insulin glulisine	Apidra
insulin lispro	Admelog, Humalog
Short Acting	
regular insulin	Humulin R*, Novolin R*
Intermediate Acting	
NPH insulin	Humulin N,* Novolin N*
Long Acting	
insulin degludec	Tresiba
insulin detemir	Levemir
insulin glargine	Basaglar, Lantus, Semglee, Toujeo

*available OTC

Thyroid Medications

As people age, their thyroid gland often stops working correctly. Thyroid hormones released by the thyroid gland have important functions that influence energy levels and metabolism, growth, body temperature, muscle strength, appetite, and the health of many organs.

Hypothyroidism occurs when the thyroid is not active enough and does not produce enough thyroid hormone. Patients with reduced thyroid function have very low energy and high levels of fatigue. Hypothyroidism is very common with age, especially in individuals assigned female at birth. Many physicians and some patients may request a brand-name drug, such as Synthroid (levothyroxine), due to higher tolerance or a more reliable therapeutic effect. If Synthroid is prescribed as *brand necessary*, it is considered a *dispense as written* (DAW) prescription when billing an insurance provider.

Thyroid replacement medications should be taken should be taken on an empty stomach to increase absorption. They must not be taken at the same time as dairy, antacids, iron, or calcium, or within two hours of ingestion of these substances.

Hyperthyroidism is the opposite condition, in which the thyroid is overstimulated and active. Hyperthyroidism is less common but more dangerous than hypothyroidism. It can lead to racing heartbeat and anxiety, bulging eyes, and even blindness. A common medication to treat overactive thyroid is methimazole (Tapazole). Patients taking methimazole should not consume alcohol, which can cause serious problems when combined with methimazole. For a list of thyroid medications described in this section, see Table 1.25.

TABLE 1.25 Thyroid Medications

Generic Name	Brand Name(s)	Route(s) of Administration	Dosage Form(s)	Common Dosage Amount(s)
Hypothyroidism				
levothyroxine	Synthroid, Levoxyl, Tirosent	oral, parenteral (IV)	capsule, tablet, solution for injection	25 mcg, 50 mcg, 75 mcg, 88 mcg, 100 mcg, 112 mcg, 125 mcg, 137 mcg, 150 mcg, 175 mcg, 200 mcg, 300 mcg
liothyronine	Cytomel	oral, parenteral (IV)	tablet, solution for injection	5 mcg, 10 mcg, 25 mcg, 50 mcg
Hyperthyroidism				
methimazole	Tapazole	oral	tablet	5 mg, 10 mg
propylthiouracil (PTU)	N/A	oral	tablet	50 mg

1.8 Respiratory Medications

Practice Tip

Patients must be reminded to keep inhalers and nebulizers clean and to rinse their mouths after using corticosteroids to prevent a fungal infection in the mouth called thrush.

Asthma, **chronic obstructive pulmonary disease (COPD)**, allergies, and coughs constrict the airways and cause inflammation, which can result in shortness of breath and wheezing, and can decrease oxygen saturation in the blood. To aid breathing, the airways may need help to relax and open.

Albuterol (ProAir, Proventil, Ventolin), levalbuterol (Xopenex), ipratropium (Atrovent), and tiotropium (Spiriva) all work in different ways to open the breathing passageways (bronchodilate) and to open the lungs of patients with asthma or COPD. Albuterol is the fastest acting bronchodilator and should be used for acute attacks. Albuterol may be prescribed as a tablet, syrup, metered-dose inhaler (MDI), propellant spray for inhaling, or sterile solution for a nebulizer, which converts it to a mist for inhalation.

The side effects of albuterol and its derivatives include increases in heart rate and blood pressure. Overuse may cause patients to develop a tolerance, and other medications need to be considered. Ipratropium and tiotropium both cause dryness of the mouth, throat, and eyes.

Many combination products are available to treat asthma and COPD. Budesonide / formoterol (Symbicort) and fluticasone / salmeterol (Advair) combine a passage-opening substance with a corticosteroid that reduces the swelling that causes difficulty breathing in asthma and COPD. Decreasing inflammation should reduce the acute attacks and the need for short-acting agents, such as albuterol.

Montelukast (Singulair)—available in tablet, chewable tablet, and granular forms—treats asthma and allergies by neutralizing and preventing the release of chemicals that cause symptoms like bronchoconstriction.

Antihistamines fight the body's histamine responses to allergies, whether severe or localized, such as itchiness, redness, nasal mucus, runny nose, swelling of airways, and coughing. First-generation antihistamines like diphenhydramine (Benadryl, which is available OTC) can be very sedating.

For less intense symptoms, physicians and pharmacists often recommend OTC, nonsedating antihistamines, such as loratadine (Claritin) or fexofenadine (Allegra). Antihistamines are also available in combination with the decongestant pseudoephedrine (Sudafed). Nasal sprays that provide intranasal steroids like fluticasone (Flonase) and mometasone (Nasonex) are used routinely to prevent seasonal allergy symptoms. Some nasal steroids are available without a prescription. For a list of respiratory medications discussed in this section, see Table 1.26.

TABLE 1.26 Respiratory Medications

Generic Name	Brand Name(s)	Route(s) of Administration	Dosage Form(s)	Common Dosage Amount(s)	Indication(s)
Bronchodilators					
aclidinium	Tudorza Pressair	inhalation	inhaler	400 mcg	COPD
albuterol	Proventil, ProAir, Ventolin	inhalation	inhaler, solution for nebulizer	90 mcg, 0.63 mg, 1.25 mg	asthma, COPD
arformoterol	Brovana	inhalation	solution for nebulizer	15 mcg	asthma, COPD
ipratropium	Atrovent HFA	inhalation	inhaler, solution for nebulizer	17 mcg	COPD
formoterol	Perforomist	inhalation	solution for nebulizer	20 mcg	asthma, COPD
glycopyrrolate	Seebri Neohaler, Lonhala Magnair	inhalation	inhaler, solution for nebulizer	15.6 mcg, 25 mcg	COPD
indacaterol	Arcapta Neohaler	inhalation	inhaler	75 mcg	COPD
levalbuterol	Xopenex	inhalation	inhaler, solution for nebulizer	45 mcg, 0.31 mg, 0.63 mg, 1.25 mg	asthma, COPD
olodaterol	Striverdi Respimat	inhalation	inhaler	2.5 mcg	COPD
revefenacin	Yupelri	inhalation	solution for nebulizer	175 mcg	COPD
salmeterol	Serevent Diskus	inhalation	inhaler	50 mcg	asthma, COPD

continues

TABLE 1.26 Respiratory Medications—*Continued*

Generic Name	Brand Name(s)	Route(s) of Administration	Dosage Form(s)	Common Dosage Amount(s)	Indication(s)
Bronchodilators					
tiotropium	Spiriva HandiHaler, Spiriva Respimat	inhalation	inhaler	1.25 mcg, 18 mcg	asthma, COPD
umeclidinium	Incruse Ellipta	inhalation	inhaler	62.5 mcg	COPD
Inhaled Corticosteroids					
beclomethasone	Qvar RediHaler	inhalation	inhaler	40 mcg, 80 mcg	asthma
budesonide	Pulmicort, Pulmicort Flexhaler	inhalation	inhaler, solution for nebulizer	90 mcg, 180 mcg	asthma
ciclesonide	Alvesco	inhalation	inhaler	80 mcg, 160 mcg	asthma
fluticasone	Flovent HFA, Flovent Diskus, Arnuity Ellipta	inhalation	inhaler	44 mcg, 50 mcg, 100 mcg, 110 mcg, 200 mcg, 220 mcg	asthma
mometasone	Asmanex, Asmanex HFA	inhalation	inhaler	50 mcg, 100 mcg, 110 mcg, 200 mcg, 220 mcg	asthma
Combination Products					
aclidinium / formoterol	Duaklir Pressair	inhalation	inhaler	400 mcg/12 mcg	asthma, COPD
budesonide / formoterol	Symbicort	inhalation	inhaler	80 mcg/4.5 mcg, 160 mcg/4.5 mcg	asthma, COPD
fluticasone / salmeterol	Advair Diskus, Advair HFA, Wixela	inhalation	inhaler	45 mcg/21 mcg, 100 mcg/50 mcg, 115 mcg/ 21 mcg, 230 mcg/21 mcg, 250 mcg/50 mcg, 500 mcg/50 mcg	asthma, COPD
fluticasone / vilanterol	Breo Ellipta	inhalation	inhaler	100 mcg/25 mcg, 200 mcg/25 mcg	asthma, COPD
fluticasone / umeclidinium / vilanterol	Trelegy Ellipta	inhalation	inhaler	100 mcg/62.5 mcg/25 mcg	COPD
glycopyrrolate / formoterol	Bevespi Aerosphere	inhalation	inhaler	9 mcg/4.8 mcg	COPD
ipratropium / albuterol	Combivent Respimat	inhalation	inhaler, solution for nebulizer	20 mcg/100 mcg, 0.5 mg/2.5 mg	COPD

continues

TABLE 1.26 Respiratory Medications—*Continued*

Generic Name	Brand Name(s)	Route(s) of Administration	Dosage Form(s)	Common Dosage Amount(s)	Indication(s)
Combination Products					
indacaterol / glycopyrrolate	Utibron Neohaler	inhalation	inhaler	27.5 mcg/ 15.6 mcg	COPD
mometasone / formoterol	Dulera	inhalation	inhaler	100 mcg/5 mcg, 200 mcg/5 mcg	Asthma
tiotropium / olodaterol	Stiolto Respimat	inhalation	inhaler	2.5 mcg/2.5 mcg	COPD
umeclidinium / vilanterol	Anoro Ellipta	inhalation	inhaler	62.5 mcg/25 mcg	COPD
Leukotriene Inhibitors					
monetelukast	Singulair	oral	granules, tablet, chewable tablet	4 mg, 5 mg, 10 mg	asthma, allergies
zafirlukast	Accolate	oral	tablet	10 mg, 20 mg	asthma
Antihistamines					
cetirizine*	Zyrtec	oral	capsule, liquid, tablet	5 mg, 10 mg, 5 mg/5 mL	allergies
desloratadine	Clarinex	oral	tablet, disintegrating tablet	2.5 mg, 5 mg	allergies
diphenhydramine*	Benadryl	oral, parenteral (IV)	capsule, oral liquid, tablet, solution for injection	25 mg, 50 mg, 12.5 mg/5 mL, 50 mg/mL	allergies, severe allergic reaction
fexofenadine*	Allegra	oral	liquid, tablet	60 mg, 180 mg, 30 mg/5 mL	allergies
levocetirizine*	Xyzal	oral	liquid, tablet	5 mg, 10 mg, 5 mg/mL	allergies
loratadine*	Claritin	oral	liquid, tablet	5 mg, 10 mg, 5 mg/5 mL	allergies
Nasal Steroids					
budesonide*	Rhinocort	transmucosal (intranasal)	nasal spray	32 mcg	allergies
fluticasone*	Flonase	transmucosal (intranasal)	nasal spray	27.5 mcg, 50 mcg	allergies
mometasone	Nasonex	transmucosal (intranasal)	nasal spray	50 mcg	allergies
triamcinolone*	Nasacort	transmucosal (intranasal)	nasal spray	55 mcg	allergies

*available OTC

1.9 Gastrointestinal Medications

The digestive system, or the gastrointestinal (GI) system, includes the esophagus, stomach, small intestine, and large intestine. The GI system often develops common ailments for which many frequently prescribed medications exist.

Gastrointestinal agents are used to treat conditions such as heartburn, indigestion, nausea and vomiting, diarrhea, constipation, ulcers, and inflammatory bowel disease.

One commonly prescribed class of gastrointestinal agents is the **proton pump inhibitor (PPI)** class. PPIs work to prevent stomach acid production, and they include esomeprazole (Nexium), lansoprazole (Prevacid), omeprazole (Prilosec), and pantoprazole (Protonix). Taken with nonsteroidal anti-inflammatory drugs (NSAIDs). PPIs treat heartburn and acid reflux, and prevent NSAID-induced ulcers. Also, drugs that suppress acid secretion given with multiple antibiotics will effectively treat *Helicobacter pylori* infections that cause ulcers. Some PPIs are available OTC.

A family of drugs known as **histamine-2 antagonists (H₂ blockers)**, such as famotidine (Pepcid), work to slow the release of acid in the stomach.

PPIs and H₂ blockers are usually well tolerated, with only occasional reports of side effects like headache and dizziness. However, PPIs such as omeprazole can interfere with beneficial effects of the blood-clotting prevention drug clopidogrel (Plavix). These drugs should not be taken together, even if they are spaced 12 hours apart.

Long-term use of PPIs has been reported to increase bone loss, especially in older patients assigned female at birth, so an OTC calcium supplement may be recommended to accompany these drugs.

Metoclopramide (Reglan) is used to treat heartburn and slow stomach emptying in patients with diabetes, as well as severe nausea and vomiting resulting from chemotherapy. It is commonly given 30 minutes prior to each meal and at bedtime; it can cause abnormal muscle movement with long-term use. Ondansetron (Zofran), which is also used for chemotherapy-induced nausea, is available as an oral disintegrating tablet (ODT), a solution, and an injection for pediatric patients or others who cannot swallow tablets. Promethazine (Phenergan), a dopamine antagonist, is commonly used in tablet, liquid, injection, or suppository forms for the treatment of nausea and vomiting from viral illness or migraine headache.

Irritable bowel syndrome (IBS) is a common disorder that affects the large intestine. Signs and symptoms include cramping, pain, bloating, gas, diarrhea, and constipation. Medications for IBS include linaclotide (Linzess) and lubiprostone (Amitiza), which treat constipation. Eluxadoline (Viberzi) treats diarrhea associated with IBS. Other medications for constipation include polyethylene glycol (MiraLAX) and docusate (Colace). Medications for diarrhea include loperamide (Imodium) and diphenoxylate with atropine (Lomotil).

Treatment of IBS involves GI drugs that work locally, such as sulfasalazine (Azulfidine), olsalazine (Dipentum), and mesalamine (Asacol, Canasa, Pentasa). Related to sulfa drugs, these agents work in the colon to treat and prevent ulcerative colitis. Patients may also receive corticosteroids orally or rectally via enema or suppository. Common side effects include headache, nausea, fatigue, and skin rash.

Severe ulcerative colitis may need to be treated with biological response modifiers like infliximab (see the Section 1.14 on biotechnology drugs for more information). For a list of GI medications discussed in this section, see Table 1.27.

Pharm Fact

Ondansetron and related drugs block serotonin and have the suffix -*setron*.

Study Idea

Mesalamine, related to sulfa drugs, should not be prescribed for a patient with an allergy to sulfonamides.

TABLE 1.27 Gastrointestinal Medications

Generic Name	Brand Name(s)	Route(s) of Administration	Dosage Form(s)	Common Dosage Amount(s)
Proton Pump Inhibitors (PPIs)				
dexlansoprazole	Dexilant	oral	tablet	30 mg, 60 mg
esomeprazole*	Nexium	oral, parenteral (IV)	capsule, oral granules, solution for injection	20 mg*, 40 mg
lansoprazole*	Prevacid	oral	capsule, disintegrating tablet	15 mg*, 30 mg
omeprazole*	Prilosec	oral	delayed-release capsule, delayed-release tablet	20 mg*, 40 mg
pantoprazole	Protonix	oral, parenteral (IV)	oral granules, delayed-release tablet, solution for injection	20 mg, 40 mg
rabeprazole	Aciphex	oral	tablet	20 mg
Histamine-2 Antagonists (H2 blockers)				
cimetidine*	Tagamet, Tagamet HB	oral	solution, tablet	200 mg*, 300 mg, 400 mg, 800 mg, 300 mg/5 mL
famotidine*	Pepcid	oral, parenteral (IV)	tablet, suspension for reconstitution, solution for injection	10 mg*, 20 mg*, 40 mg, 40 mg/5 mL
nizatidine*	Axid, Axid AR	oral	capsule, solution, tablet	75 mg*, 150 mg, 300 mg, 15 mg/mL
Antiemetics				
ondansetron	Zofran	oral, parenteral (IV)	oral solution, tablet, solution for injection	4 mg, 8 mg, 4 mg/ 5 mL, 4 mg/2 mL
prochlorperazine	Compazine	oral, transmucosal (rectal)	tablet, suppository	5 mg, 10 mg, 25 mg
promethazine	Phenergan	oral, parenteral (IV), transmucosal (rectal)	oral solution, tablet, disintegrating tablet solution for injection, suppository	12.5 mg, 25 mg, 50 mg, 6.25 mg/ 5 mL, 25 mg/mL, 50 mg/mL
Irritable Bowel Syndrome (IBS) Medications				
eluxadoline	Viberzi	oral	tablet	75 mg, 100 mg
dicyclomine	Bentyl	oral, parenteral (IV)	capsule, oral solution, tablet, solution for injection	10 mg, 20 mg, 10 mg/mL, 10 mg/5 mL
linaclotide	Linzess	oral	capsule	72 mcg, 145 mcg, 290 mcg

continues

TABLE 1.27 Gastrointestinal Medications—*Continued*

Generic Name	Brand Name(s)	Route(s) of Administration	Dosage Form(s)	Common Dosage Amount(s)
Inflammatory Bowel Disease Medications				
lubiprostone	Amitiza	oral	capsule	8 mcg, 24 mcg
mesalamine	Asacol, Canasa, Pentasa, others	oral, transmucosal (rectal)	capsule, tablet, suppository	250 mg, 375 mg, 400 mg, 1000 mg, 4 g/60 mL
olsalazine	Dipentum	oral	capsule	250 mg
sulfasalazine	Azulfidine	oral	tablet, delayed-release tablet	500 mg
Diarrhea				
diphenoxylate-atropine	Lomotil	oral	solution, tablet	2.5 mg/0.025 mg, 2.5 mg/0.025 mg/5 mL
loperamide*	Imodium	oral	capsule, liquid, tablet	2 mg, 1 mg/5 mL
Constipation				
bisacodyl*	Dulcolax	oral, transmucosal (rectal)	tablet, suppository	5 mg, 10 mg
docusate*	Colace	oral	capsule, tablet	50 mg, 100 mg
lactulose	Enulose, Kristalose	oral	oral packet, solution	10 g, 10 g/15 mL
polyethylene glycol 3350*	Miralax	oral	powder for solution	17 g
senna*	Senokot	oral	tablet	8.6 mg, 17.2 mg
Prokinetic				
metoclopramide	Reglan	oral, parenteral (IV)	oral solution, tablet, solution for injection	5 mg, 10 mg, 5 mg/mL, 5 mg/5 mL

*available OTC

1.10 Musculoskeletal Medications

℞ Put Down Roots

Analgesia comes from the Greek word *algein*, "to feel pain," with the prefix *an-*, meaning "not." It means to not feel pain or to result in painlessness.

The musculoskeletal system is made up of the bones of the skeleton, muscles, cartilage, tendons, ligaments, joints, and other connective tissue that supports and binds tissues and organs together. This section discusses medications to treat pain and inflammation, muscle spasms, osteoporosis, and gout.

Analgesic, Anti-Inflammatory, and Muscle Relaxant Medications

Analgesic medications are used to relieve or reduce pain, whereas anti-inflammatory drugs work to reduce pain, inflammation, and swelling. Many analgesic drugs are narcotics, which can substantially affect mood and behavior. Narcotics have significant contraindications and restrictions since they can cause insensibility or stupor.

Study Idea

Opiates often end in the suffix -*in* or -*ine*, as in morphine, The names of synthetic opiates end similarly, such as in OxyContin. Opioids often end in -*one*, as in *hydrocodone* and *oxycodone*.

Safety Alert

Many forms of fentanyl are involved in Risk Evaluation and Mitigation Strategy (REMS) programs, such as the Transmucosal Immediate-Release Fentanyl (TIRF) program.

Safety Alert

Oxycodone is available as both an immediate-release generic drug and an extended-release brand-name drug (OxyContin). Technicians should be aware of these differences to avoid medication errors.

All narcotics are listed by the DEA as controlled substances because of their abuse potential—they can cause greater tolerance (a need for higher doses for the same effects), physical and psychological dependence, and addiction. This, and the regulation of controlled substances, will be discussed in detail in Chapter 2.

Analgesic Medications

Common analgesics include **opiates**, which are drugs derived from the opium poppy plant, including heroin (illegal), morphine, and codeine (note the suffix -*ine*).

Opioids are synthetic narcotics that offer opium-like effects of reduced perception of and reaction to pain, and increased pain tolerance. Opioids often include opium substances but are chemically designed to have varied or extended opium-like effects. Medications that fall into this category include: hydrocodone, oxycodone, and other related drugs (note the suffix -*one*).

Opioids are Schedule II (C-II) controlled substances with no refills permitted. Opioids should not be taken with CNS depressants or alcohol.

Prescription drug abuse is the number one drug problem in the United States, and hydrocodone-combination drugs (e.g., Vicodin) are the most frequently prescribed narcotic drugs. Hydrocodone is the generic ingredient name for a powerful opioid narcotic pain reliever. Oxycodone (OxyContin, Roxicodone) also offers strong, narcotic pain relief. Many hydrocodone, oxycodone, and codeine preparations contain acetaminophen, which increases their analgesic effects.

No refills are permitted for C-II narcotics, such as oxycodone or morphine. Methadone (Dolophine) is another opioid used for pain, but it is also used for detoxification in individuals with opioid dependencies. Suboxone is a combination drug (buprenorphine / naloxone) that is primarily used to treat narcotic addiction.

In the hospital setting, injections of morphine or hydromorphone (Dilaudid) are commonly used for temporary relief of severe pain; they are also C-II controlled substances. For terminal hospice or cancer patients, around-the-clock narcotics, administered via infusion pumps, liquids, or controlled-release solid dosage forms or patches are commonly used to provide comfort and pain relief.

Narcotic analgesics can cause stomach upset and constipation. It is recommended that these medications be taken with food, and stool softeners or short-term laxatives are often recommended for the common side effect of constipation.

TAKE NOTE

Prescription drug abuse is a national epidemic, and technicians are on the front lines of the struggle to save lives. Prescription drug misuse likely played a part in the deaths of celebrities Prince, Michael Jackson, Corey Haim, Heath Ledger, Anna Nicole Smith, and Whitney Houston. But everyday people are also affected by this—each year, prescription medication addiction and/or abuse contributes to thousands of deaths.

A 2015 Boston Medical Center study showed that over 90% of patients who experienced opioid overdoses received a refill or new opioid prescription immediately afterwards. Part of the problem is that there is no system to alert prescribers of a patient's overdose.

Narcotic analgesics are generally considered CNS depressants, and they can cause drowsiness. It is best to avoid using them with other CNS depressants, such as psychiatric medications, OTC sleeping medications, or alcohol. **Adjuvant medications** are helper medications. They are not strictly used for pain, but they aid pain management and may be prescribed along with a pain reliever. Some common adjuvants are antidepressant and antiseizure medications, muscle relaxants, sedatives, and sleep-enhancing drugs.

Non-narcotic analgesics, often found in OTC medications, are used for milder pain conditions, such as **acetyl-para-aminophenol (APAP)**, also known as acetaminophen (Tylenol). APAP is a non-narcotic analgesic found in many prescription and OTC products. It is used for children and adults as a fever reducer and pain reliever (e.g., for headache and arthritis) that will not upset the stomach. Acetaminophen is considered safe to use during pregnancy. However, high daily doses can damage the liver, especially if used chronically or combined with alcohol. When acetaminophen is therapeutically combined with a narcotic, the therapy often offers better relief for pain than either drug alone, and allows for lower dosing of the narcotic.

Anti-Inflammatory Medications

Some of the most commonly prescribed medications are **nonsteroidal anti-inflammatory drugs (NSAIDs)**. They include ibuprofen and naproxen. If a patient is allergic to aspirin, NSAIDs should not be dispensed. NSAIDs come in a variety of common prescription and OTC forms. They are used to treat not only short-term pain and headaches, but also chronic conditions, such as rheumatoid arthritis, migraines, back pain. Many NSAIDs (e.g., ibuprofen [Advil, Motrin]) are effective at reducing both swelling and pain, and thus can be used to treat conditions in which swelling and pain are linked.

NSAIDs are nonnarcotic but can cause serious GI bleeding if taken in large doses for an extended period, especially in older individuals. It is recommended that NSAIDs always be taken with food, milk, or a snack. Be aware that NSAIDs may increase the blood-thinning effects of aspirin when taken at the same time. Celecoxib (Celebrex) is less likely to cause GI side effects and bleeding, but it is much more expensive than other NSAIDs. If a patient is allergic to sulfa drugs (drugs containing sulfur derivatives), Celebrex is contraindicated.

Anesthetic Analgesics and Muscle Relaxants

The local anesthetic lidocaine is a localized pain reliever that can numb an area, and is an option for non-narcotic pain relief. The brand-name form of lidocaine, Lidoderm, is a patch that is worn for 12 hours and then removed for 12 hours.

Muscle relaxants, which reduce muscle strain and pain, include carisoprodol (Soma), cyclobenzaprine (Flexeril), and tizanidine (Zanaflex). These drugs are commonly prescribed along with narcotic analgesics and antianxiety drugs. They are indicated for short-term treatment of muscle spasms; however, they are often used long term. The combination of muscle relaxants and narcotic analgesics increases the risk of sedation and respiratory depression, and must be monitored. For a list of analgesic, anti-inflammatory, anesthetic analgesic, and muscle relaxant medications, see Table 1.28.

Study Idea

Technicians should remember that large doses of acetaminophen can damage the liver. The maximum daily dose is 4,000 mg, or 4 g, per day, though some experts recommend a lower maximum daily dose of 3,000 mg (3 g) per day. The antidote to acetaminophen overdose is acetyl-cysteine (Acetadote).

Study Idea

Carisoprodol (Soma) is a C-IV controlled substance and has limited prescribing and refill capabilities

TABLE 1.28 Analgesic, Anti-inflammatory, Anesthetic Analgesic, and Muscle Relaxant Medications

Generic Name	Brand Name(s)	Route(s) of Administration	Dosage Form(s)	Common Dosage Amount(s)
Narcotic Analgesics				
buprenorphine / naloxone	Suboxone	oral (buccal, SL)	buccal film, SL film, SL tablet	2 mg/0.5 mg, 4 mg/1 mg, 8 mg/2 mg, 12 mg/3 mg
codeine	N/A	oral	tablet	15 mg, 30 mg, 60 mg
fentanyl	Duragesic, Actiq, others	oral, parenteral (IV), topical (transdermal)	lozenge, solution for injection, patch	200 mcg, 400 mcg, 600 mcg, 800 mcg, 1,200 mcg, 1,600 mcg, 12.5 mcg/hr, 25 mcg/hr, 50 mcg/hr, 75 mcg/ hr, 100 mcg/hr
hydrocodone / acetaminophen	Vicodin, Vicodin ES	oral	tablet	5 mg/300 mg, 5 mg/325 mg, 7.5 mg/300 mg, 7.5 mg/325 mg, 10 mg/300 mg, 10 mg/325 mg
hydromorphone	Dilaudid	oral, parenteral (IV)	oral liquid, tablet, solution for injection	2 mg, 4 mg, 8 mg, 12 mg, 16 mg, 24 mg, 32 mg, 1 mg/ mL, 2 mg/mL, 4 mg/ mL, 10 mg/mL
methadone	Dolophine	oral, parenteral (IV, IM)	oral solution, tablet, solution for injection	5 mg, 10 mg, 40 mg, 5 mg/5 mL, 10 mg/5 mL, 10 mg/mL
morphine	Roxanol	oral, parenteral (IV, IM)	oral solution, tablet, solution for injection	15 mg, 30 mg, 10 mg/5 mL, 10 mg/5 mL, 1 mg/mL, 5 mg/mL, 10 mg/mL, 50 mg/mL
morphine ER	Avinza, Kadian, MS Contin	oral	extended-release tablet	15 mg, 30 mg, 50 mg, 60 mg, 90 mg, 100 mg, 120 mg, 200 mg
oxycodone	OxyContin, Roxicodone	oral	solution, tablet, extended-release tablet	5 mg, 10 mg, 15 mg, 20 mg, 30 mg, 40 mg, 60 mg, 80 mg, 5 mg/5 mL
oxycodone / acetaminophen	Percocet	oral	solution, tablet	2.5 mg/325 mg, 5 mg/325 mg, 7.5 mg/325 mg, 10 mg/ 325 mg, 5 mg/325 mg/5 mL
tramadol	Ultram, Ultram ER	oral	tablet	50 mg, 100 mg, 200 mg, 300 mg

continues

TABLE 1.28 Analgesic, Anti-inflammatory, Anesthetic Analgesic, and Muscle Relaxant Medications —*Continued*

Generic Name	Brand Name(s)	Route(s) of Administration	Dosage Form(s)	Common Dosage Amount(s)
Narcotic Analgesics				
tramadol / acetaminophen	Ultracet	oral	tablet	37.5 mg/325 mg
Non-Narcotic Analgesic				
acetaminophen*	Tylenol, others	oral, parenteral (IV), transmucosal (rectal)	caplet, capsule, oral liquid, oral tablet, solution for injection, suppository	80 mg, 120 mg, 160 mg, 325 mg, 500 mg, 650 mg, 160 mg/5 mL, 10 mg/mL
Non-Steroidal Anti-Inflammatory Drugs (NSAIDs)				
celecoxib	Celebrex	oral	capsule	50 mg, 100 mg, 200 mg, 400 mg
diclofenac*	Voltaren	oral, topical	tablet, gel	25 mg, 50 mg, 75 mg, 100 mg, 1%, 3%
ibuprofen*	Advil, Motrin	oral, parenteral (IV)	capsule, oral suspension, tablet, solution for injection	200 mg, 400 mg, 600 mg, 800 mg, 100 mg/5 mL, 400 mg/5 mL, 800 mg/200 mL
indomethacin	Indocin	oral, transmucosal (rectal)	capsule, oral suspension, suppository	25 mg, 50 mg, 75 mg, 25 mg/5 mL
ketorolac	Toradol	oral, parenteral (IV, IM)	tablet, solution for injection	10 mg, 15 mg/mL, 30 mg/mL
meloxicam	Mobic	oral	tablet	7.5 mg, 15 mg
naproxen*	Aleve, Naprosyn	oral	suspension, tablet, extended-release tablet	220 mg, 250 mg, 375 mg, 500 mg, 125 mg/5 mL
Anesthetic Analgesic				
lidocaine*	Lidoderm	topical (transdermal)	patch	5%
Muscle Relaxants				
carisoprodol	Soma	oral	tablet	250 mg, 350 mg
cyclobenzaprine	Flexeril	oral	tablet	5 mg, 7.5 mg, 10 mg
metaxalone	Skelaxin	oral	tablet	800 mg
methocarbamol	Robaxin	oral, parenteral (IV, IM)	tablet, solution for injection	500 mg, 750 mg, 100 mg/mL
tizanidine	Zanaflex	oral	capsule, tablet	2 mg, 4 mg, 6 mg

*some dosage forms/strengths available OTC

Medications for Osteoporosis

Osteoporosis, or bone loss, often occurs in postmenopausal individuals and in patients assigned male at birth over the age of 75 who do not receive enough calcium. Bisphosphonates, such as alendronate (Fosamax), are one type of medication to treat bone loss. **Bisphosphonates** slow down the cells that break down bone, and they are commonly taken once a week or once a month. Only water (not a caffeinated beverage) should be taken with them. To increase absorption and minimize esophageal erosion, bisphosphonates must be taken in the morning, on an empty stomach, and not while a patient is in a reclining position. Patients should take bisphosphonates with a full glass of water and remain upright for 60 minutes after taking each dose.

Other medications for osteoporosis include calcitonin (Fortical, Miacalcin), raloxifene (Evista), and teriparatide (Forteo). Calcitonin is administered as a nasal spray and inhibits the breakdown of bone. Patients should be monitored for allergic reactions and nosebleeds. Raloxifene works as an estrogen agonist to prevent bone loss and has a boxed warning because it increases the risk of blood clots. Teriparatide is administered subcutaneously using a pen device and stimulates the cells that build new bone. See Table 1.29 for common osteoporosis medications.

TABLE 1.29 Osteoporosis Medications

Generic Name	Brand Name(s)	Route(s) of Administration	Dosage Form(s)	Common Dosage Amount(s)
Bisphosphonates				
alendronate	Fosamax	oral	solution, tablet	5 mg, 10 mg, 35 mg, 70 mg, 70 mg/75 mL
ibandronate	Boniva	oral	tablet	2.5 mg, 150 mg
risedronate	Actonel	oral	tablet	5 mg, 30 mg, 35 mg, 150 mg
Other Osteoporosis Medications				
calcitonin	Fortical, Miacalcin	transmucosal (intranasal)	nasal spray	200 units/kg
raloxifene	Evista	oral	tablet	60 mg
teriparatide	Forteo	parenteral (SubQ)	pen injector	20 mcg

Medications for Gout

Gout is a type of arthritis caused by the buildup of uric acid in the blood. When uric acid is in excess, it forms urate crystals in the joints, which result in pain, stiffness, and swelling. Medications to treat gout focus on reducing uric acid levels. Allopurinol (Zyloprim) is a xanthine oxidase inhibitor that prevents the formation of painful urate crystals. Probenecid works to increase the elimination of uric acid via the kidneys. For the acute symptoms of gout, colchicine (Colcrys) and NSAIDs are used to treat inflammation and pain. Colchicine (Colcrys) may cause gastrointestinal upset. For a list of gout medications, see Table 1.30.

TABLE 1.30 Gout Medications

Generic Name	Brand Name	Route of Administration	Dosage Form(s)	Common Dosage Amount(s)
allopurinol	Zyloprim	oral	tablet	100 mg, 300 mg
colchicine	Colcrys	oral	capsule, tablet	0.6 mg
febuxostat	Uloric	oral	tablet	40 mg
probenecid	N/A	oral	tablet	0.5 g

1.11 Renal and Genitourinary Medications

The renal system, or urinary system, includes the kidneys, bladder, ureters, and urethra. The genitourinary system includes both the genital reproductive system and the urinary tract. Complications of the renal and genitourinary systems vary across sexes. For all sexes, the most frequently prescribed renal and genitourinary agents are diuretic drugs. Drugs for overactive bladder are most often prescribed for patients assigned female at birth, and drugs that address erectile dysfunction (ED) and prostate problems are most frequently prescribed for patients assigned male at birth.

Diuretic Medications

Diuretics, sometimes called *water pills*, work with the kidneys to eliminate excess salt and water from the body by dilating (widening) blood vessels. They are used to treat swelling from water retention, high blood pressure, and heart failure. Diuretics should be taken in the morning or early evening. Most can cause potassium loss, which can result in muscle cramps or, in severe cases, irregular heart rates. Potassium loss can be offset by consuming potassium-rich foods, such as fresh citrus fruits and bananas, or by taking potassium supplements. Hydrochlorothiazide (Hydrodiuril) and furosemide (Lasix) act at different sites of the kidney, and their onset, duration of action, and potency differ. Diuretics that contain triamterene (Dyazide, Maxzide) or spironolactone (Aldactone) are considered potassium-sparing, meaning that they maintain healthier levels of potassium.

Many antihypertensive drugs listed in Table 1.10 are available in combination with a diuretic. However, diuretics must be used with caution with ACE inhibitors, digoxin, and lithium. The pharmacist must assess the potential for drug interactions. For a list of diuretic medications, see Table 1.31.

TABLE 1.31 Diuretic Medications

Generic Name	Brand Name(s)	Route(s) of Administration	Dosage Form(s)	Common Dosage Amount(s)
Loop Diuretics				
bumetanide	Bumex	oral, parenteral (IV, IM)	tablet, solution for injection	0.5 mg, 1 mg, 2 mg, 0.25 mg/mL

continues

TABLE 1.31 Diuretic Medications—*Continued*

Generic Name	Brand Name(s)	Route(s) of Administration	Dosage Form(s)	Common Dosage Amount(s)
Loop Diuretics				
furosemide	Lasix	oral, parenteral (IV, IM)	oral solution, tablet, solution for injection	20 mg, 40 mg, 80 mg, 10 mg/mL, 40 mg/5 mL
torsemide	Demadex	oral	tablet	5 mg, 10 mg, 20 mg, 100 mg
Potassium-Sparing Diuretics				
eplerenone	Inspra	oral	tablet	25 mg, 50 mg
spironolactone	Aldactone	oral	tablet	25 mg, 50 mg, 100 mg
triamterene	Dyrenium	oral	capsule	50 mg, 100 mg
triamterene / hydrochlorothiazide	Dyazide, Maxizide	oral	capsule, tablet	37.5 mg/25 mg, 75 mg/50 mg
Thiazide Diuretics				
chlorthalidone	Hygroton	oral	tablet	25 mg, 50 mg
hydrochlorothiazide	Hydrodiuril	oral	capsule, tablet	12.5 mg, 25 mg, 50 mg
indapamide	Lozol	oral	tablet	1.25 mg, 2.5 mg
metolazone	Zaroxolyn	oral	tablet	2.5 mg, 5 mg, 10 mg

Medications for Overactive Bladder

Overactive bladder can lead to urinary incontinence (loss of bladder control), varying from slight urine loss after sneezing to a complete lack of control over urination. Urinary incontinence is a common problem.

Medications to treat urinary incontinence prevent the bladder from contracting. Common medications to treat urinary incontinence include anticholinergics like oxybutynin (Ditropan) and tolterodine (Detrol LA). Oxytrol for Women is an OTC version of oxybutynin that is available as a transdermal patch. Common side effects of anticholinergics include drowsiness, dizziness, blurred vision, and dry mouth. Anticholinergics should be used with caution in older individuals.

Mirabegron (Myrbetriq) is another medication for urinary incontinence that aids bladder relaxation. Because it can cause increased blood pressure, blood pressure should be monitored in patients taking mirabegron.

For a list of medications for overactive bladder, see Table 1.32.

TABLE 1.32 Medications for Overactive Bladder

Generic Name	Brand Name(s)	Route(s) of Administration	Dosage Form(s)	Common Dosage Amount(s)
darifenacin	Enablex	oral	tablet	7.5 mg, 15 mg
mirabegron	Myrbetriq	oral, transdermal	extended-release tablet	25 mg, 50 mg
oxybutynin*	Ditropan, Ditropan XL, Gelnique, Oxytrol	oral	tablet, gel, transdermal patch	3.9 mg/24 hr, 5 mg, 10 mg, 15 mg, 10%
solifenacin	VESIcare	oral	tablet	5 mg, 10 mg
tolterodine	Detrol, Detrol LA	oral	capsule, tablet	1 mg, 2 mg, 4 mg

*some dosage forms/strengths available OTC

Medications for Erectile Dysfunction

Phosphodiesterase inhibitors for erectile dysfunction include the well-known drugs sildenafil (Viagra) and tadalafil (Cialis). These drugs vary by onset and duration of action. Rare side effects include changes in blue/green color vision and prolonged painful erections (priapism). A life-threatening drop in blood pressure (hypotension) can occur if these agents are used with any nitrate. For a list of phosphodiesterase inhibitors, see Table 1.33.

TABLE 1.33 Phosphodiesterase Inhibitors

Generic Name	Brand Name(s)	Route of Administration	Dosage Form(s)	Common Dosage Amounts
avanafil	Stendra	oral	tablet	50 mg, 100 mg, 200 mg
sildenafil	Viagra	oral	tablet	25 mg, 50 mg, 100 mg
tadalafil	Cialis	oral	tablet	5 mg, 10 mg, 20 mg
vardenafil	Levitra, Staxyn	oral	tablet, disintegrating tablet	2.5 mg, 5 mg, 10 mg, 20 mg

Medications for Prostate Problems

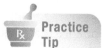

Practice Tip

Pharmacy technicians who are pregnant or trying to become pregnant, should not handle finasteride.

Benign prostatic hyperplasia (BPH), or an enlarged prostate not due to cancer, is treated with tamsulosin (Flomax) and finasteride (Proscar). Tamsulosin is a common **alpha-adrenergic blocker**, which blocks alpha receptors in the prostate and bladder and helps improve the outflow of urine. A common side effect of tamulosin is first-dose syncope (a drop in blood pressure that causes fainting), so it is usually prescribed as a bedtime dose. Finasteride is a 5-alpha-reductase inhibitor that blocks the conversion of testosterone. Finasteride can decrease hair loss and may also decrease sexual function. Some patients complain the side effects last for a sustained period after ceasing use of finasteride. In addition, finasteride can pass in the semen and may harm a fetus. It should not be used when trying to conceive, or if the individual taking finasteride is sexually active with a person who can become pregnant, and they are not using contraceptives. For a list of medications used to treat BPH, see Table 1.34.

TABLE 1.34 Medications for Benign Prostatic Hyperplasia

Generic Name	Brand Name	Route of Administration	Dosage Form	Common Dosage Amount(s)
Alpha-Adrenergic Blockers				
alfuzosin	Uroxatral	oral	tablet	10 mg
silodosin	Rapaflo	oral	capsule	4 mg, 8 mg
tamsulosin	Flomax	oral	capsule	0.4 mg
5-Alpha-Reductase Inhibitors				
dutasteride	Avodart	oral	capsule	0.5 mg
finasteride	Proscar	oral	tablet	5 mg

1.12 Reproductive System Medications

The reproductive system is a collection of internal and external organs that work together for the purpose of sexual reproduction. The reproductive system of most individuals assigned male at birth consists of two major parts: the testes, where sperm are produced, and the penis. The reproductive system of most individuals assigned female at birth consists of these major internal organs: vagina, the uterus, and the ovaries. There are many important hormones that affect the reproductive system, and many of the drugs in this section relate to those hormone systems. Agents that treat erectile dysfunction (ED) were discussed in Section 1.11 on renal and genitourinary medications.

Hormone Replacement Medications

In menopausal and postmenopausal patients or in patients who have had a hysterectomy, reproductive hormone production drops dramatically, often causing hot flashes, insomnia, and emotional imbalance. Hormone-replacement therapy (HRT) with estrogen is often used to reduce the symptoms. HRT is available in many dosage forms, including oral tablets, vaginal creams, and transdermal patches. The major side effect of estrogens is nausea, and they may increase in the risk of stroke and cancer with long-term (over five years) use. Testosterone is prescribed as replacement therapy for patients who have low testosterone levels. HRT, testosterone, and other hormonal agents are also prescribed to transgender patients undergoing medical transition. For a list of hormone replacement medications, see Table 1.35.

TABLE 1.35 Hormone Replacement Medications

Generic Name	Brand Name(s)	Route(s) of Administration	Dosage Form(s)	Common Dosage Amount(s)
conjugated equine estrogens	Premarin	oral, parenteral (IV, IM), transmucosal (intravaginal)	oral tablet, solution for injection, vaginal cream	0.3 mg, 0.45 mg, 0.625 mg, 0.9 mg, 1.25 mg, 0.625 mg/g, 25 mg
conjugated equine estrogens / medroxyprogesterone	Prempro	oral	tablet	0.3 mg/1.5 mg, 0.45 mg/1.5 mg, 0.625 mg/2.5 mg, 0.625 mg/5 mg
estradiol	Estrace	oral, transmucosal (intravaginal)	oral tablet, vaginal cream	0.1 mg/g, 0.5 mg, 1 mg, 2 mg
estradiol	Vagifem	transmucosal (intravaginal)	vaginal tablet	10 mcg
estradiol	Alora, Climara, Estraderm, VivelleDot	topical (transdermal)	transdermal patch	0.025 mg/24 hr, 0.0375 mg/24 hr, 0.05 mg/24 hr, 0.06 mg/24 hr, 0.075 mg/24 hr, 0.1 mg/24 hr
estradiol / norethindrone	Activella, CombiPatch	oral, topical (transdermal)	oral tablet, transdermal patch	0.5 mg/0.1 mg, 1 mg/0.5 mg, 0.5 mg/0.14 mg, 0.5 mg/0.25 mg
testosterone	AndroGel, Depo-Testosterone, Testim	parenteral (IM), topical	solution for injection, topical gel	100 mg/mL, 200 mg/mL, 1%

Hormonal Contraceptives

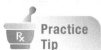

Practice Tip

Patients must be reminded that antibiotics may interfere with birth control.

Safety Alert

If patients mention severe side effects from birth control, such as intense depression or breakthrough bleeding, recommend that they consult the pharmacist and their provider.

There are many prescription birth control medications on the market. Most contain reproductive hormone combinations of **estrogen** and a progestin (a synthesized **progesterone**) to simulate pregnancy and, thereby, prevent ovulation. Common side effects include weight gain and depression.

Most birth control therapies include three weeks of active medication and one week of placebo or iron tablets. Some birth control pills, such as Seasonique (ethinyl estradiol / levonorgestrel), are available in 84-day supply packs that can reduce menstruation to once every three months.

NuvaRing (ethinyl estradiol / etonogestrel) is a once-a-month birth control device (in place for three weeks, removed for one week) through which hormones are slowly released intravaginally via a self-inserted ring dispenser; this drug should be refrigerated when stored. Xulane (ethinyl estradiol / norelgestromin) is a birth control patch that slowly releases hormones over seven days. Xulane is about the size of a Band-Aid and is worn on the inside of the upper arm or hip; it is changed once a week.

In patients over age 35 who smoke, birth control medications may increase the risk of a stroke. The FDA mandates that manufacturers provide, and pharmacists dispense, a Medication Guide with each birth control prescription.

Levonorgestrel (Plan B One-Step, Take Action, Next Choice) is an OTC medication marketed as an emergency contraceptive for use after unprotected sex and may be obtained by individuals of any age. The treatment is most effective if taken within 72 hours of intercourse. Ulipristal acetate (Ella) is another medication (available by prescription) used for emergency contraception. It is effective if taken within five days of unprotected sex. For a list of hormonal contraceptives, see Table 1.36.

TABLE 1.36 Hormonal Contraceptives

Generic Name	Brand Name(s)	Route(s) of Administration	Dosage Form(s)
Oral Contraceptives			
ethinyl estradiol / desogestrel	Apri, Desogen, others	oral	tablet
ethinyl estradiol / drospirenone	Ocella, Yasmin, Zarah, others	oral	tablet
ethinyl estradiol / levonorgestrel	Aviane, Larissia, Lutera, Seasonique, others	oral	tablet
ethinyl estradiol / norethindrone	Loestrin 21, Loestrin Fe, Migrogestin, Microgestin Fe, others	oral	tablet
ethinyl estradiol / norgestimate	Tri-Sprintec, Tri-Sprintec Lo, others	oral	tablet
ethinyl estradiol / norgestrel	Lo/Ovral 28, Low-Ogestrel 28, others	oral	tablet
norethindrone	Camila, Jolivette, Ortho Micronor, others	oral	tablet
Other Contraceptives			
ethinyl estradiol / etonogestrel	NuvaRing	transmucosal (intravaginal)	vaginal ring
ethinyl estradiol / norelgestromin	Xulane	topical (transdermal)	transdermal patch
medroxyprogesterone	Depo-Provera	parenteral (IM, SubQ)	suspension for injection
Emergency Contraceptives			
levonorgestrel*	Plan B One-Step, Take Action, Next Choice	oral	tablet
ulipristal acetate	Ella	oral	tablet

*available OTC

1.13 Hematologic Medications

Hematologic drugs include those that address problems with blood cell production, quality, and clotting. The hematological agents discussed in this section will focus on drugs used to treat thromboembolic (blood clot) disorders. Biotechnology drugs used for hematologic diseases are discussed in Section 1.14, and vitamins are discussed in Section 1.17 on alternative medicine and dietary supplements.

Safety Alert

The list of drug interactions for warfarin is long, so great care must be taken with the medication profile and any nonprescription drugs and supplements.

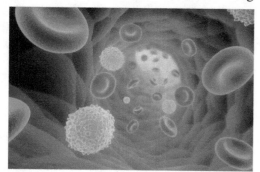

Warfarin and heparin work to prevent blood clots, but they can also cause excessive bleeding in the case of an injury. They often cause adverse drug reactions, and they interact with many other drugs.

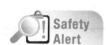

Safety Alert

In the event of dabigatran (Pradaxa) overdose, there is an antidote called Praxbind.

Warfarin (Coumadin) is a drug that is used both short and long term to prevent blood clots in high-risk patients. Patients taking warfarin are less likely to clot but more likely to bleed profusely. With blood thinners like warfarin and heparin, toxic levels are not far from therapeutic levels. So, patients must be closely and routinely monitored via blood tests that measure the international normalized ratio (INR), which shows how well the blood clots. The therapeutic level for warfarin is between 2.0 and 3.5, depending on indication. Warfarin causes serious adverse reactions when taken with many other drugs and supplements, so technicians and pharmacists must be careful to watch for drug utilization review (DUR) alerts and have them resolved by the pharmacist. Because of this, technicians should pay extra attention to all warfarin (Coumadin) questions on a certification exam. Technicians should the pharmacist if they notice that a warfarin patient is picking up any OTC item, like St. John's wort, that could cause a drug reaction.

Because blood thinner levels are so difficult to modulate some prescribers write Coumadin as *brand necessary (DAW)*. This drug (and other blood thinners) is highly susceptible to drug interactions, such as with aspirin (a mild blood thinner) and many herbal supplements (e.g., ginger, ginkgo, and ginseng). When new medications are added to a patient's regimen, or when dosages are adjusted, the pharmacist must assess the potential for serious interactions.

Warfarin works by inhibiting vitamin K–dependent clotting factors. Vitamins and diets that are high in vitamin K can impair the pharmacological effect of warfarin. Newer agents to prevent clot formation and treat blood clots include dabigatran (Pradaxa) and rivaroxaban (Xarelto), which are faster acting and do not require regular blood testing. One disadvantage to these new agents is their high cost. Clopidogrel (Plavix) often works to decrease the risk of blood clots by inhibiting the production of platelets in the blood. Diet does not affect this drug, but the use of proton pump inhibitor (PPI) medications can interfere with its therapeutic effect.

Heparin (generic only) is an anticlotting drug that is administered via IV or SubQ injection to treat and prevent blood clots. It is used in hospital settings to treat and prevent blood clots, especially in the legs and lungs. Frequent blood tests are required for IV heparin patients to monitor against its major side effect—excessive bleeding.

Enoxaparin (Lovenox) is delivered via SubQ injection to prevent blood clots. It is often used in high-risk surgeries or for **bridging therapy** to prevent blood clots after surgery, while waiting for slow-acting warfarin to take effect (usually in one week). Enoxaparin has been shown to be as effective as heparin, and it requires no blood tests and causes less bleeding.

Patients who come to the emergency department with an acute myocardial infarction (heart attack) or acute ischemic stroke may be given an IV injection dose of a fibrinolytic, such as alteplase (Activase), reteplase (Retavase), or tenecteplase (TNKase), to dissolve the clot. The major risk with these drugs is bleeding or hemorrhagic stroke. Combining these drugs with heparin can increase the risk of bleeding. For a list of common hematologic medications, see Table 1.37.

TABLE 1.37 Common Hematologic Medications

Generic Name	Brand Name(s)	Route(s) of Administration	Dosage Form(s)	Common Dosage Amount(s)
Vitamin K Antagonist—Prevention of Blood Clots				
warfarin	Coumadin	oral	tablet	1 mg, 2 mg, 2.5 mg, 3 mg, 4 mg, 5 mg, 6 mg, 7.5 mg, 10 mg
Direct Thrombin Inhibitor—Prevention and/or Treatment of Blood Clots				
dabigatran	Pradaxa	oral	capsule	75 mg, 110 mg, 150 mg
Factor Xa Inhibitors—Prevention and/or Treatment of Blood Clots				
apixaban	Eliquis	oral	tablet	2.5 mg, 5 mg
rivaroxaban	Xarelto	oral	tablet	2.5 mg, 10 mg, 15 mg, 20 mg
Antiplatelet—Prevention of Blood Clots				
clopidogrel	Plavix	oral	tablet	75 mg, 300 mg
Heparin and Low Molecular Weight Heparins—Prevention and/or Treatment of Blood Clots				
dalteparin	Fragmin	parenteral (SubQ)	solution for injection	10,000 units/mL, 2,500 units/0.2 mL, 5,000 units/0.2 mL, 7,500 units/0.3 mL, 10,000 units/0.4 mL, 12,500 units/0.5 mL, 15,000 units/0.6 mL, 18,000 units/0.72 mL
enoxaparin	Lovenox	parenteral (SubQ)	solution for injection	30 mg/0.3 mL, 40 mg/0.4 mL, 60 mg/0.6 mL, 80 mg/0.8 mL, 100 mg/mL, 120 mg/0.8 mL, 150 mg/mL
heparin	N/A	parenteral (IV, SubQ)	solution for injection	2,000 units, 12,500 units, 25,000 units, 1,000 units/mL, 5,000 units/mL, 10,000 units/mL, 20,000 units/mL
Thrombolytic Agents—Treatment of Acute Ischemic Stroke/Myocardial Infarction				
alteplase	Activase	parenteral (IV)	solution for injection	50 mg, 100 mg
reteplase	Retavase	parenteral (IV)	kit for injection	10 units
tenecteplace	TNKase	parenteral (IV)	kit for injection	50 mg

1.14 Biotechnology Medications

Pharm Fact

Infliximab (Remicade, Inflectra) is an IV biologic drug used for treating autoimmune and inflammatory diseases like Crohn's disease and rheumatoid arthritis.

Numerous drugs developed through biotechnology are used for a variety of medical conditions: (1) to treat anemia from chronic kidney disease or cancer chemotherapy, (2) to boost white and red blood cell counts for those at risk of an infection or experiencing severe fatigue, and (3) to treat inflammatory diseases.

Infliximab (Remicade, Inflectra), adalimumab (Humira), and etanercept (Enbrel) have a wide spectrum of uses, including treatment of severe rheumatoid arthritis, GI inflammatory diseases, such as Crohn's disease, and severe psoriasis that is unresponsive to conventional therapy. These drugs block tumor necrosis factor (TNF), which is a substance in the body that causes inflammation. Patients with autoimmune diseases like rheumatoid arthritis have too much TNF in the blood. This leads to inflammation and painful symptoms like joint swelling. TNF-blocking agents, or TNF blockers, suppress the activity of TNF and help reduce inflammation.

Except for adalimumab (Humira) and etanercept (Enbrel), community pharmacy technicians may not be exposed to these biological agents, but hospital technicians likely will.

Also available are biotechnology drugs that stimulate the production of white blood cells (WBCs), which are needed to boost immunity, and red blood cells (RBCs) which carry oxygen. Patients with chronic kidney disease (CKD) often have low RBC counts. Cancer, chemotherapy, and radiation therapy can all cause damaging effects to WBCs, RBCs or both. Low WBC counts increase the risk of infections, and low RBC counts increase the risk of fatigue.

Technicians working in a hospital or in a cancer or dialysis clinic need to be familiar with bone marrow colony-stimulating factors, such as darbepoetin alfa (Aranesp), epoetin alfa (Epogen, Procrit), and filgrastim (Neupogen). These are lifesaving drugs for patients undergoing chemotherapy, which can depress the bone marrow and subsequent immune system function. For a list of common biological and immunological biotechnology medications, see Table 1.38.

TABLE 1.38 Biological and Immunological Biotechnology Medications

Generic Name	Brand Name(s)	Route(s) of Administration	Dosage Form(s)	Common Dosage Amount(s)
TNF-Blocking Agents				
adalimumab	Humira	parenteral (SubQ)	pen injector kit, prefilled syringe kit	40 mg/0.4 mL, 40 mg/0.8 mL, 80 mg/0.8 mL, 10 mg/0.1 mL, 10 mg/0.2 mL, 20 mg/0.2 mL, 20 mg/0.4 mL
etanercept	Enbrel	parenteral (SubQ)	autoinjector, cartridge, prefilled syringe	25 mg/0.5 mL, 50 mg/mL
infliximab	Remicade, Inflectra	parenteral (IV)	solution for injection	100 mg

continues

TABLE 1.38 Biological and Immunological Biotechnology Medications—*Continued*

Generic Name	Brand Name(s)	Route(s) of Administration	Dosage Form(s)	Common Dosage Amount(s)
Erythropoiesis-Stimulating Agents				
darbepoetin alfa	Aranesp	parenteral (IV, SubQ)	solution for injection, prefilled syringe	25 mcg/mL, 40 mcg/ mL, 60 mcg/ mL, 100 mcg/mL, 200 mcg/mL, 300 mcg/mL
epoetin alfa	Epogen, Procrit	parenteral (IV, SubQ)	solution for injection	2,000 units/mL, 3,000 units/mL, 4,000 units/mL, 10,000 units/mL, 20,000 units/mL, 40,000 units/mL
White Blood Cell-Stimulating Agents				
filgrastim	Neupogen	parenteral (IV, SubQ)	solution for injection, prefilled syringe	300 mcg/mL, 480 mcg/1.6 mL, 300 mcg/0.5 mL, 480 mcg/0.8 mL
pegfilgrastim	Neulasta	parenteral (SubQ)	prefilled syringe kit	6 mg/0.6 mL

 TAKE NOTE

There are FDA-mandated boxed warnings for several injectable biotechnology drugs, including Enbrel, Remicade, and Humira. These drugs work by suppressing the immune system, thus increasing patient susceptibility to rare but serious bacterial and fungal infections. These TNF-blocking agents also increase the risk of malignancies like lymphoma.

1.15 Miscellaneous Medications

There are a number of other commonly used drugs that are used for a variety of conditions. These include corticosteroids, emergency medications, and drugs used for smoking cessation. These drugs are discussed in this section.

Corticosteroids

Cortisol is a hormone produced by the adrenal glands that helps the body deal with stress and inflammation. Corticosteroids—including dexamethasone (Decadron), prednisone (Deltasone), and methylprednisolone (Medrol)—resemble cortisol and are used to treat a variety of inflammatory diseases, such as rheumatoid arthritis, asthma, allergic reactions, poison ivy or poison oak, ulcerative colitis, Crohn's disease, and gout.

Corticosteroids should be taken with food and may interfere with blood sugar or blood-thinning medications. Corticosteroids are usually prescribed for short-term use because prolonged use can increase the risk of high blood pressure and elevated blood sugar, appetite and weight gain, muscle weakness and bruising, glaucoma or cataracts, stomach ulcers, and hallucinations. It is important to note that corticosteroids are not the same types of steroids as the anabolic steroids used illegally by some athletes. Some patients with chronic inflammatory conditions may be on lifelong therapy or may use high doses of corticosteroids for a short time for acute flare-ups.

Skin conditions like eczema, psoriasis, allergic reactions to bug bites, and dermatitis from poison ivy are often treated with topical corticosteroids (those applied on the skin). Triamcinolone (Kenalog) is a topical corticosteroid and is the most frequently prescribed topical drug, available in different strengths as an aerosol, cream, and ointment. Triamcinolone is more potent than the topical OTC hydrocortisone. For a list of common corticosteroids, see Table 1.39.

TABLE 1.39 Corticosteroids

Generic Name	Brand Name(s)	Route(s) of Administration	Dosage Form(s)	Common Dosage Amount(s)
dexamethasone	Decadron	oral, parenteral (IV, IM)	oral solution, tablet, solution for injection	0.5 mg, 0.75 mg, 1 mg, 1.5 mg, 2 mg, 4 mg, 6 mg, 0.5 mg/ 5 mL
hydrocortisone*	Cortizone, Anucort-HC, others	topical, transmucosal (rectal)	cream, ointment, topical solution, suppository	1%, 2.5%, 25 mg
methylprednisolone	Medrol	oral	tablet	4 mg
prednisolone	Orapred, Pediapred	oral	solution	15 mg/5 mL
prednisone	Deltasone, others	oral	solution, tablet	1 mg, 2.5 mg, 5 mg, 10 mg, 20 mg, 5 mg/ 5 mL, 5 mg/mL
triamcinolone	Kenalog	parenteral (IV, IM), topical	solution for injection, cream, ointment, topical aerosol	0.025%, 0.05%, 0.1%

*some strengths/dosage forms available OTC

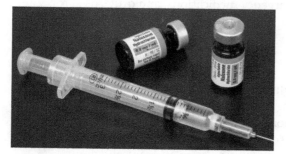

Naloxone can be delivered as an injection to treat opioid overdose.

Emergency Medications

There are several medications available to use in emergency situations. Once such medication is naloxone (Narcan, Evzio), which is indicated to treat an opioid-associated, life-threatening emergency such as an overdose. Naloxone can be administered as an injection or through the nose by first responders or family, friends, and caregivers of the individual experiencing an opioid-associated emergency. Many pharmacists are trained to administer naloxone, and some can even dispense it without a prescription, depending on state law. Narcan is a naloxone nasal spray and Evzio is a naloxone autoinjector. After the use of naloxone, the patient should receive prompt follow-up care by a medical professional.

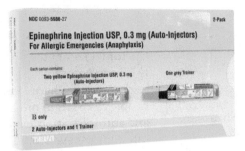

People with severe allergies—such as to bee stings—often carry emergency doses of epinephrine in the form of an Epi Pen so they can self-inject when symptoms start

Epinephrine is another medication used in emergency situations. Epinephrine is used to treat anaphylaxis, or life-threatening allergic reactions. This drug acts on the body to shut down the allergic response; it constricts blood vessels, increases blood pressure, and decreases swelling. This allows the airways to relax and open. Patients with serious allergies or a history of anaphylactic reactions may be prescribed epinephrine to keep on hand or with their caregivers. There are several brand-name epinephrine autoinjectors intended for use by patients and caregivers. They include the EpiPen, EpiPen Jr, and Auvi-Q. After the use of an epinephrine autoinjector, the patient should receive prompt follow-up care by a medical professional.

Smoking Cessation

Medications for smoking cessation are intended to help patients stop using tobacco products. There are a variety of products available, including nicotine replacement therapy and oral medications. Some nicotine replacement therapies are available OTC. Bupropion (Zyban) is an antidepressant medication that helps reduce craving for nicotine. It can lower the seizure threshold and may cause insomnia. Varenicline (Chantix) is a nicotine receptor agonist that prevents stimulation from nicotine. It can cause nausea, seizures, depression, and suicidal ideation, so patients must be carefully monitored during therapy. For a list of smoking cessation medications, see Table 1.40.

TABLE 1.40 Smoking Cessation

Generic Name	Brand Name(s)	Route(s) of Administration	Dosage Form(s)	Common Dosage Amount(s)
bupropion	Zyban	oral	tablet	150 mg
nicotine*	NicoDerm CQ, Nicotrol, Nicorette	oral, topical (transdermal), transmucosal (nasal)	gum, lozenge, transdermal patch, nasal spray	7 mg, 14 mg, 21 mg, 10 mg/mL
varenicline	Chantix	oral	tablet	0.5 mg, 1 mg

*Some dosage forms/strengths available OTC

1.16 Over-the-Counter Medications

Practice Tip

Technicians should remind customers that most OTC drugs should be used for seven days or less.

Customers often seek counsel from pharmacy personnel to select the appropriate OTC product for a specific condition. Technicians should direct them to a pharmacist's counsel. Pharmacists are the only pharmacy personnel who can legally direct people to the right medication for a medical purpose or indication, the right dosage and administration, expected therapeutic effects, side effects, contraindications, and interactions—even for OTC drugs and vitamins. However, you can help customers find the brands and types of medications they are looking for. Technicians can also help customers understand the OTC product labels, which include product name and therapeutic purpose, directions for dosage and frequency of administration for different age groups, active and inactive ingredients (such as dyes), expiration dates, precautions or warnings, and special storage requirements.

Common Over-the-Counter Medications

Safety Alert

OTC cough and cold products are generally not suitable for children under age six.

Commonly requested OTC drugs are listed in Table 1.41. Many popular OTC drugs, such as hydrocortisone (Cortizone) and ibuprofen (Advil, Motrin), once required a prescription. The active ingredients are the same as those found in the prescription formulations but are present in lower strengths and dosages. For example, OTC ibuprofen is available in a strength of 200 mg, whereas the prescription strengths are 400 mg, 600 mg, and 800 mg.

Pharmacy technicians should also be aware that some OTC drugs are in the refrigerated area of the pharmacy—in particular, fast-acting regular insulins like Novolin R and Humulin R.

Manufacturers typically provide a toll-free number if consumers have additional questions or concerns about an OTC medication when they get home. Technicians may point this out.

TABLE 1.41 Common OTC Drugs and Their Indications

Brand Name	Generic Name	Indications/Uses
Abreva	docosanol	cold sores
Advil/Motrin	ibuprofen	headache, pain
Afrin	oxymetazoline	nasal decongestant
Aleve	naproxen	headache, pain
Align	*Bifidobacterium longum*	probiotic
Allegra	fexofenadine	allergy
Alli	orlistat	weight loss
Benadryl	diphenhydramine	allergy
Bonine	meclizine	motion sickness
Claritin	loratadine	allergy
Colace	docusate sodium	stool softener

continues

TABLE 1.41 Common OTC Drugs and Their Indications—*Continued*

Brand Name	Generic Name	Indications/Uses
Cortizone	hydrocortisone	itching, inflammation
Culturelle	*Lactobacillus rhamnosus*	probiotic
Debrox	carbamide peroxide	ear wax removal
Delsym	dextromethorphan	cough
Dramamine	dimenhydrinate	motion sickness
Dulcolax	bisacodyl	constipation
Excedrin	acetaminophen / aspirin / caffeine	headache, migraine
Fleet Glycerin Suppositories	glycerin	constipation
Flonase	fluticasone	allergy
Gas-X	simethicone	gas
Gyne-Lotrimin	clotrimazole	vaginal yeast infection
Humulin R, Novolin R	regular insulin	diabetes
Imodium AD	loperamide	diarrhea
Lactaid	lactase	lactose intolerance
Lamisil AT	terbinafine	topical fungal infection
Lotrimin AF	clotrimazole	topical fungal infection
Mylanta	magnesium / aluminum / simethicone	heartburn
Miralax	polyethylene glycol	constipation
Monistat	miconazole	vaginal antifungal
Mucinex, Robitussin	guaifenesin	expectorant
Nasacort	triamcinolone	allergy
Neosporin	neomycin / polymyxin B / bacitracin	topical anti-infective
Nexium	esomeprazole	heartburn
Nix	permethrin	head lice
NoDoz	caffeine	stimulant
Orajel	benzocaine	oral anesthetic
Pepcid	famotidine	heartburn
Pepto-Bismol	bismuth subsalicylate	indigestion, diarrhea
Plan B	levonorgestrel	emergency contraception
Prevacid	lansoprazole	heartburn
Prilosec	omeprazole	heartburn

continues

TABLE 1.41 Common OTC Drugs and Their Indications—*Continued*

Brand Name	Generic Name	Indications/Uses
RID	piperonyl / pyrethrins	head lice
Rogaine	minoxidil	hair growth
Rolaids	calcium / magnesium	heartburn
Senokot	senna	constipation
Sudafed	pseudoephedrine	decongestant
Sudafed PE	phenylephrine	decongestant
Tagamet	cimetidine	heartburn
Tinactin	tolnaftate	topical fungal infection
Tums	calcium carbonate	heartburn
Tylenol	acetaminophen	pain
Visine-A	naphazoline / pheniramine	ocular antihistamine
Zostrix	capsaicin	nerve pain
Zyrtec	cetirizine	allergy

Note: Drugs in table are listed by brand name first, as these are the names more often requested by customers at the pharmacy.

Consumer Cautions

Technicians may remind patients that, when the dosages recommended by the manufacturer are exceeded, OTC medications can be very dangerous. For instance, products containing the cough suppressant dextromethorphan (DM), like Delsym, can cause auditory and visual hallucinations in high doses. Because DM products have a history of abuse among adolescents, consumers must be age 18 or older to buy these products and must present an ID to purchase them.

In addition, technicians can make patients aware that the FDA discourages giving any child under the age of six OTC cough and cold products because the risk of adverse reactions is greater than the potential benefits.

Consumers should be reminded that OTC products should be used for a restricted period—usually less than seven days—unless otherwise directed by a physician. (For example, a physician may direct an adult patient to take a low-dose aspirin on a long-term, daily basis to lower a patient's risk of heart disease.) If a patient has self-medicated with an OTC drug for seven or more days without resolution, they should be referred by the pharmacist to the appropriate healthcare professional.

1.17 Alternative Medicine and Dietary Supplements

Holistic medicine looks at the whole person when deciding how to improve health. Holistic medicine practitioners can include partnerships between traditional, western medical practitioners and those who practice alternative medicine. This partnership, using prescribed conventional treatments and alternative medicine, is called

integrative medicine and may involve, for example, recommending acupuncture to a cancer patient receiving chemotherapy.

The term **alternative medicine** applies to non-western medical practices, sometimes considered "nonconventional" treatments, such as specialized diets, acupuncture, deep breathing and relaxation techniques, guided imagery, exercise movements like yoga and Pilates, meditation, massage therapy, and chiropractic manipulations. Alternative medicine also includes using natural products as medications, including homeopathic remedies and dietary supplements, like vitamins and minerals, herbals, nutritional supplements, and probiotics.

For the purposes of this certification course, technicians should be familiar with natural products their customers might use, as some consumers will assume that a natural product is safe by virtue of being "natural." It is important to realize that natural products could have side effects or problematic interactions with prescription drugs, even when used appropriately. The rest of this section will describe natural products in more detail, starting with homeopathic remedies.

Homeopathic Remedies

Pharm Fact

Because many homeopathic medications are diluted so much, up to 1,000 times, only trace amounts of the desired ingredients remain. Skeptics say these traces are not enough to provoke any medicinal effect.

Homeopathy is based on the philosophy that the body can heal itself if the immune system can be stimulated in targeted ways through the concept of "like cures like." According to proponents of homeopathy, introducing highly diluted natural substances that create minor symptoms can activate an immune system response to help overcome illnesses with the same symptoms. The trigger substances can be plant- or animal-derived (or from diseased tissues), or from metal, chemical, and mineral substances. The science behind homeopathy is lacking, and manufacturers of homeopathic remedies are not required to provide safety and efficacy data for their products.

Dietary Supplements

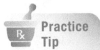

Practice Tip

Most consumers do not realize that dietary supplements, including vitamins and minerals, are not regulated by the FDA in the same manner as are OTC and prescription drugs.

A **dietary supplement** can be a vitamin, mineral, or an herbal product that is considered useful for nutrition, illness prevention, or alleviation or reduction of an illness's symptoms.

The Dietary Supplement Health and Education Act (DSHEA) states that supplements must be safe and accurately labeled. As with other food products, the label of a supplement indicates the recommended serving size rather than a dose. The label provides far less product information than an OTC drug label.

Dietary supplements are subject to restrictions on labeling. If a label contains a promise of a medical cure or effective treatment, the FDA can act to remove the supplement from the market for the reason of false advertising since no proof of the label's claims has been submitted to the FDA. The FDA can also remove any dietary supplement that is deemed dangerous. It is best to steer consumers toward products with the seal of the USP verified on them. The pharmacy technician must not counsel customers regarding the therapeutic uses of dietary supplements but refer patients to the pharmacist. For a list of dietary supplements and their indications/uses, see Table 1.42.

TABLE 1.42 Common Dietary Supplements and their Indications

Dietary Supplement	Indications/Uses
aloe vera	burn and wound healing
cascara	laxative
calcium / vitamin D	improves bone strength
echinacea	boosts the immune system
ferrous sulfate	iron deficiency, anemia
feverfew	headaches
garlic	has antibacterial and antiviral action; maintains healthy cholesterol
ginger	nausea, motion sickness, and morning sickness
ginkgo	improves memory; treats tinnitus and peripheral vascular disease
goldenseal	colds and respiratory infections; GI disorders
glucosamine / chondroitin	reduces joint pain
lactobacillus (a bacterium)	improves digestion; helps prevent diarrhea
lutein	maintains eye health
melatonin	insomnia, especially in shift workers or time-zone travelers
omega-3 fatty acids (fish oil)	lowers triglyceride levels
policosanol	maintains healthy cholesterol levels
red yeast rice	maintains healthy cholesterol levels
saw palmetto	benign prostatic hyperplasia (BPH)
St. John's wort	mild depression
soy	menopause; bone health; cardiovascular health
tea tree oil	alleviates skin ailments, such as acne, athlete's foot, and boils
turmeric	anti-inflammatory
vitamin C	prevention of common cold, viral illness
zinc	boosts the immune system; helps in the treatment of the common cold and wound healing

Vitamins and Minerals

There are many OTC vitamin and mineral products on the market that range from multivitamins to the doses of specific minerals and vitamins like B complex, A, C, D, and E. Listed on the label of each is the proportion of active substance contained as compared to the **recommended daily allowance (RDA)**. The RDA is the average intake level needed to meet the daily nutrient requirements of most (97% to 98%) healthy people. Children or adults may need daily vitamin supplements just to reach

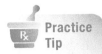

the minimum RDA. Pregnant individuals are encouraged to consume a daily prenatal vitamin (prescription or OTC) to promote fetal health and prevent birth defects. Technicians can be helpful by directing patients to both brand-name and generic vitamins, including those in chewable, gummy, and liquid formulations for children and other consumers who need them.

Some consumers take short-term high doses of individual vitamins for different indications, such as vitamin C to build immunity and fight the common cold, vitamin E for heart health, and lutein for eye health. However, research has found that habitual high doses of certain vitamins can be harmful to health. For instance, very high doses of vitamin E may interfere with blood clotting or increase the risk of heart disease. High supplement doses of vitamin A and other vitamins absorbed by fat can build up in the body and cause toxicity, liver damage, birth defects, and problems in the central nervous system.

Popular mineral supplements include iron and calcium. In many cases, these may be prescribed or recommended by a physician. Vegans and vegetarians, menstruating and pregnant individuals, and postsurgical patients may require extra iron to prevent anemia. Calcium combined with magnesium and vitamin D is recommended to keep bones strong and prevent osteoporosis. Since the salt combinations of iron and calcium in different products contain variable amounts of active minerals, questions should be referred to the pharmacist for proper product selection.

Herbal and Medicinal Plants

Though considered "natural drugs," **herbals** are also regulated as dietary supplements rather than as drugs by the FDA. The most popular herbals are echinacea, ginger, garlic, ginkgo, St. John's wort, and soy. Their indications were also listed in Table 1.42. Herbals are also dosed in serving sizes like food.

Herbals can cause drug interactions or affect the absorption, distribution, and elimination of other drug substances, including prescription and OTC drugs and other supplements. Like OTC drugs, herbal medications have side effects and can cause allergic reactions—not just the first time they are used but even after sustained use. Some herbals can accumulate in the body or cause an immune response to build up gradually.

Goldenseal has a high potential for adverse herbal-drug interactions. Concentrated and prolonged ingestion of ginger, garlic, and ginkgo should not occur with blood thinners and must be discontinued a week prior to surgery. St. John's wort should not be used with a wide range of prescription drugs, such as antidepressants, birth control medications, antiseizure drugs, cyclosporine (an organ-rejection prevention drug), digoxin (a heart medication), and warfarin, along with other blood thinners.

Protein Shakes and Nutritional Supplements

Physicians often recommend protein shakes and nutritional supplements to patients who do not eat well and are losing weight, such as seniors or patients undergoing cancer treatments who need to replenish or build up their systems. Protein sources include milk, whey, casein, egg, rice and soy (plant proteins). Some processed supplements are high in sugar, so caution must be exercised with patients with diabetes. Ensure is a brand of nutritional supplement that is available in various flavors. Like other brands, it supplies needed calories containing protein, minerals, and vitamins without fat, and it can be used as a meal supplement or replacement. Thick-It is a supplement requested by many older adult customers. When added to water, juices, tea, milk, or protein shakes, Thick-It helps with swallowing and digestion.

Probiotics

Probiotics work to build up the "good" or "friendly" microorganisms in the body, especially the positive-acting bacteria in the digestive system. Since antibiotics often destroy the bacteria causing the infection as well as the positive bacteria in the gastrointestinal (GI) tract (stomach and intestines), common side effects of antibiotic therapy include diarrhea and vaginal yeast infections. Physicians often advise patients taking antibiotics to eat yogurt that contains live bacteria cultures of *Lactobacillus acidophilus* or ingest a probiotic sold in the pharmacy. Patients who are lactose (milk sugar) intolerant often use probiotic supplements to combat digestive issues when they drink milk or eat cheese and other dairy products.

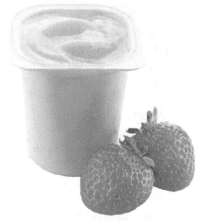
Yogurt can be a great source of probiotics that aid digestion.

Common probiotics contain various strains of *Lactobacillus* and *Bifidobacterium*, which can restore the balance of microorganisms in the GI tract. Some brand name probiotics include Culturelle, Align, and Lactinex (the latter is found in the pharmacy's refrigerator). Probiotics may also be used to treat the abdominal pain, cramping, and bloating associated with IBS. Some scientific research is now finding that probiotics can help heal skin conditions, such as eczema, prevent allergies and colds, and improve oral health.

1.18 Vaccines and Immunization

Immunization is the process whereby a person acquires immunity or resistance to an infectious disease through vaccination. **Vaccination** is the treatment with a vaccine to provide immunity against a disease. Vaccination is a proven tool for the prevention and elimination of infectious diseases. Various types of vaccines are available (see Table 1.43). Live attenuated vaccines use living but weakened pathogens to induce an immune response. Inactivated vaccines use pathogens that have been killed with chemicals, heat, or radiation.

Common side effects of vaccines include fever, headache, injection-site irritation, mild skin rash, and irritability. These symptoms are related to a systemic immune response, which makes a person feel tired and achy. There are certain contraindications to immunization. Severely immunocompromised individuals should not receive live vaccines, and live vaccines are typically contraindicated in pregnancy.

TABLE 1.43 Common Vaccines and Storage

Generic Name(s)	Brand Name(s)	Route of Administration	Storage
diphtheria and tetanus toxoids (Td)	Tenivac	parenteral	refrigerator
diphtheria, Td, and pertussis (DTaP, Tdap)	Daptacel, Infarix (DTaP) Adacel, Boostrix (Tdap)	parenteral	refrigerator
Haemophilus influenzae type B (Hib)	ActHIB, PedvaxHIB, Hiberix	parenteral	refrigerator
hepatitis A	Havrix, Vaqta	parenteral	refrigerator

continues

TABLE 1.43 Common Vaccines and Storage—*Continued*

Generic Name	Brand Name	Route of Administration	Storage
hepatitis B	Energix-B, Recombivax HB, Heplisav-B	parenteral	refrigerator
hepatitis A and hepatitis B	Twinrix	parenteral	refrigerator
zoster	Shingrix, Zostavax	parenteral	refrigerator (Shingrix), freezer (Zostavax)
human papillomavirus (HPV)	Gardasil	parenteral	refrigerator
influenza, inactivated (IIV)	Afluria, Fluad, Flublok, Flucelvax, FluLaval, Fluarix, Fluvirin, Fluzone, Fluzone High-Dose	parenteral	refrigerator
influenza, live attenuated (LAIV)	FluMist	transmucosal (intranasal)	refrigerator
measles, mumps, and rubella (MMR)	M-M-R II	parenteral	refrigerator
Measles, mumps, rubbella, and varicella (MMRV)	ProQuad	parenteral	freezer

Note: A full listing of US-approved vaccines can be found at https://www.cdc.gov/vaccines/vpd/vaccines-list.html.

In the United States, the Centers for Disease Control (CDC) publishes a schedule for childhood and adult vaccines. Pharmacy technicians should be informed of immunization schedules and be certain that they are up to date on their immunizations. Working in health care without being properly vaccinated increases an individual's risk of exposure to diseases and promotes disease transmission. It is important for patients to be up to date on their immunizations, and community pharmacists are an important provider of vaccines.

1.19 Drug Stability and Storage

Drug stability refers to the extent to which a dosage form retains its properties and characteristics over time. Drug stability directly affects the safety and efficacy of drug products. Degradation of a dosage form may cause loss of efficacy and adverse effects. Manufactured drug products will have an **expiration date**, which is the date beyond which a drug's stability and potency cannot be guaranteed. Compounded and reconstituted drug products will have a **beyond-use date (BUD)**, which is determined based on the date that the product is compounded.

Physical and chemical incompatibilities can affect drug stability. *Physical incompatibility* is the failure of a drug product to combine properly. Physical incompatibilities cause interactions between two or more substances that produce observable changes in color, odor, taste, or appearance. Chemical incompatibility occurs due to undesired chemical reactions between substances being combined. The resulting product may be toxic or inactive. Incompatibilities may occur during the process of compounding, or during reconstitution of a manufactured drug product.

Proper storage of medications is also important to drug stability. All medications have specific storage conditions as determined by the manufacturer. These conditions include the temperature at which the drug is to be stored, whether the drug is to be protected from light, and whether the drug must be dispensed in the original container. Medications stored outside of recommended temperature ranges may experience a loss of physical integrity or effectiveness. Drugs may lose potency if exposed to light or moisture. For this reason, drug products that are particularly sensitive to light or moisture should always be stored and dispensed in their original containers.

Vaccines also have specific storage requirements. While most vaccines require refrigeration, some vaccines need to be stored in the freezer, including Varivax, ProQuad, and Zostavax.

Technicians should inform customers how to appropriately store medications at home. For example, a reconstituted antibiotic suspension is stable for a limited time, about 10 days, and should be discarded once the treatment is complete. Penicillin-based solutions need to be stored in the refrigerator after they have been reconstituted. Other antibiotics such as azithromycin, clarithromycin, and cefdinir are stored at room temperature, which is generally considered to be below 86° F, or 30° C. Some temperature variation may occur during a short-term power outage, but any long-term storage above room temperature can affect medications, and patients should contact the pharmacy or manufacturer for more information.

Patients need to be made aware that if an insulin vial or syringe is frozen or left in the heat of a car or in light, the medication should not be used and should be discarded. In warm climates, or in the summer, patients may be advised to transport their insulin in a cooler, especially if they are not returning home immediately.

Once opened, most insulins have a BUD of 28 days, though newer agents may be good for up to 60 days. Check the package insert for the manufacturer-recommended BUD. Patients need to be instructed that insulin should be stored in the refrigerator until first use, and then discarded after the BUD. Patients do not need to refrigerate a vial or insulin pen after first use.

A more detailed discussion of medication and vaccine storage can be found in Chapter 8.

1.20 Final Thoughts on Medications

This chapter has introduced many medications, as well how suffixes and some prefixes in generic names relate to medication classifications. To learn the many drug families and their similarities, it is helpful to memorize drug suffixes and prefixes for quick recognition. Table 1.44 provides a list of many common drug suffixes and prefixes to help with memorization.

TABLE 1.44 Drug Suffixes and Prefixes

Suffix or Prefix	Classification	Generic Drug Examples
-prazole	proton pump inhibitor (PPI)	omeprazole, lansoprazole
-tidine	histamine-2 antagonist	ranitidine, famotidine
-statin	HMG CoA reductase inhibitor	lovastatin, simvastatin

continues

TABLE 1.44 **Drug Suffixes and Prefixes**—*Continued*

Suffix or Prefix	Classification	Generic Drug Examples
-ine	opiate analgesic	codeine, morphine
-one	opioid analgesic or corticosteroid	hydrocodone, hydromorphone or prednisone, triamcinolone
-pam or -lam	benzodiazepine (BZD)	diazepam, alprazolam
-triptan	serotonin agonist for migraine headaches	sumatriptan, zolmitriptan
-olol	beta-adrenergic blocker	propranolol, metoprolol
-pril	ACE inhibitor	lisinopril, quinapril
-sartan	angiotensin receptor blocker (ARB)	losartan, olmesartan
-dipine	dihydropyridine calcium channel blocker	nifedipine, amlodipine
-cillin	penicillin antibiotics	ampicillin, ticarcillin
ceph- or cef-	cephalosporin antibiotic	cephalexin, ceftazidime
-oxacin	fluoroquinolone antibiotic	ciprofloxacin, levofloxacin
sulf-	sulfonamide antibiotic	sulfamethoxazole, sulfasalazine
-penem	beta-lactam antibiotic	meropenem, imipenem
-omycin	macrolide antibiotic	erythromycin, clarithromycin
-cycline	tetracycline antibiotic	doxycycline, minocycline
-vir	antiviral (may be flu, herpes, or HIV infection)	acyclovir, ritonavir
-azole	antifungal	fluconazole, miconazole
-caine	Topical anesthetic	lidocaine, prilocaine
-gliptin	DPP-4 inhibitor	sitagliptin, saxagliptin
-ide	sulfonylurea	glipizide, glyburide
-glitazone	thiazolidinediones	pioglitazone, rosiglitazone
-dronate	bisphosphonates	alendronate, risedronate
-terol	beta-2 agonist for respiratory disease	albuterol, salmeterol
-tropium	anticholinergic for respiratory disease	ipratropium, tiotropium
-parin	thrombin inhibitors	heparin, enoxaparin
-mab	monoclonal antibody-biotech drug	infliximab, rituximab

Auxiliary labels help patients understand how to take their medications and prevent side effects. The computer may print off more labels than can fit on the prescription vial; technicians should check with the pharmacist to identify which are most important and must be on the vial prior to dispensing to the patient. Table 1.45 lists the most used auxiliary labels and common drugs that need them.

TABLE 1.45 Auxiliary Labels

Auxiliary Label	Common Drugs and Classifications Requiring Label
Avoid exposure to sunlight	antibiotics, antifungals, amiodarone, carbamazepine, ibuprofen, isotretinoin, loop diuretics, naproxen, spironolactone, sulfonylureas, thiazide diuretics, trazodone
Discolors urine or feces	cefdinir, ferrous sulfate, phenazopyridine, nitrofurantoin, rifampin
Do not drink alcohol when taking medication	antidepressants, antipsychotics, CNS depressants, disulfiram, metronidazole, narcotics, NSAIDs, oral contraceptives, phenytoin, sulfonylureas
Do not take if pregnant, nursing, or trying to conceive	isotretinoin, finasteride, statins, oral contraceptives
Do not take with dairy products, antacids, or iron preparations	ciprofloxacin, doxycycline, gabapentin, levothyroxine, sucralfate
Do not take with grapefruit juice	statins
Do not smoke when taking medication	hormonal contraceptives
Finish all medication as prescribed	all antibiotics, antifungals, and antivirals
Interferes with contraceptives	antibiotics
May cause dizziness	anticonvulsants, pregabalin antidiabetic agents, opioid analgesics, many antibiotics
May cause drowsiness	antidepressants, antipsychotics, benzodiazepines, hypnotics, muscle relaxants, narcotics, opioid analgesics, tramadol
Take at bedtime	alpha blockers, nicotinic acid, statins
Take on an empty stomach, 1 hour before meals, or 2 hours after a meal	bisphosphonates, captopril, sucralfate, penicillin, levothyroxine
Take with food	antibiotics (azithromycin, erythromycin), corticosteroids, metformin, narcotics, nicotinic acid, non-narcotic analgesics, NSAIDs, oral contraceptives, potassium chloride
Take with a full glass of orange juice or eat a banana daily	loop diuretics, thiazide diuretics
Take with water	potassium chloride, sulfa drugs, phenazopyridine, bisphosphonates, NSAIDs

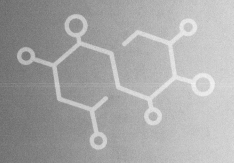

Review and Assessment

STUDY SUMMARY

The study of medications requires a great deal of memorization. Study the drugs in families to get to know them well. With study, flashcards, and practice, the information about medications will become second nature.

- Memorize different kinds of drug agents based on bodily systems and the drug families based on chemical composition and action.

- Use flashcards to study generic to brand and brand to generic names.

- Get to know the common indications, contraindications, side effects, warnings, and typical auxiliary labels.

ADDITIONAL RESOURCES

For more in-depth explanations, check out *Pharmacology for Technicians* Seventh Edition, from Paradigm Education Solutions. To master and extend the material presented in this chapter, take advantage of the resources available through the eBook resources links. These include digital supplements, study resources, and a practice exam generator with 1,000+ exam-style questions. End-of-chapter tests are accessible through the eBook for individuals using the self-study course and through Cirrus for individuals enrolled in the instructor-guided course.

Federal Requirements

2

Learning Objectives

1 List landmark legislation important to the practice of pharmacy. (Section 2.1)

2 Describe the Health Insurance Portability and Accountability Act requirements for safeguarding the confidentiality of protected health information. (Section 2.1)

3 List organizations pertinent to the practice of pharmacy. (Section 2.2)

4 Describe federal requirements for handling and disposal of hazardous drugs, nonhazardous waste, and hazardous waste. (Section 2.3)

5 Identify Food and Drug Administration recall classifications and procedures. (Section 2.4)

6 Describe elements of Risk Evaluation and Mitigation Strategies. (Section 2.5)

7 Identify federal requirements for controlled substance prescriptions and Drug Enforcement Administration controlled substances schedules. (Section 2.6)

8 Describe federal requirements for controlled substances including receiving, storing, ordering, labeling, dispensing, reverse distribution, take back programs, and loss/theft. (Section 2.6)

9 Identify pharmacy technician duties as dictated by state laws. (Section 2.7)

 Access eBook links for resources and an exam generator, with 1,000+ questions.

The practice of pharmacy is governed by numerous laws and regulations. The pharmacy technician needs to be familiar with these laws and regulations and their effect on various issues, such as patient privacy and counseling, product and ingredient safety, and controlled substances. This chapter covers these topics and discusses special requirements for handling controlled substances, including storage, record keeping, inventory control, safety, and abuse potential. It also outlines the professional standards for products, services, and personal behavior. These are topics addressed in domain 2 of the Pharmacy Technician Certification Exam (PTCE) and domain 1 of the Exam for the Certification of Pharmacy Technicians (ExCPT).

2.1 Pharmacy Oversight

Pharmacy technicians must practice within federal laws and the laws of their state, as recommended by their state's board of pharmacy (BOP) and passed by their state and municipal lawmakers. When federal and state laws are in conflict, the strictest law always prevails.

Some of these laws require specific actions on the part of the technician, such as the laws and regulations governing the dispensing, ordering, inventory, disposal, and documentation of controlled substances (covered in depth later in the chapter). An overview of the key federal laws affecting pharmacy that may be covered in a certification exam can be seen in Table 2.1, and in the sections that follow.

TABLE 2.1 Pharmacy-Related Federal Laws

Law	Year Passed	Significance to Pharmacy Practice
Pure Food and Drug Act	1906	first law to regulate the development, compounding, distribution, storage and dispensing of drugs; prohibits the inclusion of false or misleading labeling about drug strength or purity and interstate transport or sale of adulterated or misbranded drugs
Harrison Narcotics Tax Act	1914	regulated and taxed the production, importation, and distribution of opiates and coca products
Food, Drug, and Cosmetic Act (FDCA)	1938	created the US Food and Drug Administration (FDA); clearly defines *adulteration* and *misbranding*; requires that products be safe for human use and that manufacturers include product inserts
Durham-Humphrey Amendment to the FDCA	1951	distinguishes between prescription and nonprescription drugs; requires amendments to FDCA that all drug products have adequate usage directions or bear the legend "Caution: Federal Law Prohibits without Prescription" that all over-the-counter (OTC) drugs have a label that includes a list of active ingredients; allows verbal prescription and refill requests to pharmacies by telephone
Kefauver-Harris Amendments to the FDCA	1962	requires that drugs be safe and effective and that pharmaceutical manufacturers file an Investigational New Drug Application (INDA) before starting clinical trials on human subjects to win FDA approval
Comprehensive Drug Abuse Prevention and Control Act (Controlled Substances Act [CSA])	1970	established the federal Drug Enforcement Administration (DEA); identified drugs that have the potential for abuse and/or addiction and categorized them into five schedules
Poison Prevention Packaging Act (PPPA)	1970	requires child-resistant containers for most prescription and OTC drugs to prevent accidental ingestion and poisoning
Occupational Safety and Health Act	1970	created the Occupational Safety and Health Administration (OSHA), whose charge is to reduce hazards in the workplace in order to create a safe and healthy workplace for all employees; requires reporting of job-related injuries and illnesses
Drug Listing Act	1972	requires National Drug Code (NDC) numbers be assigned to every marketed drug

continues

TABLE 2.1 Pharmacy-Related Federal Laws—*Continued*

Law	Year Passed	Significance to Pharmacy Practice
Resource Conservation and Recovery Act	1976	governs the disposal of solid waste and hazardous. waste; established "cradle-to-grave" standards for the generation, transportation, treatment, storage, and disposal of hazardous waste
Orphan Drug Act	1983	provides tax incentives for developing and marketing drugs used to treat rare conditions (those that affect less than 200,000 people); established longer exclusive licensing and tax incentives for manufacturers that develop orphan drugs
Drug Price Competition and Patent Term Restoration Act (a.k.a. the Hatch-Waxman Amendments)	1984	streamlined the FDA approval process for marketing generic drugs; extended the terms of patents for companies that develop new drugs
Omnibus Budget Reconciliation Act of 1987 (OBRA-87) (a.k.a. the Federal Nursing Home Reform Act)	1987	set standards of care and established rights for those under managed care in nursing home
Prescription Drug Marketing Act (PDMA)	1987	prohibits the reimportation of drugs to the United States, except by the manufacturer
Anabolic Steroids Control Act	1990	redefined anabolic steroids as Schedule III (C-III) controlled substances
Omnibus Budget Reconciliation Act (OBRA-90)	1990	requires pharmacists to engage in drug utilization reviews (DURs) and offer Medicaid patients the option of free prescription counseling
Prescription Drug User Fee Act (PDUFA)	1992	allowed the FDA to collect fees from manufacturers to speed up the drug approval process; reduced the time for the FDA to review new drug approvals (NDAs) by half
Dietary Supplement Health and Education Act (DSHEA)	1994	classified herbal supplements as food products rather than drugs; prohibits manufacturers of herbs and dietary supplements from making claims that their products treat or cure any specific disease or illness
Health Insurance Portability and Accountability Act (HIPAA)	1996	addressed patient privacy concerns by requiring signing of a confidential annual HIPAA form outlining who has access to patient information; allows employees to easily move their health insurance from one job to another; resulted in privacy protection practices for the communicating, collecting, storing, disclosing, and disposing of patient data
Comprehensive Methamphetamine Control Act	1996	established methamphetamine as a dangerous addictive drug requiring legislative oversight and control of the exportation, importation, and manufacturing of methamphetamine substances and its precursor chemicals
FDA Modernization Act (FDAMA)	1997	allowed the previous federal legend to be abbreviated with the statement "Rx Only"; allowed pharmacists to compound for individual patients any product not commercially available ; reauthorized the PDUFA for an 5 additional years

continues

TABLE 2.1 Pharmacy-Related Federal Laws—*Continued*

Law	Year Passed	Significance to Pharmacy Practice
Medicare Modernization Act (MMA)	2003	provided a voluntary prescription drug plan (Part D) for Medicare patients for an additional cost; created health savings accounts (HSAs); allows pharmacists to get reimbursed for medication counseling and therapy management
Combat Methamphetamine Epidemic Act (CMEA)	2005	restricts sales of OTC drugs used in making methamphetamines (pseudoephedrine, ephedrine, and phenylpropanolamine); requires that these drugs be stored behind the counter and sales monitored sales be monitored, only by the pharmacist)
Patient Safety and Quality Improvement Act (PSQIA)	2005	promotes mechanisms for patient safety and continuous quality improvement; encouraged creation of Patient Safety Organizations (PSOs) to collect confidential information on medical errors to detect systematic changes to improve patient safety
Biologics Price Competition and Innovation Act (BCPI)	2009	created an abbreviated pathway for the approval of biological products that are proven to be biosimilar or interchangeable with an FDA-approved reference biological product
The Food and Drug Administration Amendments Act (FDAAA)	2007	gave the FDA the authority to require a Risk Evaluation and Mitigation Strategy (REMS) from manufacturers to ensure that the benefits of a drug or biological product outweigh its risks
Patient Protection and Affordable Care Act (ACA)	2010	comprehensive health care reform law; established health insurance exchanges; provides catastrophic coverage for high-cost illness; prohibits insurers from refusing coverage to those with preexisting conditions
Drug Quality and Security Act (DQSA)	2013	Title I a.k.a. the (Compounding Quality Act) established regulations for compounding pharmacies and outsourcing facilities and encourages regulation of all outsourcing facilities. Title II a.k.a. the (Drug Supply Chain Security Act) established a national database to track and trace drug products through the supply chain from the manufacturer to the dispensing pharmacy

Poison Prevention Packaging Act

Study Idea

Remember that certain drugs are exempt from the PPPA, such as nitroglycerin SL and oral birth control tablets in memory packs. More information can be found at the CPSC website.

The Poison Prevention Packaging Act (PPPA) of 1970 was passed to prevent accidental childhood drug poisonings. This act, enforced by the Consumer Product Safety Commission (CPSC), requires that most over-the-counter (OTC) and prescription drugs be packaged in child-resistant containers (containers which cannot be opened by 80% of children under age 5 but can be opened by 90% of adults). Upon request from a patient, a drug may be dispensed in a non–child-resistant container. In fact, the patient—not the prescriber—can make a blanket request that all their drugs be dispensed with non–child-resistant containers.

Omnibus Budget Reconciliation Act of 1990

The Omnibus Budget Reconciliation Act of 1990 (OBRA-90), mandates that pharmacies complete a drug utilization review (DUR) for medication dispensing to identify potential drug or supplement interactions or allergy warnings. The pharmacy technician should not override these types of alerts or warnings. The pharmacist must evaluate the warning and decide on the correct action. OBRA-90 requires that free counseling from a pharmacist be offered to all Medicaid patients. State boards of pharmacy (BOP) and private insurers have adopted this policy as well, and it has now become the standard of care in all US community pharmacies.

Counseling mandated under OBRA-90 must, at minimum, include the following items: name and description of medication, route of administration (ROA), dosage form, dosage, duration of therapy, directions and precautions, adverse events, interactions, contraindications, self-monitoring instructions, proper storage, refill information, and instructions about handling missed doses. OBRA-90 also requires pharmacies to obtain, record, and maintain appropriate patient profiles that include the patient's name, address, telephone number, date of birth. Each patient profile must contain the patient's medical and prescription history.

Health Insurance Portability and Accountability Act

Established in 1996, the Health Insurance Portability and Accountability Act (HIPAA) mandates the confidentiality of all health records, under penalty of law. All new pharmacy patients must be given a copy of the pharmacy's notice of privacy practices (NPP), which explains the patient's rights with respect to their personal information in clear, easily understood language. Patients must sign an acknowledgment of the receipt of this information. This document must be scanned into the patient's profile and stored for six years after the last affiliation with the patient.

HIPAA mandates the protection of **protected health information (PHI)**, which is any information that can be used to identify the patient, including name, address, names of relatives, names of employers, Social Security number, date of birth, telephone numbers, email addresses, payment information, and other health- or identity-related information. Pharmacies must have policies in place to safeguard and prevent the unauthorized release of PHI.

Technicians must be careful when dispensing and discussing patient prescriptions, so that the patient's confidential information is not overheard by other patients or staff. PHI cannot be shared or discussed with others who are not directly involved in patient care because this violates the confidentiality of the patient in question. All labels and printed documents must have patient-specific information blacked out or be shredded before disposal. Personnel who violate HIPAA can be fined and may lose their jobs.

Combat Methamphetamine Epidemic Act

Established in 2005, the Combat Methamphetamine Epidemic Act (CMEA) limits and tracks the sale of OTC products that contain pseudoephedrine, ephedrine, and phenylpropanolamine, which can be used in the production of methamphetamine. OTC products with these active ingredients must be stored behind the counter in the pharmacy, and sales are restricted to 3.6 g per week and 9 g every 30 days. Pharmacy technicians working under the direction of the pharmacist may handle the sale of pseudoephedrine. All required purchaser information must be documented in an electronic or hard-copy log that is kept for two years. This log must contain the drug name and quantity, customer name and home address, date purchased and time, and customer's signature, completed with presentation of a legal photo ID with signature. Purchasers must be at least 16 years of age.

Medicare Modernization Act

Pharmacy technicians must be aware of prescription drug plans (Medicare Part D) developed because of the Medicare Modernization Act of (MMA) of 2003. This act also created the use of health savings accounts (HSAs) for patients. The Centers for Medicare & Medicaid Services (CMS) regulates Medicare Part D prescriptions and dictates the documentation and patient counseling requirements under the MMA.

Drug Quality and Security Act

The Drug Quality and Security Act (DQSA) of 2013 was passed following an incident in which the New England Compounding Center produced an injectable steroid product contaminated with bacteria. Patients in 19 states were harmed, and distribution of the product was difficult to trace. The DQSA consists of two acts: the Compounding Quality Act and the Drug Supply Chain Security Act. The DQSA aims to decrease the number of counterfeit drugs and provide more safety oversight for compounding facilities. It required that a national database be established to track and trace drug products through the supply chain from the manufacturer or compounding facility to the patient. DQSA documentation is required when a manufactured or compounded product is delivered to a wholesaler and again when that product is delivered by the wholesaler to a pharmacy for dispensing or to a healthcare facility for administration. Technicians involved in inventory management must understand the pharmacy documentation requirements.

2.2 Oversight and Abuse

National and state agencies and governing bodies were established to oversee the laws. Reference Table 2.2 for some of the key federal agencies that provide oversight.

TABLE 2.2 Federal Oversight Agencies

Agency	Duties
Centers for Disease Control and Prevention (CDC)	works to fight infectious diseases, to stop epidemics (regional widespread contagious diseases) and pandemics (globally widespread epidemics), sexually transmitted infections, (STDs) food-borne diseases, and other contagious illnesses
Occupational Safety and Health Administration (OSHA)	works to ensure the safety and health of US workers by establishing and enforcing workplace regulations and standards; provides training, outreach, and education; encourages continual improvement in workplace safety and health
Drug Enforcement Administration (DEA)	responsible for enforcing the laws regarding all controlled substances, both illegal and legal
Food and Drug Administration (FDA)	responsible for protecting public health by ensuring the safety, efficacy, and security of human and veterinary drugs, biological products, and medical devices

continues

TABLE 2.2 Federal Oversight Agencies—*Continued*

Agency	Duties
Health Care Financing Administration (HCFA) of the Department of Health & Human Services (HHS)	provides oversight of the Medicare program, the federal portion of the Medicaid program, and related quality assurance activities
Center for Medicare & Medicaid Services (CMS)	has authority over reimbursement under the Medicare and Medicaid government drug insurance programs
Federal Trade Commission (FTC)	has authority over business practices like direct-to-consumer drug advertising

Pharmacy practice is also overseen and/or guided by professional organizations, which can be reviewed in Table 2.3.

TABLE 2.3 **Professional Oversight Organizations**

Organization	Description/Duties
United States Pharmacopeial Convention (USP)	an independent, nonprofit scientific organization that decides quality standards for prescription drugs, OTC drugs, and dietary supplements
The Joint Commission (TJC)	a nongovernmental, nonprofit professional healthcare association that sets high standards of care for hospitals and other healthcare institutions
National Association of Boards of Pharmacy (NABP)	the only professional organization that represents all 50 state boards of pharmacy (BOP)
American Pharmacists Association (APhA)	establishes professional practice standards and addresses the problem of varying qualities and recipes of imported drugs
American Society of Health-System Pharmacists (ASHP)	represents the interests of pharmacists and pharmacy technicians for best practice in hospitals, health maintenance organizations, long-term care facilities, home health care, and other components of health care
National Pharmacy Technician Association (NPTA)	an advocacy organization that updates its members on relevant news and provides online continuing education courses specific to pharmacy technician practice
American Association of Pharmacy Technicians (AAPT)	provides leadership and represents the interests of its members to the public as well as to healthcare organizations
Pharmacy Technician Educators Council (PTEC)	an organization of instructors dedicated to developing and sharing pharmacy technician program curricula, educational materials, and instructional materials; advocates for greater education, training, certification, and responsibilities for technicians across the United States
Institute for Safe Medication Practices (ISMP)	the only 501(c) (3) nonprofit organization devoted entirely to preventing medication errors

In addition to the laws, rules, and guidelines from these sources, each community and institutional pharmacy creates a policy and procedures (P&P) manual that the technicians and pharmacists must follow.

Fraud, Waste, and Abuse

Healthcare fraud is a growing problem and a major target of government enforcement efforts. Medicare fraud occurs every year in the form of false claims for unnecessary services or goods and services that were never provided to the patient. Pharmacies that participate in Medicare and Medicaid must have compliance programs in place to prevent, detect, and correct noncompliance as well as fraud, waste, and abuse. The definitions of fraud, waste and abuse are as follows:

- **Fraud**—knowingly submitting false or misrepresented claims to obtain a payment one is not otherwise entitled to, such as submitting a claim for prescriptions that will not be dispensed to the patient
- **Waste**—practices that result in unnecessary costs to the Medicare program, such as prescribing and dispensing unnecessary quantities of medication
- **Abuse**—also results in unnecessary costs to the Medicare program, but the provider does not knowingly misrepresent facts to obtain payment (e.g., a pharmacy unknowingly bills for a brand-name drug but dispenses a generic).

Enforcement efforts aimed at reducing fraud, waste, and abuse are supported by several laws, including the False Claims Act (FCA), the Physician Self-Referral Law (Stark law), and the Federal Anti-Kickback Statute (AKS). These laws exist to protect the public and taxpayer dollars from being squandered. Violations of these laws may result in a variety of penalties, including civil monetary penalties, civil prosecution, criminal conviction and fines, exclusion from participation in federal healthcare programs, imprisonment, and the loss of professional licensure.

2.3 Federal Requirements for Handling and Disposal of Hazardous Drugs, Nonhazardous Waste, and Hazardous Waste

Medications are made of chemical compounds that not only affect the patients who take them, but may also have unintended effects on the personnel who handle them. Pharmacy personnel must be trained in the safe handling of hazardous drugs and in the appropriate disposal of all types of pharmaceutical waste.

Hazardous Drugs

According to the National Institute of Occupational Safety and Health (NIOSH), drugs may be identified as hazardous or potentially hazardous based on at least one the following criteria:

- **Carcinogenicity**—any agent that promotes the formation of cancer
- **Teratogenicity**—any agent that can disrupt the development of an embryo or fetus
- **Reproductive toxicity**—any agent that interferes with normal reproduction

- **Organ toxicity in low doses**—any agent that damages organ structure or function
- **Genotoxicity**—any agent that damages genetic information within a cell causing mutations
- new drugs that mimic existing hazardous drugs in structure or toxicity.

NIOSH also maintains a list of hazardous drugs (HDs) used in health care, including cisplatin, ethinyl estradiol, etoposide, fluorouracil, ganciclovir, methotrexate, and tamoxifen. The complete list can be found at CertExam5e.paradigmeducation.com/NIOSH.

Pharmacy personnel are at risk for unintentional exposure to HDs. Possible routes of entry include dermal and mucosal absorption, inhalation, injection, and ingestion. For instance, during receipt of HDs, personnel may encounter HD residue present on drug containers. Potential opportunities for exposure are listed in Table 2.4.

TABLE 2.4 Example of Potential Opportunities for HD Exposure Based on Activity

Activity	Potential Opportunity for HD Exposure
receipt	• contact with HD residue on containers, dosage units, work surfaces, or floors
dispensing	• counting or repackaging tablets and capsules
compounding	• crushing tablets or opening capsules • pouring liquids from one container to another • weighing or mixing • constituting or reconstituting powdered or lyophilized drugs • withdrawing or diluting injectable HDs from parenteral containers • expelling air or HDs from syringes • contact with HD residue on personal protective equipment (PPE) or other garments • deactivating, decontaminating, cleaning, and disinfecting areas that are or may be contaminated with HDs • maintenance activities for potentially contaminated equipment or devices
spills	• spill generation, management, and disposal
transport	• moving HDs within a healthcare setting
waste	• collection and disposal of hazardous waste

All pharmacy personnel should be trained in the receipt, handling, dispensing, storage, compounding, and disposal of HDs, and this training must occur before the pharmacy staff member works with HDs. After initial training, retraining must occur every twelve months. Personnel must undergo training to learn which HDs are used in the facility and their risks, proper use of personal protective equipment (PPE), proper use of equipment and devices, spill management, proper disposal procedures, and what may occur in the event of exposure to HDs.

Personnel working with HDs should don PPE, which includes chemotherapy gloves, a disposable gown, a head and/or hair cover, and shoe covers. PPE must be worn during receiving, storing, transporting, compounding, and during spill management. During spill management, personnel should also wear eye, face, and respiratory protection.

Storage of HDs should occur away from patients, visitors, and employee break areas. Storage should be appropriately secure to prevent breakage and spills. Some HDs may be stored with regular medications, but others must be stored separately.

Pharmacies that prepare HDs must have appropriate environmental and engineering controls, including a negative pressure room. Engineering controls for the preparation of HDs must be separate from engineering controls used for non-hazardous preparations. Biological safety cabinets are used for the preparation of HDs. A sink and eye-wash station must be readily available.

Each facility must have emergency procedures to cover spills or accidental release of HDs. Spills should be cleaned up immediately using a HD spill kit and using proper HD clean-up procedure, which includes deactivation, decontamination, cleaning, and disinfection. If personnel are exposed to HDs, they should immediately remove gloves and/or gown and clean the affected skin with soap and water. If eyes are affected, they should be flooded for 15 minutes using an eyewash station or isotonic eyewash. Necessary medical attention should be obtained, and the exposure documented in the employee's medical record.

Nonhazardous Waste

Most pharmaceutical waste and medications are nonhazardous. Nonhazardous pharmaceutical waste includes OTC medications, antibiotics, and other medications. Nonhazardous pharmaceutical waste can be disposed of in designated bins (usually blue or white) or in the regular trash if it will be incinerated. Glass and used needles must be disposed of in appropriate sharps containers. Personnel must follow all applicable state and local laws and regulations when disposing of nonhazardous waste.

Hazardous Waste

There are several types of hazardous waste, including solid waste, hazardous material, and infectious waste. Waste is considered hazardous if it is specifically listed on one of four lists (F, K, P, and U). Pharmaceutical wastes are usually included on the P and U lists. Waste can also be classified as hazardous based on certain characteristics, which include ignitability, corrosivity, reactivity, and toxicity.

Disposal of hazardous waste must follow all EPA, federal, state, and local laws and regulations. Discarded gloves, gowns, and other disposable materials should be contained in thick, leak-proof plastic bags that are colored differently than other hospital trash bags. Disposal containers for hazardous drug waste must be clearly labeled "Hazardous Drug Waste Only," and they should be sealed when at capacity. There should be at least one such disposal container in every area where hazardous waste is generated.

Safety Data Sheets

A Safety Data Sheet (SDS) is a document written by the manufacturer of hazardous chemicals, which provides information about the properties of the chemicals, their associated hazards, and proper handling and cleanup, including appropriate PPE.

SDSs should be stored near the location in which hazardous chemicals are used and can be consulted in the event of an accidental exposure. SDSs contain information in the following 16 categories:

1. identification
2. hazard(s) identification
3. composition/information on ingredients
4. first-aid measures
5. fire-fighting measures
6. accidental release measures
7. handling and storage
8. exposure controls/personal protection
9. physical and chemical properties
10. stability and reactivity
11. toxicological information
12. ecological information
13. disposal considerations
14. transport information
15. regulatory information
16. other information.

For more information on hazardous drug compounding, see Chapter 7.

2.4 FDA Drug Labels and Recalls

Since its creation, the FDA has had the power to force manufacturers to adhere to specific labeling requirements or face the consequences of having their products pulled from the shelves. A summary of the major labeling requirements can be found in Table 2.5.

TABLE 2.5 Drug Label Requirements (Legal and USP Standards)

Label	Requirements
prescription drug label	name and address of patient; name of prescriber; name, address, and phone number of dispensing pharmacy; name or initials of dispensing pharmacist or technician, prescription number and ℞; name, strength, and quantity of drug and instructions for use; date filled; BUD or expiration date; refill information; for select drugs, a package insert; for controlled substances, the statement "federal law prohibits transfer of this drug to any person other than the patient for whom it was prescribed"
OTC label	name and address of manufacturer; name of product; all ingredients (active and inactive); net contents; directions for use, including the product's purpose, dosage amount and frequency, symptoms, and ROA; caution/warning labels; contraindications
unit dose label and repackaged drug label	name of manufacturer; name, strength, and dosage form of drug; lot number; beyond use date (BUD); bar code
medication order label	name and address of patient; name of drug; dosage strength, amount, timing, and frequency; lot number; BUD or expiration date; bar code

continues

TABLE 2.5 Drug Label Requirements (Legal and USP Standards)—*Continued*

patient package insert	name, description, indications, and pharmacology of drug, and instructions for use; dosage and administration information; contraindications; precautions; warnings; adverse reactions; drug abuse information (e.g., "habit forming"; "tolerance/dependence"; "addiction"); overdose information; how the drug is supplied; date of most recent label revision
	must be distributed with the following drug classes: oral contraceptives and other estrogen-containing hormone products, intrauterine contraceptive devices, diethylstilbestrol products, and metered-dose inhalers
nonsterile compounded product label	all labeling requirements of prescription drug labels
	name or initials of dispensing pharmacist; name of preparation; date of compounding; internal ID or lot number; instructions for use; storage requirements; BUD
sterile compounded product label	name of patient and prescriber; name or initials of dispensing pharmacist; name and strength of preparation; dosage and administration information, including time of and instructions for administration; solution and volume; storage requirements; date of compounding; BUD
	infusion rate may also be needed
hazardous drug label	All drugs containing hazardous agents must include the proper labeling appropriate to the product, as noted previously, but also the yellow caution label
	A safety sheet on administration instructions and cleanup must also be included
National Drug Code (NDC)	Each drug produced by a manufacturer is identified with a specific 11-digit NDC number*. The FDA requests, but does not require, the NDC on each label, but the NDC makes the product trackable for community and hospital use, so manufacturers include it
	The NDC number is composed of three sets of numbers, which identify the manufacturer, drug strength, and package size

*The first five numbers of any NDC indicate the drug manufacturer. The next four numbers designate the specific drug and its strength. The last two numbers indicate the package size.

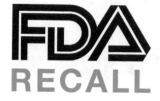

Drug Recall Classifications and Procedures

When an official **drug recall** is released by the manufacturer and/or the FDA, the wholesaler will typically email or mail the drug recall information to the pharmacy, which includes: drug name, dose, National Drug Code (NDC), lot number, expiration date, as well as the date and type of recall. The FDA can either mandate the recall if the threat to the public is severe enough or request a voluntary drug recall by the manufacturer, wholesaler, and pharmacy. Three classes of response levels of drug recalls exist, with class I being the most urgent and dangerous. The FDA determines the class based on the healthcare situation, manufacturer actions, and customer data from MedWatch and other sources. Table 2.6 describes the response-level classes of drug recalls.

TABLE 2.6 Recall Classes for Drugs

Class	Risk	Action Response
I	**Urgent, immediate danger**—A reasonable probability exists that the product will cause or could result in serious harm or death	All patients who have received or purchased this product should be notified
II	**Moderate danger**—A probability exists that the product could cause adverse health events, but the events would be medically reversible or temporary	Pharmacists and/or physicians must decide the best practice about notifying patients
III	**Least danger**—The product will probably not cause an adverse health event, but there is a product quality problem	Pharmacists and/or physicians must decide the best practice about notifying patients

Study Idea

Memorize the difference between class I, II, and III drug recalls.

For all drug recalls, the technician must check the drug inventory and the retail shelves for each recalled item, pull it from inventory immediately to protect patients, and notify the pharmacist, who signs a recall form. This form is then returned to the wholesaler with any recalled drug stock items. The pharmacist should also designate the appropriate plan to notify patients who have received recalled drugs: notification in class I is required; notification in the cases of class II and III recalls and of manufacturer withdrawal are up to the pharmacist's or physician's judgment. Cash register and insurance transaction reports are essential for finding customers who purchased the recalled items. If patients have specific questions about what to do to counteract any medication problems from the recalled drug, the technician must connect them with the pharmacist.

After a recall is complete, the FDA makes sure that the product is destroyed or suitably reconditioned (recategorized with new conditions for sale), investigates why the product was defective, and determines any actions that should be taken. The FDA posts weekly reports on drug recalls that pharmacy personnel should read (found here: PharmPractice7e.ParadigmEducation.com/SafetyReport1).

To prevent problems before drugs are officially classified as recalled, the FDA also posts two pages of drugs pending recall classification: the Human Drug Product Recalls Pending Classification (found here: PharmPractice7e.ParadigmEducation.com/SafetyReport2) and the Non-Blood Product On-Going Recalls (found here: PharmPractice7e.ParadigmEducation.com/SafetyReport3). These sites should be checked regularly to keep patients informed.

At times, pharmacists and technicians may see that a drug has been recalled or is pending recall classification. When a product has been identified on either list, it should be immediately pulled from the shelves, and the manufacturer should be notified that a return and credit are desired. Consumers can also return a recalled drug for refund or credit, per pharmacy or drug wholesaler policy.

2.5 FDA Risk Evaluation and Mitigation Strategies

The Food and Drug Administration Amendments Act (FDAAA) of 2007 gave the FDA the authority to require a Risk Evaluation and Mitigation Strategy (REMS) from manufacturers to ensure that the benefits of a drug or biological product outweigh its risks. REMS are drug safety programs for certain medications with serious safety concerns, and are intended to reinforce medication use behaviors and actions that support the safe use of medications.

REMS include a risk mitigation goal and are comprise information communicated to and/or required activities that must be carried out by those who prescribe, dispense, or take the medication. Each REMS is set up to address specific safety concerns. Elements of a REMS can include one or more of the following:

- *Communicating to patients*—REMS may require the drug manufacturer to develop material for patients, such as Medication Guides, which are handouts for patients distributed with many prescription medications. Medication Guides are written in patient-friendly language and give patients information about how to use the medication and avoid serious adverse events; they are usually provided each time the drug in question is dispensed.
- *Communicating to healthcare providers, pharmacists and healthcare settings*—REMS may require the drug manufacturer to communicate directly to various healthcare providers and provide information about a specific serious risk with a medication and how to reduce that risk.
- *Required activities or clinical interventions*—REMS may require participants to take certain steps that support the safe use of the medication. Sometimes, this must be done before the medication can be prescribed, dispensed, or received.
- *Required certifications and actions*—REMS require prescribers and pharmacists become certified in specific REMS and agree to carry out a set of activities to reduce the risk of the drug.
- *Required documentation of safe use condition*—REMS may require documentation of a safe use condition (such as a monthly lab test) before the drug can be dispensed to the patient.
- *Required patient actions*—REMS may require the patient take certain actions to remain on the treatment.

REMS can be required for a single drug or an entire class of drugs. The FDA can require a REMS before or after a drug is approved for marketing. While drug manufacturers are responsible for developing the REMS program, the FDA must review and approve all REMS programs. Important REMS for technicians to know are discussed in Chapter 3.

2.6 Controlled Substances Regulations

The Drug Enforcement Administration (DEA) is the federal agency responsible for supervising and enforcing laws related to the use and sale of legal (and illegal) controlled substances. A controlled substance is defined as a substance that has the potential for abuse and physical or psychological dependence. The DEA monitors and tracks the flow of controlled substances from manufacturer to wholesaler to pharmacy to patient.

Study Idea

Methadone for opioid detoxification and maintenance may only be administered at specially licensed clinics and hospitals.

Pharmacies, physicians and other prescribers, manufacturers, and wholesalers are required to register with the DEA to dispense, prescribe, produce, or distribute controlled substances. Pharmacy technicians assist pharmacies in maintaining their legal dispensing status by following the dispensing and documentation regulations. The DEA, working alongside state drug agencies, investigates unauthorized prescribing and dispensing and conducts unannounced inspections of pharmacies.

Clinics that dispense narcotic drugs that are used in the treatment of substance abuse (e.g., methadone clinics) must complete a separate DEA registration annually. Suboxone (buprenorphine / naloxone) and Subutex (buprenorphine) require a special DEA number beginning with the letter X in order to dispense at a local community pharmacy. These drugs are used commonly as alternatives to methadone in the treatment of opioid/narcotic dependency. The use of methadone for opioid treatment may only administered by specially licensed clinics and hospitals; however, it is allowed to be dispensed at community and hospital pharmacies if it is being prescribed for pain management.

Drug Classifications

Practice Tip

Because C-I drugs are illegal, there will never be a stock bottle with a C-I label.

The 1970 Controlled Substances Act (CSA), as part of the Comprehensive Drug Abuse Prevention and Control Act, established the classification system for drugs with potential for abuse. The CSA categorized these drugs into schedules denoted by Roman numerals. The lower the schedule number, the higher the risk of abuse (see Table 2.7). For a list of the classifications of commonly prescribed controlled substances, see Appendix B. Schedule I drugs, such as heroin, have the highest risk of abuse and dependence, and are, therefore, illegal.

Stock bottles of all controlled substances must be clearly marked with a Roman numeral and with the uppercase letter C, denoting the schedule of the drugs contained within.

- C-II or Schedule II
- C-III or Schedule III
- C-IV or Schedule IV
- C-V or Schedule V

TABLE 2.7 Controlled Substance Schedule Restrictions

Schedule	Manufacturer's Label	Potential for Abuse	Accepted Medical Use	Examples
Schedule I	C-I	highest potential for abuse—illegal	for research only; must have license to obtain; no accepted medical use in the United States	heroin, lysergic acid diethylamide (LSD), marijuana
Schedule II	C-II	high potential for abuse, which can lead to severe psychological or physical dependence	dispensing severely restricted; cannot be prescribed by telephone except in an emergency or hospice; no refills on prescriptions	morphine, oxycodone, meperidine, hydromorphone, fentanyl, methylphenidate, dextroamphetamine, hydrocodone with aspirin or acetaminophen
Schedule III	C-III	lower potential for abuse and dependence than C-II	prescriptions can be refilled up to five times within six months if authorized by physician	testosterone or other anabolic steroids, buprenorphine/naloxone, buprenorphine, acetaminophen with codeine
Schedule IV	C-IV	lower potential for abuse than C-II and C-III; associated with limited physical or psychological dependence	same as for Schedule III	benzodiazepines, zolpidem, eszopiclone (Lunesta), phenobarbital, carisoprodol, tramadol

continues

TABLE 2.7 Controlled Substance Schedule Restrictions—*Continued*

Schedule	Manufacturer's Label	Potential for Abuse	Accepted Medical Use	Examples
Schedule V	C-V	lowest potential for abuse	Certain drugs in this schedule are considered exempt narcotics by some state laws and, as such, can be sold without a prescription. In these situations, purchasers must be over 18, have a valid drivers license, and are required to sign a log to obtain the drug.	liquid codeine combination cough preparations, diphenoxylate / atropine

Study Idea

When there is a disparity between federal, state, and local laws, the strictest rule must be applied to your practice.

Controlled substances must be prescribed for legitimate medical needs, and any controlled substance dispensed must include a transfer warning label that reads, "Caution: Federal law prohibits the transfer of this drug to any person other than the patient for whom it was prescribed."

Based on the public use and abuse of drugs on the market, the DEA and individual states have the option to reevaluate and reclassify any drug. As noted, when there is a disparity between state and federal regulation of a drug, the strictest regulation is applied. For example, many states classified carisoprodol (Soma) as a Schedule IV (C-IV) drug before the DEA approved the change to C-IV in 2011.

Schedule I

Marijuana, which is a Schedule I (C-I) drug, has been made legal for specific purposes in certain states. However, the strictest law still applies in pharmacy, so DEA licensed pharmacies cannot dispense marijuana even if the state laws allow it.

Schedule II

Study Idea

Pharmacists may order C-II drugs with either a paper DEA Form 222 or electronically using CSOS.

Schedule II (C-II) drugs can be legally prescribed and dispensed but are carefully regulated because of the high risk for abuse and dependence. Many of the top 200 prescribed drugs are in this category, including morphine, oxycodone / acetaminophen (Percocet), oxycodone (OxyContin), dextroamphetamine / amphetamine (Adderall), and methylphenidate (Ritalin). The most dispensed C-II drug in community pharmacy is hydrocodone / acetaminophen (Vicodin, Vicodin ES).

Unlike other drugs that technicians can order for stock inventory, C-II drugs must be ordered and purchased by the pharmacist. The order must be submitted on a DEA Form 222 (see Figure 2.1). For a list of other required DEA forms, see Table 2.11. Some states permit electronic ordering of C-II drugs through a specially encrypted system, the Controlled Substance Ordering System (CSOS), administered by the DEA. Controlled substance prescriptions from a foreign physician (such as from Canada or Mexico) cannot be filled because foreign physicians do not have a DEA license and number. Some pharmacies are not permitted to fill C-II prescriptions from out-of-state providers.

The pharmacist must verify the inventory receipt of all C-II drugs, including type and quantity. C-II drugs must be stored in a safe or in a locked cabinet.

FIGURE 2.1 DEA Form 222

When ordering C-II controlled substances, the pharmacist must complete and sign this form.

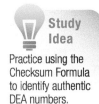

Dispensing of C-II drugs is tightly regulated. In most pharmacies, the pharmacist is the only person allowed to dispense a C-II drug. In the hospital, narcotics are stored in a locked unit at the nursing station. Access is limited to a nurse with the appropriate key or lock code.

In community and hospital pharmacies, each dosage unit of a C-II drug must be accounted for by a computerized or manual perpetual inventory record (see Figure 2.2). A shortage of a C-II drug triggers an immediate investigation. In hospitals and institutions, secure dispensing machine stations (e.g., Pyxis) automatically update inventory any time a drug is dispensed. Technicians, pharmacists, and nurses must continually check that the amounts documented as being filled and dispensed match with the quantities in the automated station. Nurses also do periodic blind counts of the contents of secure dispensing cabinets to verify that the quantity of C-II drugs match that which the cabinet is tracked to store.

The technician must review every prescription carefully for completeness and authenticity, and especially prescriptions for C-II drugs. They must check the authenticity of the DEA number by using the DEA Checksum Formula (see the Take Note on the previous page), and verify that the letters at the beginning of the DEA number are appropriate.

Study Idea

Practice using the Checksum Formula to identify authentic DEA numbers.

FIGURE 2.2 Perpetual Inventory Record

A perpetual inventory record accounts for each unit of a C-II drug dispensed or received. This should match the information that is tracked electronically during prescription filling.

The Corner Drug Store – C-II Perpetual Log

Drug Name: _Methylphenidate 5mg Tabs_   **NDC:** _0123-4567-10_

Prescription No.	Dispense Date	QTY Dispensed	Inventory	RPh Initials
Starting	Inventory	– – – – –	380	– – – – –
2001415	01/22/20XX	–30	350	JPS
2001423	02/07/20XX	–90	260	RJA
INV. 55874	02/08/20XX	+200	460	RJA
2001439	02/10/20XX	–120	340	CA
2001445	02/15/20XX	–30		

Electronic prescriptions for controlled substances are allowed by the DEA if the prescriber and pharmacy meet strict electronic security requirements. The prescriber identity must be authenticated and protected by at least two of the following:

- a password or response to a security question
- a biometric, such as a fingerprint or eye scan
- a hard token that serves as a cryptographic or onetime password device.

TAKE NOTE

Although most pharmacies today have a computer system that verifies a physician's DEA number, it is possible to verify the number by hand using the DEA verification formula known as the **DEA Checksum Formula**.

Step 1: Add the first, third, and fifth digits of the DEA number.

Step 2: Add the second, fourth, and sixth digits of the DEA number.

Step 3: Double the sum obtained in Step 2.

Step 4: Add the results of Steps 1 and 3. The last digit of the sum should match the last digit of the DEA number.

Example 1

Check the validity of Dr. Jones' DEA number: BJ2243551.

Step 1: 2 + 4 + 5 = 11

Step 2: 2 + 3 + 5 = 10

Step 3: 10 × 2 = 20

Step 4: 11 + 20 = 31

The last digit of the sum in Step 4 matches the last digit of the DEA number. The number is valid.

A hard-copy prescription for a C-II drug must be complete, written in indelible black on tamper-proof paper, and signed by the prescribing physician. There may be no alterations. The pharmacist should recognize the prescriber's signature. The date on the prescription is important; some states limit the amount of time a C-II prescription is valid (e.g., from 72 hours to 60 days). No refills are allowed on C-II drugs, and most pharmacies are not allowed to file these prescriptions for future use.

However, since many children (and some adults) take methylphenidate (Ritalin, Concerta) and other stimulants like dextroamphetamine / amphetamine (Adderall) daily to control attention deficit hyperactivity disorder (ADHD), the DEA and most states allow the prescriber to provide prescriptions for future use with the notation, "Do not fill until XX/XX/20XX" with the correct date. The combined fills may not be for more than a 90-day supply of medication.

All prescriptions for C-II drugs must be filed separately from other prescriptions and must be readily retrievable. Each prescription must be signed and dated by the pharmacist. Federal law requires pharmacies to keep C-II prescriptions for a minimum of two years; state laws may require such prescriptions be kept on file for up to five years. In practice, most pharmacies keep all prescription records indefinitely for legal reasons.

Individual states may have additional regulations for C-II drugs. Some states allow a C-II prescription to be submitted by phone in an emergency, provided the prescriber mails a hard copy to the pharmacy within a specified amount of time (usually 72 hours to 1 week). The pharmacist must verify the authenticity of the prescriber's DEA number, reduce the verbal order to writing, and document the nature of the emergency on the back of the prescription. Some states also allow prescribers to order a C-II prescription for a hospice patient via fax or phone; most pharmacies treat this situation as an emergency and require the prescriber to mail a hard copy of the prescription within a week.

Schedule III–IV

Schedule III and Schedule IV (C-III and C-IV) medications have less risk for abuse and dependence, but the risk is present, especially if these medications are used in high doses over a long period of time. Prescriptions for C-III and C-IV drugs can be refilled a maximum of five times, and refills must be dispensed within six months of the original date of the prescription.

The DEA also limits the transfer of C-III and C-IV medications between pharmacies. Patients may request the transfer of a prescription to another pharmacy for convenience, during a vacation, or if the patient has a second home in another community. In most states, only the pharmacist can legally transfer a prescription for a controlled substance. A patient may request that the receiving pharmacy call to request the transfer from the pharmacy that holds the hard copy of the prescription. However, a prescription for a C-III and C-IV drug can only be transferred one time. The patient cannot then refill the prescription again at the original pharmacy; instead, a new prescription must be requested from the prescriber. In transferring the prescription, the originating pharmacy must close the prescription for the transferred drug so that no additional refills can be obtained from that location. Documentation must include the name and phone number of the receiving pharmacy and the receiving pharmacist, as well as the DEA numbers of both pharmacies.

Prescriptions for C-III and C-IV drugs are less likely to be forged than C-II drugs but are more likely to be refilled early. The pharmacy technician must review the date of the last refill and the days supply. For example, a prescription for "acetaminophen with codeine 300 mg/30 mg #90 with signa: 1 tab PO TID PRN" written on November 1, should last until around December 1. If the patient tries to refill the prescription on November 20th, the technician may have to tell the patient that the prescription cannot be refilled early. Each pharmacy has a policy regarding how far in advance (usually 24 to 48 hours) it will provide refills of C-III and C-IV drugs.

Most C-III and C-IV drugs do not have to be kept in a safe or in a locked cabinet and are generally stored with the inventory of nonscheduled drugs. No special DEA forms are needed to order C-III and C-IV, and a senior pharmacy technician may be responsible for ordering them. The pharmacist is often responsible for verifying and signing for the receipt of all C-III and C-IV drugs; these signed inventory receipts are kept on file.

Prescriptions must be readily accessible for inspection. If not separated from other prescriptions, C-III and C-IV prescriptions must be marked for easy identification with a large (at least one inch high) red C for control in the lower right corner.

Schedule V

Schedule V (C-V) drugs have the lowest potential for abuse and dependence and include prescription cough syrups that contain codeine (such as Robitussin AC) as well as diphenoxylate / atropine (Lomotil) for diarrhea, and pregabalin (Lyrica) for neuropathic pain.

Some states—and many pharmacies—require a prescription to dispense these medications. Insurance companies will not cover the cost of these medications without a prescription. C-V prescriptions are generally filed with the prescriptions for C-III and C-IV drugs for easy retrieval.

Federal law and many states allow pharmacists to dispense certain C-V drugs such as codeine-containing cough syrups without a prescription if certain restrictions and record-keeping requirements are met. Restrictions for the sale of C-V medications include:

- Drugs must be stored behind the counter in the prescription area (or can be locked with other controlled substances).
- The amount of cough syrup sold to a single customer is generally limited to a specific volume (such as 120 mL or 4 fl oz) within a 48-hour period.
- Only the pharmacist (or the pharmacy technician under direct supervision) can make the sale.
- The purchaser must be 18 years of age or older and have proof of identity.

If the state allows sale of C-V drugs without a prescription, the pharmacy technician or pharmacist must legally record all sales in a record book or computerized database and include the following information:

- name and address of the purchaser
- date of birth of the purchaser
- date of purchase
- name of the drug and quantity sold
- name and initials of the pharmacist handling or approving the sale.

To apply C-II to C-V regulations properly, students must learn and remember the most commonly prescribed controlled substances, as shown in Appendix B.

Restricted Sale of Certain Over-the-Counter Products

Certain OTC products also have specific restrictions and procedures that must be followed during consumer purchases. These products include OTC C-V drugs, such as the OTC cough medications containing codeine and products containing ephedrine and pseudoephedrine. These OTC products must be stored behind the counter, and technicians must follow the same sales restrictions and documentation procedures as mentioned previously for C-V prescriptions. These drugs are often referred to as behind-the-counter medications.

Due to the Combat Methamphetamine Epidemic Act (CMEA), the number of OTC products containing pseudoephedrine and ephedrine that can be purchased at one time or within one month is limited. These restricted OTC products include cold and sinus medications, ephedrine containing tablets, and certain metered dose inhalers (MDIs). Some states limit the purchase of these products to prescription only, and several states require that only pharmacists conduct the sales. Violations of the state or federal laws may result in the loss of the pharmacist's license or the pharmacy's business license.

Technicians must legally document the purchases and purchasers of pseudoephedrine or ephedrine in a software program or manual logbook similar to that for C-V drugs and have individuals sign for purchases. This documentation must be kept for a minimum of two years to allow for DEA and FDA tracking.

In addition, to continue offering these drugs for sale, all pharmacies must electronically submit an annual self-certification to the DEA. This certification confirms that:

- all employees have been trained in how to handle these products,
- training records are being maintained,
- sales limits are being enforced (3.6 grams a day, 9 grams every 30 days),
- products are being stored behind the counter or in a locked cabinet,
- an electronic or written logbook is being maintained.

For an example of a hard-copy log and the required information, see Figure 2.3. Many pharmacies are now using the online, real-time National Precursor Log Exchange (NPLEx), which tracks and consolidates the data on these sales and helps law enforcement see trends in areas and overlapping sales.

FIGURE 2.3 Sales Log of Restricted Products Containing Pseudoephedrine and Ephedrine

Pseudoephedrine Products Dispensing Record

Purchaser's Name	Driver's License Number	Purchaser's Address	Date of Purchase	Product Name	Quantity Purchased	Dispensed by (Initials)	Purchaser's Signature

To calculate the limits for these sales, you must take the weight of each tablet in a package and multiply it by the number of tablets to find the total amount of drug in the package. For ease in calculations, the DEA supplies tables for restricted amounts per packages, as shown in Tables 2.8 and 2.9. Know how to use these tables, but don't memorize them. Instead, memorize the general limits per day and month. Some states may have stricter or additional restrictions.

TABLE 2.8 Number of Tablets That Equal Retail Sales Limits

Drug and Form	Limits	Number per Package = 3.6 g	Number per Package = 7.5 g*	Number per Package = 9 g
Ephedrine				
Ephedrine HCl 25 mg	3.6 g per day; 9 g per month	175 tablets	366 tablets	439 tablets
Ephedrine Sulfate 25 mg		186 tablets	389 tablets	466 tablets
Pseudoephedrine (as HCl)				
Pseudoephedrine HCl 30 mg	3.6 g per day; 9 g per month	146 tablets	305 tablets	366 tablets
Pseudoephedrine HCl 60 mg		73 tablets	152 tablets	183 tablets
Pseudoephedrine HCl 120 mg		36 tablets	76 tablets	91 tablets
Pseudoephedrine (as Sulfate)				
Pseudoephedrine Sulfate 30 mg	3.6 g per day; 9 g per month	155 tablets	324 tablets	389 tablets
Pseudoephedrine Sulfate 60 mg		77 tablets	162 tablets	194 tablets
Pseudoephedrine Sulfate 120 mg		38 tablets	81 tablets	97 tablets
Pseudoephedrine Sulfate 240 mg		19 tablets	40 tablets	48 tablets

*The monthly limit for mail-order pharmacies is less, at 7.5 grams.
Note: The DEA also supplies a table listing the limits of milliliters of liquid base of products containing ephedrine and pseudoephedrine to guide sales of liquid OTC products.
Source: DEA website.

TABLE 2.9 Sales Limit of Milliliters of Liquid Base Containing Restricted Substances

Drug and Form	mL Limits per Day	mL Limits per Month
Ephedrine		
Ephedrine HCl 6.25 mg/5 mL	3,515 mL	8,788 mL
Pseudoephedrine (as HCl)		
Pseudoephedrine HCl 15 mg/1.6 mL	468 mL	1,171 mL
Pseudoephedrine HCl 7.5 mg/5 mL	2,929 mL	7,323 mL
Pseudoephedrine HCl 15 mg/5 mL	1,464 mL	3,661 mL
Pseudoephedrine HCl 15 mg/2.5 mL	732 mL	1,830 mL
Pseudoephedrine HCl 30 mg/5 mL	732 mL	1,830 mL

Drug and Form	mL Limits per Day	mL Limits per Month
Pseudoephedrine HCl 30 mg/2.5 mL	366 mL	915 mL
Pseudoephedrine HCl 60 mg/5 mL	366 mL	915 mL

Preventing Forgeries

Practice Tip

The DEA launched a texting tip line in some areas to anonymously report suspicious prescription drug activity. Type TIP411 (847-411), then type DEADRUGS or PILLTIP.

The pharmacy technician must be vigilant in reviewing narcotics prescriptions. It is not uncommon for a forged prescription to be presented by a new, supposedly out-of-state patient on a weekend or evening when the prescription cannot be authenticated. A patient who requests a brand name narcotic and offers to pay cash (instead of providing insurance information) should raise a red flag. Cash payment does not create a paper trail that could alert other pharmacies that receive a similar prescription. Table 2.10 provides a list of indicators that should alert the technician to check with the pharmacist.

TABLE 2.10 Indicators of a Potentially Forged Prescription or Drug-Seeking Behavior

- The prescription is altered (for example, a change in quantity).
- Prescription pads have been reported missing from local doctors' offices.
- The prescription is presented as a clever computerized fax and is not on tamper-proof safety paper.
- There are misspellings on the prescription.
- A refill is indicated for a C-II drug.
- A prescription from the emergency department is written for more than a #30 count or 7-day supply.
- A prescription is cut and pasted from a preprinted, signed prescription.
- A second or third prescription is added to a legal prescription written by a physician. More than one handwriting style is used.
- A patient presents a prescription containing several medications but wants the pharmacy to fill only the narcotic prescription.
- The prescription is signed with different handwriting or in different ink, or the prescription is not signed by the physician.
- The DEA number is missing, illegible, or incorrect.
- The prescription is written by an out-of-state physician or a physician practicing in an area far from the pharmacy. This event is particularly suspicious if the prescription is received at night or on the weekend when it would be difficult to confirm the prescription.
- An individual other than the patient drops off the prescription. Pharmacy personnel should require a driver's license or other photo ID and document this information.
- A new patient specifies a brand name narcotic.
- A new patient wants to pay for the prescription with cash, even though they have insurance. Doing so prevents a paper trail.

Most pharmacies have a computerized physician database containing DEA, National Provider Identifier (NPI), and state license numbers, in addition to general contact information. However, pharmacy technicians should learn to recognize the names and legal signatures of the local prescribers who send prescriptions to the pharmacy, especially for controlled substances, to help prevent forgeries on the spot. Insurance plans require a pharmacy to have a physician's DEA number on file to be reimbursed for prescriptions for all controlled substances. Some pharmacies fill controlled substances only for patients residing in their immediate geographical area and for prescribers who practice in their community and write their prescriptions with tamper-proof paper.

Controlled Substance Inventory

The DEA requires that all pharmacies complete a biennial (every two years) inventory that includes an exact count of all C-II drugs and an estimate of other controlled substances. If a C-II container designed to hold 1,000 or more doses has been opened, an exact count is necessary. The inventory record must contain the following information for each controlled substance:

- name of the drug
- dosage form and strength
- number of dosage units or volume in each container
- number of containers.

Many community pharmacies have a policy, or are subject to state law, that requires them also to perform an exact inventory of all C-II drugs monthly or by some other regular schedule. In the hospital, inventories of narcotics are conducted at the start of each nursing shift, typically three times per day, or perpetually if an automated drug dispensing system is in use. Inventories of C-III and C-IV drugs are checked at least annually in most community and hospital pharmacies. Upon discovery of significant loss or theft of controlled substances, DEA Form 106 must be completed.

Disposal of Controlled Substances

Disposal or destruction of any controlled substance must be recorded by a pharmacist on DEA Form 41 and witnessed and signed by another pharmacist. Expired drugs and broken dosage units are generally saved until the next visit by a state drug inspector or until the drugs are transferred to a registered reverse distributor for disposal. Disposal records must contain the following information:

- pharmacy DEA number, name, and address
- reverse distributor's DEA number, name, and address
- number of units (in finished forms and/or commercial containers) disposed of and the manner of disposal.

The records must be electronically sent to the local DEA branch (or two hard copies sent by mail) and a copy stored at the pharmacy for at least two years. The disposal record must be dated to reflect when the product was sent for destruction. Besides the DEA Form 41, the reverse distributor will fill out DEA Form 222 as the purchaser of any outdated C-II drugs, even if no value is assigned to them. This helps close the loop on the products' distribution trail. (See Table 2.11 for a more complete list of common DEA forms.)

TABLE 2.11 Commonly Used DEA Forms for Pharmacies

DEA Form	Description
224	application form for a pharmacy to dispense controlled substances or for a prescriber to prescribe them
222	controlled substance order form
41	destruction of controlled substances report and witness form
106	theft/loss of controlled substance form (required when there is a "significant loss")
Automation of Reports and Consolidated Orders System (ARCOS)	the DEA's Electronic Data Interchange (EDI); increases ease of ordering, tracking, and submitting monthly, annual, and biannual reports
Controlled Substance Ordering System (CSOS)	DEA-run system that allows for secure electronic transmission of Schedule I–V controlled substance orders without the supporting paper Form 222

Take Back Programs

Medicine take back options are the best way to safely dispose of most types of unneeded or expired prescription or OTC medications. There are generally two kinds of take back options. The first is permanent collection locations and sites, such as certain pharmacies. The second is biannual National Drug Take Back Day events sponsored by the DEA with help from local law enforcement. More information about take back programs can be found at CertExam5e.ParadigmEducation.com/TakeBack.

2.7 State Laws

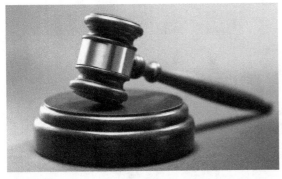

Serious violations of laws, regulations, or ethics by pharmacy technicians may result in loss of job, suspension or revocation of professional ability to practice, and/or criminal or civil penalties.

In addition to knowledge of federal laws affecting pharmacy practice, the technician must be cognizant of state laws and regulations. The pharmacy technician may be responsible for registering with their BOP, a requirement in most states, and renewing that registration as often as annually in addition to fulfilling all continuing education (CE) requirements. The BOP may also require technicians to pass a certification exam within a certain period of time. If the technician is practicing in a specialty area, such as a sterile or non-sterile compounding pharmacy or facility or a nuclear pharmacy, additional training and certification may be required. In most states, the pharmacy technician may legally perform the following duties:

- dispensing medication, record keeping, pricing, and billing
- preparing doses of a premanufactured product
- compounding sterile and nonsterile medications according to protocols
- customer service for prescriptions
- transporting medications to patient care units in the hospital
- checking and replenishing drug inventory.

In all practice locations, however, all duties must be carried out under the direct supervision of a licensed pharmacist. Some states may allow the technician to perform additional responsibilities, such as taking telephone refill requests from prescribers or assisting in drawing up medications for vaccine administration. Technicians must know what your individual BOP allows. In some states, certified pharmacy technicians can check the work of other technicians, called *tech-check-tech*. In all settings, the act of counseling a patient or providing a professional recommendation is reserved for the pharmacist.

In any given state, the state board of pharmacy (BOP) is the regulatory body that oversees the practice of pharmacy and the personnel that practice it. The role of the BOP is to protect the public by establishing standards of pharmacy practice in its state. That includes defining the roles and duties of pharmacists and pharmacy technicians. The BOP can discipline pharmacists and pharmacy technicians for violations of pharmacy laws and regulations, and for unprofessional behavior.

Review and Assessment

STUDY SUMMARY

Knowing the key laws and standards that affect your practice as a technician is essential. For taking the certification exam, study the tables in this chapter, especially those that list the laws, controlled substance levels, and types of recalls. Know pharmacy procedures and expectations codified in the laws, so you can do things legally and safely. The exam will ask questions about how to apply these laws and when. Learn common controlled substances and their schedules, which are listed in Appendix B, to know how to properly dispense them.

ADDITIONAL RESOURCES

For more in-depth explanations, check out *Pharmacy Practice for Technicians*, 7e from Paradigm Education Solutions. To master and extend the material presented in this chapter, take advantage of the resources available through the eBook resources links. These include digital supplements, study resources, and a practice exam generator with 1,000+ exam-style questions. End-of-chapter tests are accessible through the eBook for individuals using the self-study course and through Cirrus for individuals enrolled in the instructor-guided course.`

Patient Safety and Quality Assurance

Learning Objectives

1. Identify various agencies involved with patient safety, including the US Consumer Product Safety Commission, the US Food and Drug Administration), and the Institute for Safe Medication Practices. (Section 3.1)

2. Describe the three phases of the drug approval process. (Section 3.1)

3. Describe procedures and processes for reporting issues that impact patient safety such as errors and adverse events. (Section 3.1)

4. List types of prescription errors and strategies to prevent errors. (Section 3.2)

5. Identify high-risk, high-alert and look-alike sound-alike drugs. (Section 3.2)

6. Recognize issues that require pharmacist intervention to protect patient safety. (Section 3.3)

7. Elaborate on the process of continuous quality improvement. (Section 3.4)

8. Access and use references and resources as needed to perform job duties. (Section 3.5)

 Access eBook links for resources and an exam generator, with 1,000+ questions.

According to the Centers for Disease Control and Prevention (CDC), 48.7% of patients have used at least one prescription drug in the last 30 days, 21.8% have used three or more in the last 30 days, and 10.7% have used five or more in last 30 days. With each drug added, the risk for errors, drug/drug interactions, and adverse drug reactions multiplies. Pharmacy technicians have hands-on methods for providing safe medications to patients by following pharmacy procedures, rules, and standards. That is why domain 3 of the PTCE (26.25%) is dedicated to medication error prevention and patient safety questions, and these types of issues are woven throughout all of the domains of the ExCPT, especially 4.

Patient safety is a subset of the larger push in the pharmacy industry for quality control and improvement, which uses systematic approaches to analyze and reduce errors, prevent and control infection outbreaks, and improve overall safety, productivity, profitability, and patient satisfaction.

3.1 Medication Safety Systems

One of the first challenges of medication safety is ensuring that medications are safe for human use. The US Centers for Disease Control and Prevention (CDC), the Centers for Medicare and Medicaid Services (CMS), the Consumer Product Safety Commission (CPSC), the US Drug Enforcement Agency (DEA), the US Food and Drug Administration (FDA), the Federal Trade Commission (FTC), and the Occupational Safety and Health Administration (OSHA), are agencies set up by the federal government to enforce laws, conduct research, and establish prevention processes. The state boards of pharmacy (BOP) also advocate for safety laws on the state level.

The major nongovernmental agencies involved in medication safety efforts are the Institute for Safe Medication Practices (ISMP), the National Coordinating Council for Medication Error Reporting and Prevention (NCC MERP), The Joint Commission (TJC), which oversees healthcare institution accreditation, and the US Pharmacopeial Convention (USP). Within each pharmacy and compounding facility, the policy and procedures (P&P) manual lays out the safe procedure for pharmacy filling, dispensing, and compounding based on the laws, regulations, standards, and counsel from these organizations.

FDA New Drug Oversight & Approval Process

Study Idea

Brand names may only be on the prescription label if the proprietary product is dispensed. If the less expensive alternative is used, you must put the generic name on the label.

The FDA is responsible for the review and approval of all prescription and over-the-counter (OTC) medications, including generic drugs. Although the manufacture of vitamins and herbal and dietary supplements is not under FDA control, the FDA does monitor adverse reactions to and marketing claims for them.

Every new drug approved by the FDA has a chemical name, a generic or nonproprietary name, and the manufacturer's recommended brand or trade name. Table 3.1 lists the different types of names used for a common pain medication. The chemical name describes the chemical structure of the particular drug molecule. The brand name is owned by the company that develops the drug, gets FDA approval (as explained later in this chapter), and first markets it. The generic or nonproprietary name is given by the United States Adopted Names (USAN) Council and is developed to provide an identifier that is not protected by a patent. Once the original patent of the brand-name drug expires (usually 17 years or more after the patent is filed), any manufacturer can apply to the FDA with an **Abbreviated New Drug Application (ANDA)** to market a generic version, which usually sells for a reduced price.

TABLE 3.1 **Types of Drug Names**

Name Category	Drug Name
chemical	2-(4-isobutylphenyl) propionic acid
generic	ibuprofen
Brand	Advil, Motrin, Motrin IB

Investigational Drugs and New Brand-Name Drug Approvals

For all new brand-name drugs, manufacturers must file an **Investigational New Drug (IND) Application** with the results from in-depth animal studies before the new drug can be approved for testing on human subjects. In the IND application, the manufacturer must offer a compelling case for the human need for the drug, the results of the animal studies, an explanation of how the drug would be manufactured, and a detailed description of the proposed clinical studies on humans. The clinical studies must then be submitted and approved by the **Institutional Review Board (IRB)** of the university or hospital where the research will be conducted before the human clinical studies can begin. The IRB, sometimes known as the Human Use Committee, comprises scientists and practitioners from various disciplines. The committee must review, approve, and monitor all medical research involving humans. Each study participant must sign an **informed consent form**—a document that states the purpose and risks of the research in easily understandable terms.

After the IND is approved by the FDA and the IRB, non-FDA scientists conduct three phases of human clinical studies as part of the drug approval process. Phase 1 is the initial study or trial of the new drug, usually completed on a small number of healthy volunteers, and aims to test the overall safety of the medication. Phase 2 aims to evaluate the effectiveness and safety of a drug for a specific indication or disease state on a slightly larger number of unique patients. If the results of phase 1 and phase 2 studies are promising, phase 3 studies are conducted in larger clinical trials to better assess the overall benefits and risks of the investigational drug on patients (see Figure 3.1).

FIGURE 3.1
The FDA Drug Approval Process

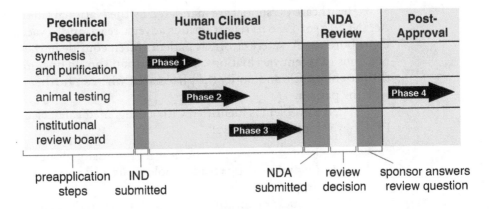

Technicians often work on the dispensing, documentation, and inventory management of the investigational drug in the studies, following all the special FDA regulations for safety and tracking. All investigational drugs must be documented and stored separately from the regular pharmacy drug inventory. The informed consent forms and documentation of each dispensing and administration of the investigational drug must also be filed.

If the investigational drug shows promise after phase 3 studies are completed, the pharmaceutical manufacturer can submit a **New Drug Application (NDA)** to the FDA. The results of the scientific studies are evaluated by an independent advisory panel of experts, and recommendations are forwarded to the FDA. If the benefit of the drug outweighs the risk, the drug is generally approved. However, the FDA may request additional studies be completed. The drug approval process takes a year or longer in most cases. After a drug is approved, measures are put in place to track and prevent serious and unexpected adverse reactions. This safety system, sometimes referred to as "phase 4" of the FDA drug approval process, is discussed in the following section.

Adverse Reaction Reporting and Tracking

Once a drug is released and a larger population of patients is using it, the probability that problems will arise increases. The FDA tracks **adverse drug reactions (ADRs)**, which are harmful or negative effects of or reactions to a particular drug on a patient, through different feedback processes. The **FDA Adverse Event Reporting System (FAERS)** is a centralized database that stores information from two separate federally sponsored reporting programs: MedWatch and VAERS. For reference, go to CertExam5e.ParadigmEducation.com/FAERS.

MedWatch and VAERS have a variety of duties, summarized below:

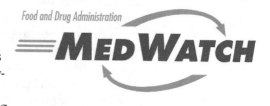

Food and Drug Administration

- **MedWatch**—Run by the FDA in collaboration with the ISMP, MedWatch is a voluntary program that offers healthcare professionals and consumers an avenue to anonymously report a serious adverse event associated with a specific drug, biologic, medical device, or any other FDA-regulated product.

- **Vaccine Adverse Event Reporting System (VAERS)**—Cosponsored by the CDC, VAERS is a safety surveillance program, collecting information from vaccination providers and from the public about adverse reactions (possible side effects) that occur after a patient has been given a vaccine approved for market release in the United States.

Healthcare personnel are mandated by the National Childhood Vaccine Injury Act (NCVIA) of 1986 to report serious adverse reactions to vaccines. Technicians may contribute to this safety effort, as patients often confide in them, and they report reactions to recent vaccinations. The technician should document the information on the patient profile and notify the pharmacist who can further discuss the reaction with the patient.

When a problem is identified with a drug, medical device, or other product, the FDA may respond in five ways:

1. Issue safety alerts to healthcare professionals or consumers on the drugs (including drug recalls), biologicals, dietary supplements, counterfeit drugs, and so on.
2. Request medication labeling changes to the product package insert, including contraindications, warnings, boxed warnings, precautions, and adverse reactions.
3. List the drug as a high-risk medication and require that it be dispensed with a Medication Guide for provider and patient education. This action may also be required before market release because of the results of clinical studies.
4. Require Risk Evaluation and Mitigation Strategies (REMS). These, too, may be required before market release.
5. Remove the product from the market in a drug recall, as described in Chapter 2.

Product Labeling Warnings

The FDA requires manufacturers to include safety information in the **package insert (PI)** attached to each stock bottle. Technicians often reference PIs for information on precautions, contraindications, warnings (including boxed warnings), and adverse reactions. This information is also published in the Prescriber's Digital Reference (PDR).

Avandia, Paxil, Adderall, and Coumadin are examples of drugs that require boxed warnings and additional communications to pharmacists and prescribers. Boxed warnings are significant warnings assigned to products approved and regulated by the FDA. These warnings must be observed and followed when dispensing these products.

The FDA can also require specialized patient container labeling. A good example is the case of new labeling for patients who may be pregnant or nursing. Until 2015, the FDA categorized the risks of taking a drug or biologic during pregnancy under a five-letter system (A, B, C, D, and X) based on what was known about that product. However, to make it easier for patients to understand, the FDA now requires the product labeling to include explanatory sentences and/or paragraphs that address the categories and subcategories listed in Table 3.2. Technicians must look for these warning descriptions on labels and recommend counseling with the pharmacist when patients seem to fall into these categories. OTC drugs are not required to have this information.

TABLE 3.2 New Labeling for Drugs that Affect Pregnant and Lactating Patients and Individuals of Reproductive Potential

pregnancy (includes patients in labor and delivery)	pregnancy exposure registry risk summary clinical considerations data
lactation (includes nursing patients)	risk summary clinical considerations data
individuals of Reproductive Potential	pregnancy testing contraception infertility

Medication Guides for High-Risk Medications

For select high-risk drugs and certain entire drug classifications used by general or vulnerable populations, such as those listed in Table 3.3, the FDA requires by law that the pharmacy provide additional information in a Medication Guide. Medication Guides are printed handouts that accompany the patient's prescription receipt for the medications that require them. They include boxed warnings, guidelines on the safe and effective use of high-risk drugs, and information about how to minimize the risk of serious adverse reactions.

TABLE 3.3 Examples of Drugs and Drug Classifications and Drug Classifications Requiring a Medication Guide

Drug	Risk Factor
isotretinoin (Accutane, Claravis, Sotret, other brand names)	causes birth defects; patients who can become pregnant must be on some form of birth control or be advised not to get pregnant while on this medication
ADHD drugs (e.g., mixed amphetamines, methylpheni-date)	may cause insomnia, loss of appetite, and changes in pulse and blood pressure; may interfere with growth and weight in children; monitor vital signs

continues

TABLE 3.3 Examples of Drugs and Drug Classifications and Drug Classifications Requiring a Medication Guide—*Continued*

Drug	Risk Factor
antidepressants (SSRIs, such as fluoxetine, sertraline, paroxetine, citalopram, escitalopram)	may be associated with increased suicide risk, especially in adolescent patients; watch for changes in behavior
ciprofloxacin (Cipro)	may cause tendon rupture
amidarone (Amidarone HCL Injection)	may cause lung/liver damage, abnormal heartbeats, and thyroid dysfunction; limited to life-threatening conditions due to its side effects; monitor vital signs and symptoms
warfarin (Coumadin)	reduces blood clotting, so patients must be careful when working with sharp objects, shaving, and participating in contact sports while taking this drug; interacts with many drugs
fentanyl transmucosal drug products (various forms)	indicated only for breakthrough pain in cancer patients tolerant of and maintained on around-the-clock opioid therapy; risk of respiratory depression and even death
NSAIDs (e.g., diclofenac, ibuprofen, naproxen)	may cause increased risk of stomach ulcers; take with food, use no longer than necessary
rivaroxaban (Xarelto)	may cause bleeding; avoid other drugs that can cause bleeding, such as aspirin, and with NSAIDs, such as ibuprofen; monitor uncontrolled bleeding of nose, gums, and so on, and discoloration of urine/stools
zolpidem (Ambien)	may cause confusion, sleepwalking, next-day sleepiness and driving issues, especially in higher doses in patients assigned female at birth and older adults; do not combine with alcohol; use lower doses in high-risk groups

Risk Evaluation and Mitigation Strategies

For some high-risk drugs, Medication Guides, alone, are insufficient. For drugs that are necessary, but also pose significant health risks, the FDA requires manufacturers develop **Risk Evaluation and Mitigation Strategies (REMS)** for providers and patients to follow. In some cases, community and institutional pharmacies and prescribers must register with the drug manufacturer or federal REMS program for each drug they will be dispensing or wholesaling and receive drug-specific REMS training. The pharmacist must review any required Medication Guides with patients and do other required counseling and monitoring activities.

REMS programs are individually designed to closely track patients on these high-risk drugs and make periodic assessment reports to the FDA on their statuses. Technicians can become familiar with these drugs at CertExam5e.ParadigmEducation.com/REMS. Technicians must know common drugs that require REMS. Study and memorize the drugs listed in the following sections.

Thalidomide

Though at first rejected for FDA drug approval, thalidomide (Thalomid) was eventually approved for treatment of leprosy or severe nerve inflammation and pain.

However, because of its known harm to fetuses in utero, or **teratogenicity**, the FDA requires the REMS program called **System for Thalidomide Education and Prescribing Safety (STEPS)**. It is intended to mitigate the risks for all patients..

Isotretinoin and the iPLEDGE Program

Study Idea

A patient has seven days from the last pregnancy test to fill their prescription for isotretinoin.

Isotretinoin (a synthetic analog of vitamin A) is a common generic drug for severe acne and other skin problems. Isotretinoin also has a very high incidence of teratogenicity. Common brands of this drug are Accutane and Claravis (see Table 3.4 for others). The **iPLEDGE program** is a REMS that was designed for isotretinoin and related drugs to prevent birth defects and to educate all patients on the drugs' risks and proper uses. All patients must be registered and agree to meet all conditions required during treatment. Pharmacies may receive the drug only from a certified wholesaler and can only dispense for written prescriptions by a certified prescriber. An assigned risk management authorization (RMA) number must be placed on each prescription, and prescribers must agree to provide contraception counseling prior to and during treatment. The prescription quantity is limited to a 30-day supply with no refills, and all pregnancies must be reported. Patients must agree not to share their medication or donate blood while taking isotretinoin and for one month after discontinuing use.

Patients who can become pregnant must commit to using two forms of contraception while on the drug and for one month after drug discontinuation. Prescribers must document the forms of contraception that patients are currently using. Patients must agree to monthly pregnancy tests and have a negative result prior to prescribers issuing a new or refill prescription. Patients must agree to pick up the prescription within a specified period (usually within seven days) or the prescription is void.

TABLE 3.4 Brand Name Drugs in the iPLEDGE Program

Available in the US and Canada	Available in Canada Only
Absorica	Epuris
Absorica LD	Isotroin
Accutane	
Amnesteem	
Claravis	
Myorisan	
Sotret	
Zenatane	

Note: Pharmacists who dispense isotretinoin and patients to whom it is prescribed must agree to the terms of the iPLEDGE program as part of its REMS.

Transmucosal Fentanyl

The REMS program for fentanyl seeks to limit access to only the appropriate opioid-dependent cancer patients or those in palliative care, and to promote patient education and safe storage to avoid accidental exposure to children. Prescribers must agree to initiate therapy with the lowest dose, follow up on efficacy of dose titration, and document any signs of misuse or abuse. Pharmacies are also responsible for training all staff, including pharmacy technicians on the REMS for fentanyl. Hospital pharmacies can dispense transmucosal fentanyl to inpatients only. Patients must review the Medication Guide, sign an agreement with the prescriber, and follow prescribed instructions exactly.

Study Idea

Special DEA licenses are issued to prescribers of buprenorphine products for treating opioid dependence. These DEA numbers begin with "X."

Study Idea

When dispensing clozapine, if the patient has not had their absolute neutrophil count (ANC) done, you cannot dispense the drug.

Buprenorphine Transmucosal Products for Opioid Dependence

These medications, including Subutex and Suboxone, are prescribed by doctors certified to treat opioid dependence. Certified physicians have DEA numbers that all start with an "X," indicating their ability to prescribe these medications. Subutex (buprenorphine HCL) is a sublingual tablet formulation commonly prescribed to pregnant patients and patients who cannot tolerate Suboxone. Suboxone is available as a film and sublingual tablet used to control relapse with opioid addiction. Other products available are Bunavail and Zubsolv. The REMS goals are to prevent accidental overdose, misuse, and abuse, and to inform patients of serious risks.

Clozapine and Olanzapine

An atypical antipsychotic drug, clozapine (Clozaril, FazaClo, FazaClo ODT, Versacloz) has been found to cause a life-threatening decrease in white blood cells. Technicians participate in documentation, facilitating patient access to the pharmacist, and any monitoring. Clozapine registry requirements state that the patient must be registered with the dispensing pharmacy and the prescribing physician. There must be appropriate laboratory monitoring of the patient's blood.

Before the long-acting injectable formulation of the antipsychotic medication olanzapine (only available as Zyprexa Relprevv) can be administered to a patient, the prescriber, healthcare facility, patient, and pharmacy must be enrolled in the Zyprexa Relprevv Patient Care Program. Post-injection delirium/sedation syndrome (PDSS) may occur in patients after administration. Patients must be monitored for at least three hours after every monthly injection. Everyone in the pharmacy involved with the process must be aware of the high risk associated with olanzapine injection.

Flibanserin

The adverse reactions for flibanserin (Addyi)—the sexual drive enhancing drug for women—include extreme hypotension and loss of consciousness (syncope) due to a drop in blood pressure when taken with alcohol. The drug poses other dangers as well. Prescribers and pharmacies, must complete training and enroll to be authorized to handle this drug. Pharmacists must counsel patients on how to properly use the drug and to avoid alcohol while taking this medication.

Drug Supply Chain Security Tracking

In 2012, the New England Compounding Center prepared a solution for injection of methylprednisolone that was provided to healthcare clinics and institutions in many states. Because the drug was contaminated, it caused at least 64 deaths and seriously injured at least 750 individuals. In 2013, Congress passed the Drug Quality and Security Act (DQSA), which includes the Drug Supply Chain Security Act (DSCSA) and the Compounding Quality Act (CQA). It aimed to establish a national database to track and trace drug products through the supply chain from the manufacturer to the pharmacy and to increase compounding safety guidelines. Requirements of the law include the following:

- verification that all trading partners and practitioners are properly licensed
- drug-tracking documentation to be completed by the compounder/manufacturer, wholesalers and distributers, pharmacies, and administering clinicians and kept on file for a minimum of six years
- inspection of all drugs upon receipt to remove any suspicious products for further investigation.

The key points of drug checks and documentation occur at delivery by the compounder/manufacturer to the wholesaler, by the wholesaler to the pharmacy, from the pharmacy to the medication administrator, and at the point of administration (for which documentation was already required by the healthcare facility). Technicians take part in the documentation at the points of drug inventory delivery and dispensing. It is important to file invoices from all wholesale purchases and only purchase from FDA-approved wholesalers and manufacturers. During the receiving process, technicians must be able to recognize signs of drug tampering and counterfeiting and know how to report all suspicious products to the FDA.

US Consumer Product Safety Commission

The Poison Prevention Packaging Act of 1970 (PPPA) is enforced not by the FDA but by the US Consumer Product Safety Commission (CPSC). The incidence of childhood deaths, emergency room visits, and calls to poison control centers has been considerably reduced since the law was enacted. Prescription and OTC drugs and common household products are subject to packaging requirements under the PPPA.

A child-resistant container is defined as one that cannot be opened by 80% of children but can be opened by 90% of adults. Exceptions include:

- prescriptions sent from a community pharmacy to a nursing home or hospital because the medication will be administered by a nurse and stored in a locked area
- certain emergency medications that require quick access, such as sublingual nitroglycerin for chest pain
- specific drugs with packaging that already limits child access, such as metered-dose inhalers (MDIs), birth control medications, and Medrol Dosepaks.

Older adult patients or patients with certain disabilities can opt out of special packaging requirements. Then the technician may dispense the medications using a non-child-resistant lid. In these cases, the pharmacy must keep on file a signed opt-out document.

Reuse of plastic prescription vials and lids on refills is also prohibited by the PPPA to prevent potential contamination and defect due to previous use.

3.2 Preventing Medication Errors

The pharmacy technician, as a member of the healthcare team, works to provide the right patient with the right drug, at the right strength, with the right route of administration (ROA) and in the right form, with the right documentation, and to deliver the right education material, all with 100% accuracy (see Figure 3.2).

Yet in 2012, 700 pharmacists from various settings responded to a survey by the ISMP and American Pharmacists Association (APhA), and 44% admitted making errors. Of these, 37% admitted that they did not report the errors they made. This shows that prescription errors are significantly underreported and underscores the need for effective checks and balances.

FIGURE 3.2 Patient *Rights* in Prescription Drug Dispensing

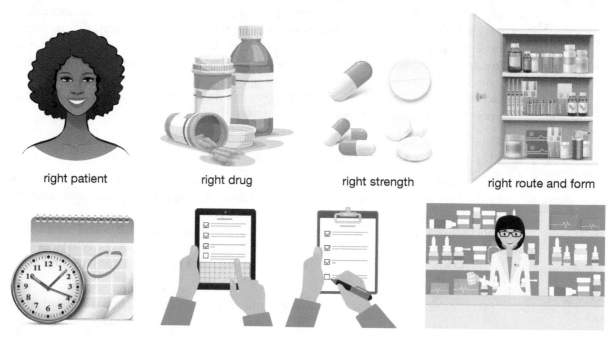

right patient   right drug   right strength   right route and form

right time   right documentation   right education

NCC MERP defines a **medication error** as "any preventable event that may cause or lead to inappropriate medication use or patient harm while the medication is in the control of the healthcare professional, patient, or consumer." A medication error often results in an ADR. It may be a short-term acute reaction, long-term injury, or even death.

Root Cause Analysis and Failure Modes and Effects Analysis

After a medication error has occurred, a root cause analysis (RCA) can help to identify the factors that led to the error. Getting to root causes often entails asking the question, "Why did this happen?" and when an answer is given, asking, "Why did that happen?" to each succeeding answer at least five times.

To proactively prevent medication errors, many independent pharmacies, chain and mail-order pharmacies, hospital and other institutional pharmacies, and compounding facilities use **failure modes and effects analysis (FMEA)**. *Failure modes* are the ways in which something can fail, and *effects analysis* looks at the results or consequences and analyzes prevention techniques. In pharmacy, root causes fall into four categories, as seen in Table 3.5.

Practice Tip

Technicians need to watch out for medications that look alike (e.g. bupropion vs. buspirone), or sound alike (e.g., Xanax vs. Zantac) or both (e.g., guanfacine vs. guaifenesin).

TABLE 3.5 Categories of Cause and Types of Medication Errors

Category	Definition	Examples
Root Causes		
manufacturing	There are issues with the drug, administration method, packaging, or educational materials provided	The packaging for one product looks nearly alike in coloring and branding to another
organizational	The rules, policies, and/or procedures are inadequate or training is insufficient. Pharmacy personnel experience an excessive workload and a culture of fear of not being productive enough or speaking up when something seems wrong	An outdated policy on sterile compounding leads to compromised sterility of an admixture. Technicians and pharmacists are too rushed to double-check calculations or selections
technical	Equipment is not calibrated or working properly	The pharmacy's automatic dispensing machine is malfunctioning. A computer glitch mixes a prescription for one patient with another patient's prescription
human	An error is caused by an individual not following procedures, missing or ignoring a step, or inadequate training	A technician pulls a bottle of medication from the shelf to fill a prescription from memory and does not read the label. Stores frequently relocate medications
Prescriber Errors		
illegible handwriting or misspelled escript	The information on a prescription is questionable due to handwriting or spelling	Look-alike drug names are highly susceptible to misspellings, especially since prescriptions commonly do not have rationales to guide selection
insufficient knowledge of drug for problematic prescription	The prescriber is not aware of special prescribing requirements of a drug	There is a REMS requirement for a drug prior to dispensing , which the prescriber did not know about
use of high-risk abbreviations and measurement notations	Abbreviations are misinterpreted	Writing "u" for units can lead to a tenfold increase in dose
Dispensing Errors		
wrong drug error	A drug that was different from the prescribed drug was selected and dispensed	A look-alike medication or one with a similar name was selected from the shelves or placed into wrong slots in the robotic dispensing machine or automated dispensing cabinet
adverse drug error	A DUR warning alert is missed or ignored	A patient on warfarin is prescribed Bactrim, and the interaction warning is overridden
wrong amount/dosage error	The dose given is 5% greater or less than the dose prescribed	Synthroid 0.025 mg is dispensed as Synthroid 0.25 mg
wrong label/mislabeling error	Incorrect data is entered on the label	Prescription data is entered into the wrong patient profile

continues

Category	Definition	Examples
Dispensing Errors		
wrong formulation error	Different dosage forms or salts are not interchangeable without prescriber authorization	The patient has an order for Ondansetron oral disintegrating tablets but is dispensed oral swallowing tablets
documentation error	Essential information is missing or incorrect	The med list in computer is not updated with recent med changes
medication education error	Proper education material is not passed on to the patient	The proper Medication Guide is not dispensed with a drug
contaminated product error	Medication that is supposed to be removed from stock is still on shelves for dispensing	Drug recall is not addressed in a timely manner
Causes of Dispensing Errors		
incomplete information	Policy is not followed when completing a patient profile	Allergies are missing from a patient profile
incorrect assumption not checked	Incorrect assumptions are made about missing or questionable information	Assuming that they can interpret the prescriber's illegible handwriting, the technician selects the wrong drug
selection error	On a pull-down menu or shelf, drugs with similar names or labeling are present, and the wrong one is selected	A look-alike or sound-alike drug is selected
capture/habit error	Error or inattention and habit cause a wrong selection or calculation	Used to dispensing the usual adult dosage for a medication, the technician fills the adult dose for a child, and the pharmacist approves it without noticing
rushed error	Pressure to meet deadlines or quotas causes an error and the double-checking is skipped	The technician cuts corners to decrease the time it takes to fill a prescription
distraction error	Interruptions during critical filling phases cause missed steps or incorrect actions	The phone is ringing, customers are demanding attention, and the technician misses a step
fear error	Fear of speaking up and bothering the pharmacist or an other technician allows medications with suspected errors to be dispensed without double-checking	The pharmacist has been angry with you in the past for asking too many questions, so you stop asking for help
Administration Errors		
omission error	The prescribed dose is not given and/or taken	A patient forgets to take a medication or a nurse neglects to administer a medication

continues

TABLE 3.5 Categories of Cause Levels and Types of Medication Errors—*Continued*

Category	Definition	Examples
Administration Errors		
extra dose(s) error	A patient receives more doses than prescribed	A nurse gives two tablets but the order is for one; a patient thinks more is better of another medication and takes an extra dose to feel better sooner
wrong dose	The calculations done are incorrect, or the weighing instruments were not calibrated properly	The dose given is 5% greater or less than the dose prescribed
wrong time	The medication is given too early or too long after the intended time of administration	A patient in the hospital is to receive an intravenous antibiotic at 8 a.m. but does not receive the medication until noon
wrong mixture with other drugs and supplements	A patient or nurse do not attend to the accompanying educational warnings	A patient takes a few drinks of alcohol while on a medication for which alcohol causes an adverse reaction; a nurse permits a patient to drink grapefruit juice while taking statins

Pharm Fact

FMEA encourages finding problems with the system instead of blaming individuals. Do not point fingers but help identify why the error happened and how it can be prevented from happening again.

Study Idea

Many times, drug names are abbreviated, such as ASA for aspirin or HCTZ for hydrochlorothiazide. Be aware of common drug abbreviations used in prescription writing.

Resources to Fight Medication Errors

In addition to the FDA's MedWatch and VAERS, several nonprofit and professional agencies track and/or work to minimize medication errors.

The ISMP tracks, collects, and disseminates information to healthcare personnel regarding safe medication practices using the following tools (among others):

- The ISMP National Medication Errors Reporting Program (ISMP MERP) is a voluntary medication error reporting program. It allows healthcare providers who have made a medication error to self-report anonymously.
- The confidential information submitted to ISMP MERP may be used as part of future case studies and for the education and training of healthcare professionals. The ISMP seeks out trends and address causes with innovations and guidance. In a study of 26,604 reports, 60% of errors occurred in the dispensing process, and pharmacy technicians were involved in nearly 40% of these errors. Major contributing factors included inexperience, distraction in the workplace, and excessive workload.
- The ISMP distributes specific lists of high-alert medications to dispense with great care in different settings: acute care, community and ambulatory healthcare, and long-term care (found here: CertExam5e.ParadigmEducation.com/HighAlertMeds.) To accompany these lists, the ISMP developed the High-Alert Medication Modeling and Error-Reduction Scorecards (HAMMERS) tool to help pharmacies track and improve their policies to reduce errors (found here: CertExam5e.ParadigmEducation.com/HAMMERS).
- The ISMP has also assembled the List of Error-Prone Abbreviations, Symbols, and Dose Designations (found here: CertExam5e.ParadigmEducation.com/ErrorProneAbbrev). It is important to study this list and HAMMERS.
- The ISMP with the FDA have also been fighting against look-alike drug names and labeling. They have established a warning list of drug names that are too close for safety and have recommended using tall man lettering (found here: CertExam5e.ParadigmEducation.com/ISMPlist).

- Tall man lettering uses capitalized bold lettering to emphasize the differences between two or more names that are too close, as with bu**PROP**ion and bus**PIR**one, or aceta**ZOLAMIDE** and aceto**HEXAMIDE**. (For the full list, go to: CertExam5e.ParadigmEducation.com/TallManLetters.)

Other agencies that track and/or work to minimize medication errors include:

Study Idea

Unsafe abbreviation "qd." can be misinterpreted as "qid." Using a "u" for units could be interpreted as a zero.

- The USP provides safety recommendations throughout the chapters of the *US Pharmacopeia–National Formulary* (USP–NF). The USP also makes recommendations to have manufacturers change formulations and packaging, such as revising the labels on Heparin Lock Flush Solution and Heparin Sodium Solution to be bright red with the warning "HIGH ALERT" on them.
- TJC publishes a Do Not Use list of abbreviations (see Table 3.6) for prescribers in the healthcare facilities that seek to gain or maintain accreditation, and this influences all prescribers (found here: CertExam5e.ParadigmEducation.com /JointCommision).
- The American Society of Health-System Pharmacists (ASHP) publishes comprehensive guidelines on the prevention of medication errors in hospitals.

TABLE 3.6 The Joint Commission's Official Do Not Use List

Do Not Use	Potential Problem	Use Instead
U, u (unit)	mistaken for "0" (zero), the number "4" (four), or "cc"	write "unit"
IU (International Unit)	mistaken for IV (intravenous) or the number 10 (ten)	write "International Unit"
Q.D., QD, q.d., qd (daily) Q.O.D., QOD, q.o.d, qod (every other day)	mistaken for each other period after the Q mistaken for "I" and the "O" mistaken for "I"	write "daily" write "every other day"
Trailing zero (X.0 mg)*	decimal point is missed	write X mg
Lack of leading zero (.X mg)	decimal point is missed	write 0.X mg
MS	can mean morphine sulfate or magnesium sulfate	write "morphine sulfate"
MSO_4 and $MgSO_4$	confused for one another	write "magnesium sulfate"

Note: This information applies to all orders and all medication-related documentation that is hand-written (including free-text computer entry) or on preprinted forms.

*Exception: A "trailing zero" may be used only where required to demonstrate the level of precision of the value being reported, such as for laboratory results, imaging studies that report size of lesions, or catheter/tube sizes. It may not be used in medication orders or other medication-related documentation.
Source: The Joint Commission

Technology and Automation Innovations

Some of the biggest innovations in medication safety have arisen from technology and innovation: eprescriptions (escripts), electronic health records (EHRs) and profiles, drug utilization reviews (DURs) and insurance adjudication, robotic and automated filling and compounding, bar-code scanning, bar-coded patient wristbands, computerized provider order entry (CPOE), and electronic medication administration records (eMARs), to mention the most common. Automated compounding is being used to prepare commonly used, complex intravenous (IV) products such as total parenteral nutrition (TPN) solutions.

Studies have shown that these automated systems decrease medication errors; however, healthcare workers need to be aware that technology may create new errors. Technicians must double-check for accuracy as they work, perform computer software updating and data storage back up, and maintain the upkeep of the equipment needed for all automated devices and technology.

Manufacturing and Dispensing Improvements

Besides implementing the recommended tall man lettering on their labels, manufacturers often offer improvements in packaging. Unit packaging for hospitals has helped patients get the right dose per day. PillPack pharmacy is an online pharmacy that delivers patient prescriptions organized into medication pouches per date and time. PillPack prescriptions come in a roll of perforated pouches and the patient merely tears off pouches for the medications needed for the day. Topi-CLICK is a patented delivery system to dose compounded hormone creams and gels accurately. These are just a few examples.

3.3 Ways Technicians Can Reduce Errors

The pharmacist is ultimately responsible for the accuracy and dispensing of prescriptions, but the pharmacy technician plays an important role in ensuring safety. The pharmacy technician has a moral and ethical obligation to raise questions to protect patient safety. It is better to err on the side of caution than to make a hasty decision and risk harming or killing a patient.

The work area should be uncluttered and well-lit, and drug stock bottles should be returned to inventory after dispensing. When dealing with look-alike sound-alike drugs, the pharmacy should separate the stock containers in the inventory so that products that look and/or sound similar are not next to each other on the shelf. Technicians must be focused—even while multitasking—to prevent errors. Personal calls or cell phones distract attention and compromise safety. Technicians need to understand and follow the P&P manual and state and federal laws.

Using NDC Numbers and Bar Codes for Safety

Technicians should verify all their drug selections with the listed NDC number and by scanning the NDC bar code on the stock label. The NDC number plays a crucial role in the prevention of medication errors. For example, if the prescription is for the antibiotic clarithromycin 500 mg but the technician inadvertently selects clarithromycin 500 mg XL. When the technician scans the label, the computer will indicate the error. See Figure 3.3 and Table 3.7 for how to find the NDC numbers on labels and scan the bar codes.

FIGURE 3.3 NDC Numbers and Bar Codes

All stock medication labels include a unique, product-specific National Drug Code (NDC) in both numeric and bar-code form. The first number set (4–5 digits) identifies the manufacturer, the second set (3–4 digits) indicates the product code, and the last set (2 digits) shows the packaging size and type. Refer to Table 3.7, below, to see the breakdown of the information contained in the NDC numbers for these particular medication labels.

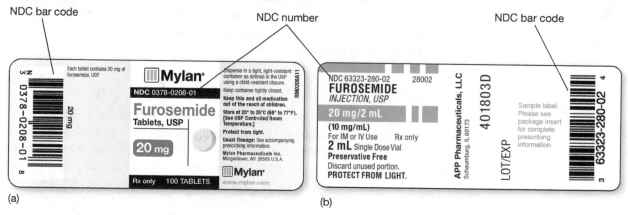

(a)   (b)

TABLE 3.7 Reading NDC Numbers

Manufacturer			Product Code			Packing Size and Type	
	NDC	Name		NDC	Product	NDC	Size
(a)	0378	Mylan Pharmaceuticals, Inc		0208	furosemide 20 mg tablet	01	100 tablets
(b)	63323	APP Pharmaceuticals, LLC		280	furosemide injection 20 mg/2mL	02	2 mL vial

Note: (a) and (b) refer to labels in Figure 3.3.

Study Idea

Know the crucial points in the filling and compounding processes when a pharmacist needs to be consulted.

Times for Pharmacist Intervention

At what point should a technician filling a prescription or medication order consult the pharmacist? Any time that the technician is unsure, it is better to ask than make a mistake. There are also key points in the processes for verification: after entering the profile and prescription, during the DUR and online adjudication if there are any alerts, after the prescription is filled but before applying the label, as well as any time there is a question.

Drug Utilization Review Issues

When alerts arise during the DUR, the technician should consult a pharmacist before proceeding. A patient's allergy list should be updated every time they present a new prescription because new allergies may have occurred since the last update. Common medication allergies include penicillin, sulfa, codeine, and common food allergies include eggs and nuts. Some pharmaceuticals, including vaccines, are grown in egg cultures, and should not be dispensed to patients with egg allergies. The pharmacist will use their professional judgment to decide whether to contact the prescriber or to fill the prescription.

Adjudication and Prior Authorization Issues

Some alerts that happen during adjudication need to be addressed by the pharmacist. Commonly, this occurs for such medications as proton pump inhibitors (PPIs), antihyperlipidemic-like statins, antidepressants, and nonsteroidal anti-inflammatory drugs (NSAIDs, like naproxen). When prior authorization is required, it is up to the prescribing physician to justify the use of the more expensive drug. The technician or pharmacist will need to contact the prescriber for review and action; the pharmacist may be able to expedite the clarification process by telephone, particularly if a delay would harm the patient (e.g., waiting for an antibiotic needed to treat an infection). Often, the prescriber will change to a comparable medication that is covered.

Counseling Issues

At the dispensing of each prescription, the technician is bound by law to offer counseling from the pharmacist. A pharmacist should always be consulted if a patient requests counseling on a prescription or OTC product. If specifically asked, the technician may point out the location of an OTC product. In some states, pharmacy technicians can consult with patients on OTC medications. In other states, technicians are permitted only to read the medication label to the patient and then refer the patient to the pharmacist for more information.

Pharmacists can recommend an OTC product for certain conditions that do not require treatment by a physician. Pharmacists do not diagnose, however, so, if the patient is unsure what is wrong, the pharmacist must advise the patient to see a physician.

Patients often have questions at the time they pick up medications or after beginning a medication. The pharmacy technician is permitted to answer questions about the price or what a tablet looks like but should not advise about issues such as missed doses or improper use of a medication. If a patient requests a therapeutic substitution, mentions a use of the medication that is incorrect, or says that a dose has been missed, the technician must ask the pharmacist to talk to the patient.

Adverse Drug Reactions

If a patient ever reports an ADR, the technician must immediately notify the pharmacist. ADRs will be assessed by the pharmacist who will determine if the reaction should be added to the patient's profile as an allergy and/or be reported to MedWatch.

Safety Processes at Every Step

Pharm Fact

All information on a prescription label needs to be in language and measurements the patient understands.

The average prescription usually takes around 15 minutes to fill. Even so, experienced technicians have built habits of safety into every step. Simple things are important, such as always scanning the bar code, using a leading zero when entering decimals below the value of 1, and not entering a zero after whole numbers (also known as *eliminating the trailing zero*). For example, .5 mg is wrong, whereas 0.5 mg is right; 5.0 mg is wrong, whereas 5 mg is right, as is explained in Table 3.6. Special attention and consideration should be built into every step of filling a prescription. Below is an overview of such processes.

1. *Reviewing Profile and Prescription*—Check each element of the patient profile against the prescription, especially noting patient allergies. Double-check the patient name and spelling (first, middle, and last), date of birth, and address to make sure the correct patient's profile is being accessed and updated. Are all the ID and contact information present for the prescriber (including DEA number)? Is the prescription complete with the date, the inscription, signa, and prescriber's signature?

2. *Entering and Checking the Drug Information*—This is where the technician must check the prescription against the computer's drug choices and spellings, available routes of administration and formulations, and the decimals and measurement units. Make sure that you avoid entering any of the dangerous measurement notations and abbreviations listed by the ISMP or TJC. Have the pharmacist check the transmitted prescription or the information you enter against the hard copy and/or profile.

3. *DURs and Adjudication*—This is where the screening for allergies, drug/drug and/or drug/supplement interactions, and formulary issues occur. Computer software used in pharmacies will alert users to these issues using colored labeling, pop-up messages, and other forms of warning sign communication. The technician and pharmacist are also responsible for remaining on the lookout for any issues having to do with the physical condition of the patient, such as with children, older adults, and pregnant or nursing individuals. See Table 3.8 for information on dealing with DURs for those special populations.

4. *Generating the Prescription Label*—Recheck the label with the original prescription to make sure everything matches up correctly.

5. *Retrieving the Proper Medication*—Scan the stock label and verify correct brand name/generic, manufacturer, strength, formulation, and ROA. If the prescription is dispensed by an automated system, the technician needs to double-check the drug dispensed by the robot or dispensing cabinet.

TABLE 3.8 DURs and Special Populations

Information to Check	Resources to Verify Information	Potential Errors Resulting from Failure to Check/Verify Information
Drug screening Does the prescribed medication interact with other conditions or medications listed on the profile?	patient, physician, family member, patient profile, interaction screening program, insurance provider electronic messages, drug information resources (e.g., books, call centers, package inserts [PIs], patient information handouts)	contraindicated drug dispensed; drug/drug or drug/disease interaction occurs
Pediatric patient dosing Is the prescribed dose and frequency of dosing in a pediatric patient consistent with manufacturer recommendations and pharmacy references?	original prescription, physician, PIs, electronic database, reference texts, pharmacist experience	serious overdose (or underdose) leading to side effects, adverse reactions, or treatment failure
Geriatric patient dosing Is the prescribed dose and frequency of dosing in a geriatric patient consistent with manufacturer recommendations and pharmacy references?	original prescription, physician, PIs, electronic database, reference texts, pharmacist experience	serious overdose (or underdose) leading to side effects or adverse reactions, or treatment failure
Pregnant (or potentially pregnant) and lactating patient dosing Is the prescribed drug indicated in patients who are pregnant or may become pregnant? Does the drug pass into the breast milk?	physician, PIs, electronic database, reference texts, questions to patient, pharmacist experience	congenital birth defects, side effects in breast-fed infants

Study Idea

Cleaning counting trays with alcohol or soap and water is necessary after dispensing penicillin or sulfa drugs.

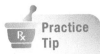

Practice Tip

To keep medication quality high, address recalled items and remove close to expiration stock in a timely and ongoing fashion.

Study Idea

Identify the times in the filling process that require pharmacist intervention or review.

6. *Filling or Compounding the Medication*—Calculations are crucial at this stage to get the right dosage and days supply. Counting cannot be done with tools or automated equipment that has been used for drugs known to induce allergic reactions, because there is a risk of residue cross-contaminating other drug products.

7. *Preparing for Pharmacist Review*—The medication, prescription, label, notes for calculations and conversions, computer screen profile, and other pertinent information must be presented in an organized fashion to facilitate clear review. The proper patient education materials (including Medication Guides and auxiliary labels) must also be included.

8. *Storing Medication Properly*—The prescribed medication must be stored in proper conditions in terms of temperature, lighting, humidity, and so on. It needs to be sufficiently separate from other patients' medications and well organized for easy retrieval.

9. *Delivering Medication to the Nurse, Patient, or Caregiver*—Before delivering or filling a unit dose cart, the technician must double-check the patient information to ensure the right patient will receive it. A bar-code scan will verify this too. The medications in dispensing cabinets and machines must be scanned as they are filled into the proper shelves and when they are removed for administration or dispensing. If the medication is dispensed directly to the patient, the patient must be offered counseling and the appropriate educational materials. If the patient asks if the medication is right, double-check the prescription. Also, if the appearance of the medication has changed since the last refill, explain this. If the patient has more in-depth questions, refer them to the pharmacist. The medication information that the patient must receive is listed in Table 3.9.

TABLE 3.9 Information Patients Must Receive with Their Medications

- brand and generic name
- medication's proper appearance
- purpose of the medication and the duration of treatment
- correct dosage and frequency and the best time or circumstances to take a dose
- how to proceed if a dose is missed
- medications or foods that interact with the prescribed medication
- whether the prescription is in addition to or replaces a current medication
- common side effects and how to handle them
- special precautions necessary for each drug therapy
- proper storage for the medication

3.4 Quality Control and Assurance

Within pharmacies and healthcare facilities, medication errors are difficult to track because there are no national laws that require pharmacy personnel errors be reported. To encourage more medical and medication error tracking and analysis by pharmacies and healthcare institutions, the federal government passed the 2005 **Patient Safety and Quality Improvement Act (PSQIA)**. The PSQIA encourages the creation of **patient safety organizations (PSOs)** that can collect confidential information on medical and medicine errors to develop systematic changes for safety. Those who report errors are legally protected from being sued or being punished in the workplace by loss of responsibilities, pay, or promotions.

In addition to PSOs pharmacies conduct their own quality assessments to ensure quality and accuracy. Quality assessments include examining product integrity and safety (patient and staff members), as well as customer service, productivity, efficiency, and profitability. In addition to safety processes outlined in a pharmacy's P&P manual, each pharmacy can set up systems to track and rate their success based on different quality-assessment criteria and seek ways to improve.

Continuous Quality Improvement

Continuous quality improvement (CQI) is a process used to evaluate systems and errors. It includes these basic steps:

- Describe the process and the sources of variation from the intended outcome.
- Conduct a team analysis to clarify the source of variation and the extent of problem.
- Discuss alternatives and make decisions on how to reduce variations.
- Implement a plan, and measure its effectiveness.

A full discussion of CQI is beyond the scope of this chapter, but it is important to note that it is a team process. The process does not stop with the initial implementation of a plan; it is a continuous process that cycles and is updated as new data becomes available or healthcare rules change. Cooperation is needed at all levels to effectively manage current errors and prevent future errors. An organizational failure happens when a hospital or employer doesn't change policies that are found likely to cause errors and harm to patient.

Hiring Quality Staff, Safety Roles, and Employee Safety and Satisfaction

The quality of the workforce is an essential component of any high-quality business. To ensure that pharmacies and institutions employ the best qualified people, an employer will validate all potential employees' credentials and employment histories. *Credentials* are the education and licensing requirements to practice a particular job. For pharmacy technicians, national certification is one of the best credentials.

Advanced Technicians in Safety Roles

An experienced technician might be given extra responsibilities to ensure medication safety. The **tech-check-tech** system, where advanced technicians check the work of less experienced technicians before the pharmacist verifies a medication, has been found to greatly reduce medication errors. Technicians who serve as medication profile specialists or medication reconciliation specialists in hospitals have also reduced many of the errors and omissions in medication histories that admitting personnel do not have the knowledge base to catch or query.

Employee Safety and Satisfaction

Pharmacies and healthcare institutions must protect the safety of their workers as well as their patients. That is why they follow OSHA regulations and USP, TJC, and CDC recommendations. Pharmacies and healthcare institutions require hand-washing standards and personal protective equipment (PPE), sharps containers, medication disposal processes, and hazardous spill kits. They also encourage or require annual flu vaccinations and implement the CDC's universal precautions against the transmission of bloodborne pathogens. (See Table 3.10.)

TABLE 3.10 Universal Precautions for Prevention of Bloodborne Infection Transmission

- Universal precautions apply to all individuals within the hospital.
- Universal precautions apply to all contact or potential contact with blood, other bodily fluids, or body substances.
- Disposable gloves must be worn when contact with blood or other bodily fluids is anticipated or possible.
- Hands must be washed thoroughly after removing gloves.
- Blood-soaked or contaminated materials (such as gloves, towels, or bandages) must be disposed of in a wastebasket lined with a plastic bag.
- Properly trained custodial personnel must be called if cleanup or removal of contaminated waste is necessary.
- Contaminated materials (such as needles, syringes, swabs, and catheters) must be placed in red plastic containers labeled for disposal of biohazardous materials. Proper institutional procedures generally involve incineration.
- A first aid kit must be kept on hand in any area in which contact with blood or other bodily fluids is possible.
- The kit should contain, at minimum, the following items:
    - ~ adhesive bandages for covering small wounds
    - ~ alcohol
    - ~ antiseptic or disinfectant
    - ~ bottle of bleach, which is diluted at the time of use to create a solution containing 1 part bleach to 10 parts water, for use in cleaning up blood spills
    - ~ box of disposable gloves
    - ~ disposable towels
    - ~ medical adhesive tape
    - ~ plastic bag or container for contaminated waste disposal
    - ~ sterile gauze for covering large wounds.

Practice Tip

Safety needles (needles that retract into the syringe or have attached sheaths) can help prevent needle sticks. All needles and other sharps must be properly disposed of in a sharps container.

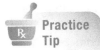

Practice Tip

HAIs are also known as nosocomial infections.

Besides safety on the job, personal satisfaction is also an important aspect of a career as a pharmacy technician. Job satisfaction is about more than earning a paycheck. Satisfaction comes from doing the best job possible every day. This includes showing commitment to the profession by continuing to improve your skills and knowledge through training and continuing education. Employers often provide avenues for advancement, including training, responsibility, position, and compensation to retain their experienced and qualified staff members, thereby putting staff skills and expertise to greater use. They also often send out employee satisfaction surveys to better understand the needs of employees to improve the worksite, and hopefully, lead to better patient care and satisfaction.

Hospital Quality and Patient Satisfaction

Hospital accreditation is a sign of quality health care for patients. TJC places a strong emphasis on patient and personnel safety and in quality healthcare service and products. It sets standards, evaluates facilities against those standards, and monitors progress toward facility and national healthcare goals. It also initiates and supports medication safety efforts, as with its Do Not Use pharmacy abbreviation list.

In hospitals, there are committees working on safety and quality control. These committees track medical and medication errors to find root causes and to improve hospital processes. A hospital Infection Control Committee (ICC) specifically works on preventing inadvertent transmission of infection and disease. It also tracks healthcare-associated infections (HAIs) to help prevent them from occurring in patients and staff in the future. The ICC ensures that hospital staff are trained in standard hygiene, infection controlling protocols, and universal precautions.

How can a healthcare provider or institution know if the patient is happy with the care provided? Many hospitals and healthcare institutions use surveys (e.g., Press Ganey) to measure patient satisfaction. Hospital pharmacies can also survey their customers—the physicians, surgeons, and nurses who order or administer the drugs. Survey results can identify trends, areas that work well, and areas that need improvement. Institutions can also use survey results to compare their own performance over time and compare their institution's performance against other institutions' performance." Such analysis can lead to improvements.

In community pharmacies, satisfaction is less likely to be measured by a formal survey. Repeat business is one measure of satisfaction. Patients who return again and again are usually content with the level of service. Magazines and newspapers in many areas can offer another means of assessing consumer satisfaction through annual "Best of" contests and surveys. These offer positive reinforcement that the institution is satisfying its clientele.

Quality assurance is an ongoing activity, and one in which the pharmacy technician has an important role to play. Only by identifying areas of weakness can pharmacy professionals and the institutions they serve become better at serving patients safely and protecting workers.

3.5 References and Resources

Accessing and analyzing information is critical to patient safety. A pharmacy technician is responsible for researching and providing information to other members of the pharmacy team. There are many references and sources of information available, and it is critical to know which to use in each situation. Knowledge of references and how to use them will increase your value as a pharmacy technician.

It is important to be familiar with both federal and state pharmacy laws as well as regulations from individual boards of pharmacy. Other federal references to be aware of include the FDA's Approved Drug Products with Therapeutic Equivalence Evaluations, which is available as an online resource. More commonly called the Orange Book, this reference documents drug products that have been approved by the FDA and information about which products are therapeutically equivalent to each other. The Orange Book can be accessed at CertExam5e.Paradigm Education.com/OrangeBook.

Study Idea

Remember that the FDA Orange Book lists the approved drugs and doses and generic substitutions.

The FDA's Purple Book lists biological products that are approved by the FDA, and references whether biological products are biosimilar to or interchangeable with other biological products. Requirements for substituting biological products for one another vary by state law, so always consult your pharmacist if you have doubts. The Purple Book can be accessed online at: https://www.fda.gov/drugs/therapeutic-biologics-applications-bla/purple-book-lists-licensed-biological-products-reference-product-exclusivity-and-biosimilarity-or

Drug Facts and Comparisons is a reference of clinical information for both prescription and OTC products. It provides important clinical and practical information for pharmacists and pharmacy technicians and facilitates the provision of important information to patients. Micromedex is another pharmacy reference that provides information on pharmaceutical products, medication management, disease and condition management, pricing and product information, and patient education. Lexi-comp, an online database, is another comprehensive source of drug-related information.

Trissel's Stability of Compounded Formulations, commonly referred to as "Trissel's," is a comprehensive reference on the compatibility, stability, pH, storage, and preparation of parenteral drugs. Trissel's is a printed and online reference intended for use by professionals who prepare and deliver parenteral medications.

Pharmaceutical monographs are reference guides that are included with each drug product. Also known as the prescribing information, the monograph contains many important facts about the associated product, including indication, usage, dosage forms, contraindications, warnings/precautions, adverse reactions, drug interactions, clinical trial information, counseling information, and additional relevant information. DailyMed is an online reference that contains labeling information and PIs for all approved drug products. DailyMed can be accessed online at CertExam5e.ParadigmEducation.com/DailyMed.

When using references, always be mindful of the quality of information being provided, and make sure you use reliable sources like the ones described in this review. The ability to locate, utilize, and interpret pharmacy-related information is a critical skill for pharmacy technicians and important to maintaining and enhancing patient safety.

Review and Assessment

STUDY SUMMARY

Medication safety and quality-assurance programs in health care are integral to containing costs and protecting patients. Pharmacy technicians need to be aware of the work being done by the FDA, ISMP, and various other organizations to protect the safety of both patients and employees.

Pharmacy technicians must always watch for potential errors and how to prevent them. They should understand the importance of the NDC, bar codes, look-alike sound-alike drug lists, high-risk high-alert medications, and policies and procedures used to correctly select medications and fill prescriptions.

Pharmacy technicians must know strategies to prevent filling errors. Be aware of the importance of having work double-checked by a pharmacist and knowing when to ask for help. Understand the importance of quality assurance and performance improvement strategies to ensure patient safety and satisfaction.

ADDITIONAL RESOURCES

For more in-depth explanations, check out Pharmacy Practice for Technicians, 7e from Paradigm Education Solutions. To master and extend the material presented in this chapter, take advantage of the resources available through the eBook resources links. These include digital supplements, study resources, and a practice exam generator with 1,000+ exam-style questions. End-of-chapter tests are accessible through the eBook for individuals using the self-study course and through Cirrus for individuals enrolled in the instructor-guided course.

4

Order Entry and Processing

Learning Objectives

1 Explain when generic drugs can be legally substituted for prescribed brand-name drugs. (Section 4.1)

2 Interpret common pharmacy abbreviations and medical terminology. (Section 4.2)

3 Describe the process of maintaining and updating patient profiles, including insurance information. (Section 4.3)

4 Identify the components of prescriptions. (Section 4.4)

5 Identify the components of medication orders, and describe how they differ from prescriptions. (Section 4.5)

6 Describe the process of online claims submission and troubleshooting rejected claims. (Section 4.6)

7 Compare and contrast the processes for filling, labeling, and verifying prescriptions and medication orders. (Section 4.7)

8 Identify the role of the pharmacist throughout the steps of the order entry and fill process. (Section 4.8)

9 Identify the medical equipment, devices, and supplies used to administer drugs, and describe their uses. (Section 4.9)

 Access eBook links for resources and an exam generator, with 1,000+ questions.

In both community and hospital pharmacies, pharmacy technicians are responsible for assessing prescriptions or medication orders for completeness and accuracy. In the community pharmacy, technicians have the added responsibility of checking the prescriptions for legality and authenticity. This chapter reviews the components of a prescriptions and medication orders, and the common notations and abbreviations used by prescribers. It also discusses the patient profile, medication history, the Drug Utilization Review (DUR), and the process of filling, packaging, labeling prescriptions, gathering patient education resources, and the final check by the pharmacist. This domain represents 21.25% of the PTCE and 45% of the ExCPT.

4.1 The Filling and Dispensing Roles of the Pharmacy Technician

In all settings, the goal of the profession of pharmacy is to provide the right patient with the right drug, at the right strength, with the right route of administration (ROA) and in the right form, with the right documentation, and to deliver the right education material, all with 100% accuracy. Though the prescribing and filling processes differ between community and institutional pharmacy settings, both prescriptions and medication orders depend upon complete patient-medication and allergy profiles and the shared language of pharmacy abbreviations, which are described in Section 4.2. (An overview of the general process for both prescriptions and medication orders is shown in Figure 4.1.)

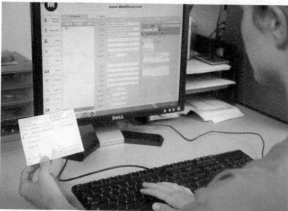

Technicians work hard to make sure prescriptions, medication orders, labels, and the computerized data match up.

Generic Substitutions for Prescribed Brand-Name Drugs

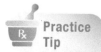

Practice Tip

On each prescription, watch for provider notes. "Brand medically necessary," "brand necessary," and "DAW" all mean the same thing—no substitutions without authorization!

Pharmacy technicians in all states are permitted (or in some cases required) to substitute the appropriate lower-cost generic drug in place of a prescribed brand-name drug without physician approval if the generic drug is considered bioequivalent. To be **bioequivalent**, the generic must be both pharmaceutically and therapeutically equivalent to the brand-name drug. To be **pharmaceutically equivalent**, the generic drug must contain the same amount of active ingredient in the same dosage form. Bioequivalent generic drug products may differ in certain characteristics, including shape, scoring configuration, packaging, inert ingredients (including colorings, flavors, and preservatives), expiration date, and—within certain limits—labeling.

Each generic drug also needs to be **therapeutically equivalent**, or provide the same medicinal benefit at the same dosage with the same degree of safety under the conditions specified in the labeling. This means that the bioequivalent generic drug enacts the same standards of safety and efficacy as the brand-name drug.

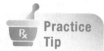

Practice Tip

If a physician writes "brand medically necessary" on a prescription, it would be indicated by "DAW1" for insurance processing.

However, since not all patients will respond similarly to a specific drug, the prescriber is permitted by law to write, **"DAW"** (dispense as written) and/or, "brand medically necessary" on the prescription. to indicate that the generic drug should not be substituted, and the prescription filled with the brand-name drug. The patient may also specifically request a brand-name drug, which would be written as **"DAW2"** on the prescription for insurance processing. This generally results in a higher copay, so the technician must make sure the patient is aware. Conversely, a patient may request a lower-cost generic, even if the physician wrote "brand necessary." In this case, a call to the physician's office is necessary to gain approval for the generic drug in place of the brand-name drug.

FIGURE 4.1 Overview of Medication Filling and Dispensing Process

Each step in the filling and dispensing processes for prescriptions and medication orders is an opportunity to do things correctly or to make an error. At each step, there is also chance to catch and correct any previous errors.

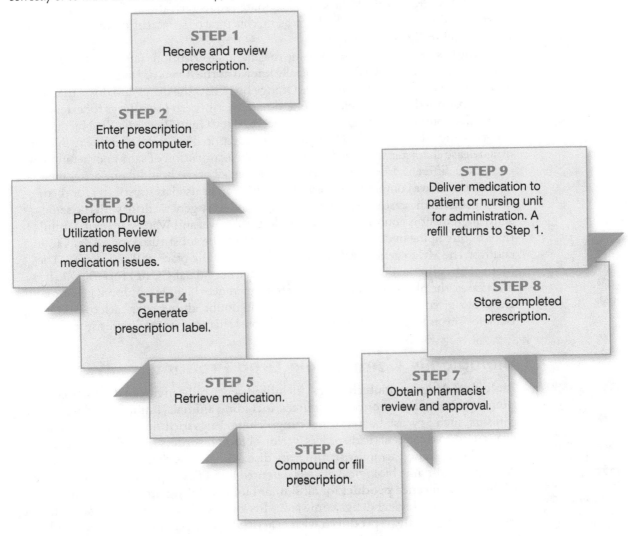

Caution Against Substitutions of Pharmaceutical Alternative Products

Study Idea

Remember that brand-name and generic drugs, though substitutable, are not exactly alike. The different formulations may affect patients differently. When dispensing refills, pass on any patient concerns about substitutions to the pharmacist.

For refills, it is important that the pharmacy technician review the patient profile to see if a brand-name or generic drug was previously dispensed so patients can remain on the same bioequivalent form of medication. Generic drugs do not exist for all brand name drugs because some drug patents have not yet expired. If a generic drug is unavailable, pharmaceutical alternative drug products can provide solutions for substitution, if allowed by a physician's approval. A pharmaceutically alternative drug is one that contains the same active therapeutic ingredients but might contain different salts (for example, hydroxyzine hydrochloride instead of hydroxyzine pamoate), or come in different dosage forms (a tablet rather than a capsule), or even have different release mechanisms (an immediate-release tablet rather than an extended-release tablet). Pharmacists are able to make recommendations for substitution of pharmaceutical alternatives, but the physician must be the one to authorize the use of such products.

Thus, if a prescription is written for 100 mg of metoprolol succinate (an extended-release formulation), a pharmacy technician cannot substitute 100 mg of metoprolol tartrate (an immediate-release formulation). Although the active ingredients and dose are identical, the salts (succinate versus tartrate) and the release characteristics of the drugs differ. For this reason, this type of substitution must not occur unless specifically prescribed.

The first reference for brand-name to generic substitutions (and pharmaceutical alternatives) is the Orange Book, officially known as the *Approved Drug Products with Therapeutic Equivalence Evaluations*. The Orange Book lists the drugs and doses that may be safely substituted. For example, two brand-name antihypertensive drugs for extended-release (24 hours) blood pressure control are Adalat CC and Procardia XL. Nifedipine is the active ingredient in both. They cannot be substituted for each other due to different drug-release characteristics. Each manufacturer's formulation of salts or other ingredients offers different drug characteristics. However, all of the brand-name drugs mentioned above have compatible generic drugs that can be used as substitutes for them.

Just as in the case of brand-name drugs, not every generic drug with the same active ingredient is equivalent. For example, the Actavis and Watson generic formulations of nifedipine in doses of 30 mg and 60 mg can be substituted for Adalat CC. In contrast, the Mylan generic nifedipine can be used in the place of Procardia XL. The Matrix Labs generic nifedipine can be used for either Adalat CC or Procardia XL. In most cases, the pharmacy software will cross-reference the FDA-approved generic equivalents of a given brand-name drug, but, when in doubt, always refer back to the Orange Book for the most current list of drugs and doses that may be safely substituted.

Biologically Comparable Drug Products

Study Idea

An interchangeable biological drug is different from a generic equivalent because the source of the biological drug is a live or once-live organism or matter.

Biological drugs, or biotech drugs (including genetically engineered drugs), come from a variety of live or once-live sources, including animals, humans, and microorganisms, such as yeast, bacteria, and fungi. These drugs include expensive injectable drugs used to treat genetic disorders, various blood disorders related to cancer or chemotherapy, and various inflammatory diseases, such as rheumatoid arthritis. When a brand-name biological drug is patented and FDA approved, it becomes the **biological reference product** for all similar biological drug products to come.

Because biological drugs come from live or once-live matter or organisms, they cannot be chemically reproduced with exactitude, so a generic version cannot be designated as pharmaceutically or therapeutically equivalent. Instead, the FDA has evaluated and approved **biosimilar drugs**, which are similar though not identical to the parent innovator drugs. They have been proven to address the same indications with the same pharmaceutical mechanisms, or precise ways that the active ingredients exert their influence on the body. Biosimilar drugs must also have the same administration routes, dosage forms, conditions of use, and levels of quality and strength as the original biological drugs.

If a biosimilar drug is tested and found to be both similar and provide similar levels of therapeutic results, the FDA can designate it as an **interchangeable biological drug**, which is both biosimilar and therapeutically effective. Once a biosimilar drug is designated by the FDA as an interchangeable biological drug, it can legally be substituted for the prescribed brand-name biological drug without contacting the physician for approval, like a brand-name to generic drug substitution.

As biosimilar and interchangeable biological drugs move through the FDA approval processes, they are included in the online Purple Book, officially known as the *Lists of Licensed Biological Products with Reference Product Exclusivity and Biosimilarity or Interchangeability Evaluations*.

Additional Resources for Drug Substitutions

The FDA also publishes a book on veterinary medications, or the Green Book, officially known as the *Approved Animal Drug Products*. Because some veterinary drugs can be purchased at pharmacies, this is also a valuable reference for pharmacists and technicians.

Additionally, pharmacy technicians should be familiar with other reference books that help identify equivalent drug products. Facts & Comparisons is available in paper and online versions and is a good reference for drug products as well as FDA-approved and unapproved indications for drugs. ASHP Drug Information is commonly used in institutional pharmacies as a drug reference. The US Pharmacopeia-National Formulary (USP–NF) also contains drug monographs.

Many references are available online with a paid subscription, including Lexicomp, Clinical Pharmacology, and Micromedex. Your employer will be required by state law to have some of these drug references.

4.2 Common Pharmacy Abbreviations

Pharmacy personnel must recognize all shorthand abbreviations used in prescriptions and medical orders. Table 4.1 lists common prescription abbreviations for amount, dosage form, and time and site of administration. Most of these abbreviations are derived from Latin. Note that weight and volume amounts borrow heavily from the measurement systems discussed in Chapter 5.

Focus and attention to detail are critical when reviewing a prescription or medication order. Note that when the units are abbreviated, there is minimal visual difference between gram (g) and grain (gr), but 1 gram is equal to 1000 milligrams and 1 grain is equal to 65 milligrams, so potential exists for a dosage error. That is why metric measurements are safest for prescribers to use.

Arabic numbers are usually used for dosage quantities. Lowercase Roman numerals are generally seen on prescriptions using apothecary measures, and they follow—rather than precede—the unit of measurement, as in "aspirin gr v," meaning *5 grains* or "tbsp iii," meaning *3 tablespoons*. However, because of frequent errors, Roman numerals are discouraged. Additionally, fractions in Roman numerals follow a different notation system (*ss* means ½), which adds another layer of confusion to a prescription.

In addition, some other traditional pharmacy abbreviations have proven dangerous. For instance, failure to differentiate the directions *q.d.* (daily) from *q.i.d.* (four times a day) can result in serious harm to a patient; often the tail of the *q* in *q.d.* (or a period between the *q* and *d*) may look like an *i* because it loops back. For this reason, the Institute for Safe Medication Practices (ISMP) recommends avoiding the use of the lowercase abbreviation *q.d.*; either use *QDay* or *daily* or *every day*.

In Table 4.1, a red line is drawn through common abbreviations the ISMP recommends should NOT be used because they come with an increased risk of misinterpretation, which could lead to a medication error. For a more a complete list of pharmacy abbreviations, see Appendix A. However, because some prescribers still use these abbreviations, Roman numerals, and nonmetric units, it is still important to study them and know their uses.

Abbreviations for dosage forms are usually straightforward. Many generic drugs are available in both capsule and tablet formulations and can be used interchangeably if they are in the same dosage strength. In some cases, the prescriber may write a prescription for tablets, but if the capsule is in stock, it can generally be substituted if approved by the prescriber. Prescriptions written for the eyes and ears may be

Safety Alert

Prescribers of controlled substances may use Roman numerals as a safety precaution. It prevents someone from illegally changing 30 tablets to 80 by completing the curves of the "3." so the prescriber may write, "xxx tablets" or, "30 (xxx)."

Safety Alert

Remember that 1 mL is equal to 1 cc and the terms used interchangeably. The ISMP recommends not using "cc" as it is easily misread.

solutions or suspensions; there is a subtle difference between these dosage forms, and they should not be interchanged without the approval of the prescriber.

TABLE 4.1 Common Prescription Abbreviations

Abbreviation	Meaning	Abbreviation	Meaning
Amount/Dosage Form		**Time of Administration—Continued**	
cc	cubic centimeter (mL)	PC, p.c.	after meals
cap	capsule	P.M., p.m.	evening, after noon
g	gram	PRN, p.r.n.	as needed
gr	grain	QN, q.n.	every night at bedtime
gtt	drop	QD, q.d.	every day
mg	milligram	QID, q.i.d.	four times a day
mL	milliliter (cc)	QOD, q.o.d	every other day
QS, q.s.	a sufficient quantity	stat	immediately
tbsp	tablespoon	TID, tid, t.i.d.	three times a day
tsp	teaspoon	t.i.w.	three times a week
MDI	metered-dose inhaler	**Site of Administration**	
SOL, sol	solution	AD, ad	right ear
SUPP, supp	suppository	AS, as	left ear
SUSP, susp	suspension	AU, au	each ear
TAB, tab	tablet	NPO, npo	nothing by mouth
UNG, ung	ointment	OD, od	right eye
#	number of, quantity	OS, os	left eye
Time of Administration		OU, ou	each eye
AC, a.c.	before meals	PO, po	oral, by mouth
AM, a.m.	morning, before noon	PR, pr, R	per rectum
BID, b.i.d.	twice a day	SL, sl	sublingual (under the tongue)
hr	hour	TOP, top	topical (skin)
HS, h.s.	at bedtime	VAG, vag	vaginally

Note: The abbreviations that are crossed out with red slashes are still in use but are discouraged by the Institute for Safe Medication Practices (ISMP).

4.3 Patient Profile

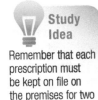
Each time a patient presents a prescription or refill at the pharmacy or hospital, the technician or admitting nurse must create or update the **patient profile**, including physical address, prescription billing, and allergies (see Table 4.2 for the components of a patient profile). The technician must ask the patient questions about allergies, alcohol use, OTC medications, and herbal, vitamin, and dietary supplements because these can also interact poorly with medications, decreasing efficacy or causing adverse medication reactions. The pharmacy software program uses the profile for processing the **Drug Utilization Review (DUR)** to provide alerts about potential adverse reactions, medication conflicts, and allergies, and the pharmacist uses the information in the profile to help counsel the patient.

The profile contains the patient's medication history, which tracks all the drugs the pharmacy has dispensed to the patient. When a patient requests a refill without the previous medication container or prescription number, the technician can retrieve the prescription information from the patient's medication history.

The profile must also include patient requests, such as for containers that are not child resistant, a 90-day supply when possible instead of a month's supply, or other necessary accommodations.

TABLE 4.2 Components of the Patient Profile

Component	Content
identifying information	patient's full name (including middle initial and any suffixes), physical street address, telephone number, birth date, and sex; increasingly, pharmacy databases enter email addresses so refill notifications and other communications can be made electronically
insurance information	information necessary for billing patient insurance
medical and allergy history	information concerning existing conditions (e.g., diabetes, heart disease), known allergies, and adverse drug reactions; pharmacy software reviews patient medical history to make sure the prescription is safe
medication and prescription history	most databases list any prescriptions filled at the individual pharmacy location; some list OTC medications as well. The new prescription is compared to previously filled prescriptions; pharmacy software reviews this information to check for adverse interactions with drugs or food
patient requests	prescription preferences (e.g., containers that are child resistant or not child resistant, generic substitutions, large-print labels, foreign language preference)
Health Insurance Portability and Accountability Act (HIPAA) and confidentiality statements	pharmacies are required by law to provide new patients with a Notice of Privacy Practices (NOPP). The action must be documented and included in the profile. This statement is for the protection of the pharmacy

Patient Privacy and Health Insurance Portability and Accountability Act Regulations

In addition to providing personal and medication information, each new patient or their guardian must sign a HIPAA form (outlining the pharmacy's privacy policy) and designate those with whom their medication history information can be shared. A scanned version of this document must be added to the patient profile. Technicians must be on guard to keep prescriptions, medication history, profile, and other patient information confidential, or they are breaking the law.

Inputting Insurance Information

After reviewing a new prescription or refill order, the technician is responsible for updating any changes to the patient's demographic and insurance information. If a patient has more than one prescription insurance plan or any coupons/manufacturer discounts, the technician needs to enter all payment data before submitting the claim. A new patient to the pharmacy must be asked to provide all payment sources prior to filling the prescription.

Verifying patient insurance information up front reduces unnecessary requests to insurers, which reduces the pharmacy's time and financial investment, and which decreases customer wait time. To begin the process, the technician asks for the customer's prescription insurance card to input the information into the computer, or to double-check it against the existing profile. For common components of an insurance identification card, see Figure 4.2.

Study Idea

Review the card information needed to process an insurance claim for a prescription.

- name of the insured person and the primary insurance carrier along with other family members covered (sometimes)
- insurance carrier
- patient identification number (sometimes known as subscriber ID)—designating the insurance holder
- person code—indicating the relationship to insurance holder
- bank identification number (BIN)—6 digits designating the pharmacy benefits manager
- processor control number (PCN)—designating the kind of plan and processing flow
- the date coverage became effective
- the amount of the copay for generic and brand-name prescriptions (and other tier payments).

FIGURE 4.2
Parts of an Insurance Identification Card

In this example, the mother is the primary insurance holder for her four children, the insurer is Central Healthcare, and the employer is UDrug.

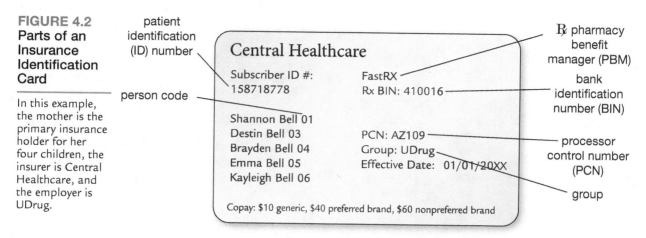

Central Healthcare

Subscriber ID #: 158718778

FastRX
Rx BIN: 410016

Shannon Bell 01
Destin Bell 03
Brayden Bell 04
Emma Bell 05
Kayleigh Bell 06

PCN: AZ109
Group: UDrug
Effective Date: 01/01/20XX

Copay: $10 generic, $40 preferred brand, $60 nonpreferred brand

patient identification (ID) number

person code

℞ pharmacy benefit manager (PBM)

bank identification number (BIN)

processor control number (PCN)

group

Each patient will have a patient identification (ID) number and will have different person codes, even for shared family plans. The primary insurance holder's person code is 01 (or 001), and their spouse's code is 02 (or 002). The person codes for dependent children would be 03 (003), 04 (004), 05 (005), and so on, generally in their birth order. Always double-check that the right person code was entered for the patient.

Insurance card formats are not standardized, so getting all the necessary information may not be easy. For repeat or returning customers, you must ask if any information has changed, insurance if the card is still up to date, and consider asking if the patient's insurance has been updated since the last time they were seen at your pharmacy. If the cardholder's employment status has changed, the drug insurance on the profile will likely have changed. A patient may also be dual eligible, having more than one insurer. If so, the information on both cards must be entered into the patient profile, designating which insurer is the primary carrier and which is the secondary (and sometimes even tertiary) carrier.

The BIN and PCN identify the correct pharmacy benefit manager (PBM) and the internal processing code for the patient's plan. Some insurance cards do not list a PCN, making the technician's job a little more difficult. Insurance and Medicaid-funded programs may switch PBMs within the calendar year without notifying patients or issuing new insurance cards, so PBM information must be identified and updated with each patient visit.

To electronically process a workers' compensation insurance claim, the technician must ask for additional information to enter into the patient profile. In addition to the BIN, PCN, and group number, the patient's Social Security number, date of injury, and name of compensating business are also required. Worker's compensation may not be billed to the same insurance as the employee's health insurance, and the technician will need to check with the employer for directions for billing the claim.

4.4 Components of a Prescription

A prescription may be submitted by computer as an electronic prescription (e-prescription), paper, phone, or fax. Table 4.3 lists the common parts of a prescription, and Figure 4.3 shows a paper version, though most are now delivered as e-prescriptions. Some state Medicaid programs require that if paper is used, it must have a security mark or other safety features that prevent copying, erasure or modification, and counterfeiting of the form.

E-prescribing can minimize forgeries and the risk of potential medication errors resulting from failure to understand a prescriber's handwriting, misinterpretation of abbreviations, and illegible faxes. E-prescribing of controlled substances must be approved by each state board of pharmacy (BOP). Controlled substances require a prescriber's Drug Enforcement Administration (DEA) number and, where permitted, can only be done via e-prescribing if the prescriber's transmission is protected with at least two of the following security measures: a password or response to security question, a biometric (fingerprint or eye scan), a password device, or a cryptographic token.

Prescriptions can be phoned in or faxed to the pharmacist and then transcribed into the patient profile. State laws also determine whether technicians can take refill prescriptions over the phone. With all refill prescriptions, technicians must check for accuracy and any changes or additions to the patient profile.

TABLE 4.3 Components of a Prescription

prescriber	name, address, telephone number, and other information identifying the prescriber, including state license number, DEA number, and National Provider Identifier (NPI)
date	date on which the prescription was written (may not be the same day the prescription was received); prescriptions are valid for one year, unless for a controlled substance, which are generally valid for six months
patient information	patient's full name, address, telephone number, and date of birth
R̥	stands for the Latin word *recipe*, meaning *take*
inscription	medication prescribed, including generic or brand name, strength, and amount
subscription	instructions to the pharmacist on dispensing the medication
signa (sig)	directions for the patient
additional instructions	any additional instructions that the prescriber deems necessary
signature	signature of the prescriber

Checking a Prescription

To be complete, check that the prescription contains all necessary information. Figure 4.3 provides an image of how these elements can be assembled in a paper prescription.

FIGURE 4.3 A Complete Prescription

patient's birth date

patient information

inscription

signa

signature of prescriber

subscription

prescriber's DEA number for controlled drug and insurance

date of prescription

NPI number

R̥ MT. HOPE MEDICAL PARK
ST. PAUL, MN (651) 555-3591

DOB 10-15-1963   DEA# AY 3456781
Pt. name *Isabella Peregrini* Date 2-16-2019
Address *10 Central Avenue Chicago, IL 60601*

Synthroid 150 mcg tablet   # thirty (30)
Take 1 tab po q AM.

Dr. _____ Dispense as written
    M. Yang
Dr. _____ Substitution permitted

_____ Fills *two* times (no refill unless indicated)
1357986420
NPI #

Accuracy

In addition to checking for completeness, the technician must review prescriptions for accuracy. Often the prescriber's name is preprinted on the prescription at the top with address, phone number, and pertinent licensing numbers. If not legible or preprinted, the prescriber's name may be identified in the pharmacy's database by telephone number or by the **National Provider Identifier (NPI)**. The prescriber's state license number is sometimes required by the state, and the NPI number is usually required by insurance for reimbursement.

If the prescription is for a controlled substance, such as a narcotic pain medication, nerve medication, sleeping medication, or weight loss meditation the prescriber must have a federal DEA number on file in the pharmacy database and on the prescription. This number differs from a state license number and the NPI. If the DEA number is not listed or available, the technician may have to call the prescriber or their nurse and request it.

Many prescribers practice in more than one physical location or clinic. In such cases, it is important to identify both the correct name and phone number of the medical office from which the prescription was written. This is necessary to clarify prescription information or request future refills on medications. The technician should also compare the signature against the prescriber's known signature to prevent forgeries.

The technician must also verify the patient's name. It is not uncommon for two patients to have the same first and last name (e.g., Rhonda Taylor and Rhonda S. Taylor). Some patients may prefer their middle names instead of their first names, making locating the patient record in the pharmacy database a challenge. Note, however, that third-party payers require claims to be submitted under the name listed with the insurer.

Asking the patient's date of birth, even if already on the prescription, is an effective way to verify that the pharmacy records match the correct patient. Write the patient's date of birth on the prescription.

Check the date the prescription was written. Do not assume that the prescription was written on the same day the pharmacy received it. If the date is missing, a follow-up call to the prescriber is necessary, or the patient may need to get a new prescription. The prescription can be filled up to one year from the date written, unless it is for a controlled substance (which is generally six months from date written).

In the **inscription**, the technician should verify that the drug name, strength, dosage form, and quantity are correct and legible. Many drugs have look-alike and sound-alike names, so the technician's focus and attention to detail are important. Many drugs come in various dosage forms—extended release and sustained release, inhalers and nebulizer solutions, and so on—so it is critical that the correct medication is entered into the patient profile in the computer.

When the prescriber writes "DAW" or "brand medically necessary," then the brand-name drug must be entered into the computer and dispensed. Brand-name drugs are commonly ordered for Coumadin, Dilantin, and Synthroid because of the narrow therapeutic index of these medications. For insurance billing they would be coded with *DAW1*. If the drug name or directions are illegible, or the drug strength or quantity is missing, a call to the prescriber is necessary. Depending on the state and pharmacy's regulations, the pharmacist may need to verify any change. It is always good practice to verify information to minimize potential medication errors.

If the drug is not available in the prescribed strength, one option is to fill the prescription with a different strength and dosage that equals the original as discussed with calculation examples in Chapter 5. For instance, with the prescription for Synthroid 225 mcg 30 tablets for 1 tablet a day (see below), one could perhaps fill the prescription with 150 mcg tablets and change the directions to "1.5 tablets per day."

> ℞   Synthroid 225 mcg tablet #30. 1 tablet every day

Another option is to enter two prescriptions of available strengths that can fulfill the prescription—one for 200 mcg and one for 25 mcg. But that would result in a higher cost to the patient and the insurer. For either change, the pharmacy technician must consult with the pharmacist. Any changes to a prescription must be reviewed and often initialed by the pharmacist, especially for a prescription for controlled substances.

The quantity to be dispensed is usually listed on the prescription. Sometimes, however, the prescriber may instead simply indicate either a one-month or three-month supply. In such cases, the pharmacy technician must calculate the quantity to be dispensed. For example, the technician would enter #180 for the quantity of tablets for the following prescription:

> ℞   Glipizide 10 mg tablet PO b.i.d. 90 days supply

Study Idea

Do not assume refills, always enter "No Refills" if the prescriber did not indicate whether the prescription should be refilled.

In some states, if a prescription is written for a 30-day supply with two refills, the pharmacy technician or pharmacist can fill a three-month supply. For example, a prescription for simvastatin 40 mg #30 with 2 refills could be filled with simvastatin 40 mg #90. The pharmacy may do this to reduce the patient's out-of-pocket costs. Many insurers charge a reduced copay for a three-month supply. This reduces the frequency of patient trips to the pharmacy to pick up their medication, which is convenient for many patients.

In other states, the medical office must approve combining a single prescription with two refills into one dispensing, and the approval must be documented on the prescription. Mail-order pharmacies, especially those connected to insurance providers, tend to provide 90-day (3-month) supplies of medications.

The **signa (sig)**, or directions for use, should be clear on the prescription, so the technician can translate the abbreviations into the proper language for label instructions. The label must be reviewed and approved by the pharmacist before the medication is dispensed to the patient.

Legality

Technicians also need to determine whether prescriptions are legal. Legal prescribers include not only doctors , but also dentists (DMD, DDS), veterinarians (DVM), podiatrists (DPM), optometrists (ODs), physician assistants (PAs), nurse practitioners (NPs), and advanced practice nurses (APNs). Legal prescribers vary state-to-state as determined by state law. PAs must practice under the direct supervision (and license) of a practicing physician. NPs have prescriptive authority and can write or sign prescriptions according to the defined protocol in their states, even for controlled substances. A registered nurse (RN) may write a prescription, but it must be signed by a licensed prescriber.

To be legal, each prescriber must also prescribe within their profession. For example, a veterinarian cannot prescribe medications for humans; an optometrist is limited to eye medications; and a dentist is restricted to prescribing appropriate medications, such as antibiotics and pain medications, in quantities limited to patients' dental needs. In some states, physicians can prescribe medications for themselves and for family members, but this privilege never applies to controlled substances.

Pharmacy technicians must know the regulations for the states in which they practice. For instance, many states (and pharmacies) require a prescription (or a diagnosis and medication requiring injections) to dispense syringes. Furthermore, each state may have different prescribing rules. Technicians may have to determine whether a PA can prescribe narcotics without the signature of their supervising physician, or whether an NP can prescribe narcotics. Technicians will also need to know things like their state's requirements for tamper-proof prescriptions.

Controlled substance prescriptions must follow all the federal requirements covered in Chapter 2. Check that the prescriptions follow these guidelines:

- Whenever state and federal regulations of controlled substances conflict, apply the more stringent regulation.
- Prescriptions for Schedule II (C-II) controlled substances require secure transmissions or a signed hard copy; the prescriber may not fax or phone in such prescriptions unless permitted by state law.
- Most—but not all—states allow the dispensing of certain Schedule V (C-V) controlled substances, such as cough syrups, without a prescription. The customer must be 18 years old or older, and they must present appropriate identification and sign a tracking log. Limited amounts are allowed for sale at one time, such as 120 mL or 4 fl. oz. of cough syrup within a 48-hour period.

Refills

The number of refills prescribed is indicated on the computerized prescription or circled on the hard copy. Generally, refills are allowed for prescriptions for up to a year from prescribing date. If the number of refills is not written or circled on the prescription, assume that no refills were ordered. Prescriptions that are more than 12 months old cannot be refilled. Refills for controlled substances are even more limited, as seen in Table 4.4.

TABLE 4.4 Controlled Substance Refill Limits

- C-II controlled substances cannot be refilled or transferred.
- C-III and C-IV controlled substances can only be transferred once and cannot be refilled early.
- C-III and C-IV controlled substances may only be refilled 5 times within 6 months of the prescribing date.
- C-V controlled substances may be refilled up to 11 times within 1 year of the prescribing date.
- Controlled substances in any schedule may be subject to even more state restrictions.

If a full supply of the drug is not available, the pharmacy can do a **partial fill**, providing a two- to five-day supply to hold the patient over until the full amount arrives. An **emergency fill** of two- to three-day supply of medication can be dispensed for essential medications for chronic conditions when it is necessary to bridge a patient over until a doctor's visit for a new prescription. Generally, emergency fills are not allowed for controlled substances. However, in extreme circumstances with terminally ill patients, an emergency fill for a controlled substance for pain relief is permissible. Emergency fills are at the discretion of the pharmacist.

For maintenance drugs, such as birth control medications, the prescriber may indicate p.r.n. or "as needed" refills for up to a year.

If patients want to transfer a prescription refill from one pharmacy to another, the pharmacists of the new and the originating pharmacy must converse on the phone or through an online secure system. The new pharmacist can request to "**transfer in**" the prescription and ask the former pharmacist to "**transfer out**" and close the prescription. For the transfers, the originating pharmacy must verify that the patient's name, birth date, contact information, prescriber, date of prescription, and the details of the prescription (including medication name, strength, dosage form, number of refills remaining, dosage, and sig) match before authorizing the prescription to be transferred out.

Chain pharmacies that share online patient profiles can do refill location changes without transferring in and out because they share the same database, considering the full chain as a single pharmacy unit. Patients may be able to order a refill online and select the location for pickup.

Authenticity and Spotting Forgeries

Study Idea

Talk to a pharmacist or pharmacy technician about their experiences identifying controlled substance prescription forgeries.

In a community pharmacy setting, the technician and the pharmacist must verify the authenticity of the prescription, especially in the case of controlled substances. Technicians must learn common techniques for spotting forged prescriptions. Has the prescription been altered in any way, especially in quantity or number of refills? Is the prescription written on tamperproof paper with a visible watermark?

Some prescriptions may be photocopies or facsimiles cleverly produced with a laser printer. Prescription blanks are sometimes stolen from doctors' offices and prescriptions forged, especially for narcotics. Be wary of prescriptions written for unusual quantities for new out-of-state patients, especially on weekends and nights when the prescription cannot be verified with the prescriber. Such "patients" often request expensive brand-name drugs and pay cash, so there is no paper trail.

It is important to know how to verify the prescriber's DEA number. This number consists of two letters (the second letter is the same as the first letter of the last name of the prescriber) plus seven numerals. A provider's DEA number can be verified using the DEA Checksum Formula, which can be reviewed in Chapter 2. However, even if the DEA number is correct, the prescription still could be forged.

4.5 Components of a Medication Order

Pharm Fact

Computerized prescriber order entry is like e-prescribing but done within a hospital or other healthcare institution.

Medication orders are used by prescribers to request pharmaceuticals for patients in hospitals and other institutional settings, including nursing homes, long-term care facilities, nurse-delivered home health care settings, and psychiatric hospitals. A medication order is typically delivered by a **computerized prescriber order entry (CPOE) system** from a handheld device or from a computer in the patient's room, operating room (OR), emergency room (ER), admittance room, or nurses' station. The prescriber transmits the order to the pharmacy or enters it into the patient's profile, and the pharmacist verifies the order for accuracy and patient safety before the technician begins the filling process.

A medication order can also be conveyed via hard copy. The information on the medication order is then reviewed by the pharmacy technician (or nurse/unit clerk and pharmacist in the hospital) and entered into the patient profile in the computer for pharmacist approval. At the time of administration, nurses reconcile the medication with the order and patient through an **electronic medication administration record (eMAR)** by scanning the bar code on the medication and the patient's wrist band before administering the first dose.

Some institutions do not have a computerized medication administration record (MAR). Medication orders must be transcribed by hand onto a paper MAR to be double-checked by a nurse. Transcription errors may occur with this process. Hospitals are moving toward having pharmacy technicians do the entry of patient medication profiles and medication reconciliation.

Differences between a Medication Order and a Prescription

There are several ways in which a medication order differs from a prescription, including:

- Instead of directly dispensed to the patient, medication orders are filled and delivered to the patient's unit to be administered by nursing personnel in a hospital, nursing home, or other medical facility.
- Medication orders come in the following kinds: **admitting order** (with home medication inclusion order), **daily order** (each day's medications), **continuation order** (periodic review of daily order to continue or modify it), **standing order** (similar order on file for all patients undergoing similar surgeries or procedures), **stat order** (emergency order), and **discharge order** (for home therapy upon leaving).
- Depending on state regulations and site policies, hospital medication orders are usually renewed every seven days. Orders for antibiotics and narcotics often have an **automatic stop order (ASO)** after a given period. The ASO requires the physician to continually review medications for each patient.
- Prescriptions are for a defined amount of medication; medication orders, except for narcotics, are dispensed until the order is changed or discontinued, or the patient is discharged.
- In the administration of the medication order, nurses provide an extra layer of professional review and expertise that helps minimize medication errors.
- Most dispensed medications from a medication order must be part of the hospital formulary, whereas a community pharmacy does not have a formulary. Specific requests for nonformulary medications must go through a process of approval and special ordering through the Pharmacy and Therapeutics (P&T) committee. If a nonpreferred or nonformulary medication is ordered by a hospital prescriber without DAW specified, the technician must follow the drug substitution policy outlined in the hospital's **policy and procedure (P&P) manual**. Typically, the hospital pharmacy can automatically substitute the ordered medication with the pharmaceutically equivalent formulary item without specific physician approval (for example, dispensing pantoprazole when omeprazole is ordered). The technician must know the formulary and institutional policies well.
- Increasingly, hospital pharmacies employ robotic devices to assist pharmacy technicians in retrieving and packaging drugs for unit dose use, filling carts, stocking nursing units, and sterile compounding.
- Hospital medication orders are often for medications administered intravenously (IV), such as parenteral and nutritional solutions, antibiotics, or other medications.
- Medication orders can also be prepared for investigational drugs through studies approved by the hospital's **institutional review board (IRB)**. Often, one or more technicians are dedicated to this task and oversee the inventory, working with the study team to ensure that the investigational drugs are stored and dispensed separately from the general hospital pharmacy.

Study
Idea

Identify the different
requirements for a
prescription and a
medication order.

Checking the Medication Order

The pharmacy technician must review the medication order for completion. A hospital medication order must include the following:

- prescriber's name and NPI (and DEA number if needed)
- patient's name, birth date, and room number
- patient's height and weight
- date and hour the order was written
- drug name, dosage form and strength, rationale for use
- site and route of administration
- administration directions, including timing
- prescriber's signature.

Prescribers in hospital and institutional settings are not as varied as those seen in community pharmacies. Prescribers within hospital and institutional settings are usually physicians, residents, interns in training under direct supervision, or NPs.

The route of administration on medication orders is usually oral (PO) for tablets, capsules, and many liquid solutions or suspensions. A few medications, such as nitroglycerin, work faster if placed *sublingually (SL)*, or under the tongue. If a patient is vomiting continuously, the prescriber may order a drug administered rectally.

In the example below, the dosage form must be part of the medication order and the sig. The *suppository (supp)* and *PR* designations indicate that the drug is to be administered per rectum. Creams and suppositories can also be prescribed vaginally or intravaginally (VAG).

> ℞ Phenergan 25 mg supp. Sig: 1 supp PR every 6h p.r.n.

Time of administration is important. For instance, if a prescriber writes the medication order, the technician should transcribe it exactly this way in the computer. Entering *b.i.d.* (twice a day) is not quite the same as entering *q12h* (every twelve hours) because the patient may take the medication six or eight hours apart in a "twice a day" order.

Some medications, like acid reducers and medications for diabetes, are best taken before meals, and this direction will be abbreviated *a.c.* Some medications that can cause stomach ulceration (like ibuprofen) are taken with food. If the prescriber writes "p.c.", the medication should be taken after meals.

If the amount of medication taken by the patient varies each day, the prescriber may use the abbreviation *q.s.* This abbreviation is interpreted as the "quantity sufficient" to fill the prescription. The technician will then need to calculate the amount of medication needed (see Example 4.1 for an overview of these processes).

Study
Idea

The abbreviation
"a.c." means "before
meals," and the
abbreviation p.c.
means "after meals."
Review commonly
used abbreviations.

Example 4.1

The pharmacy receives a prescription for:

> ℞ Orapred 15 mg/5 mL syringe
> Sig: 15 mg PO BID with food on Day 1
> 10 mg BID on Day 2
> 7.5 mg BID on Day 3
> 5 mg BID on Days 4–5
> Quantity: q.s.

Calculate the prescribed dosage of Orapred in milliliters (mL) and the number of oral syringes to be dispensed on the first day. Then, repeat those steps for the remainder of the days until you have the total number of milliliters required to fill the prescription.

Step 1 Calculate the volume in milligrams (mg) per oral syringe and the number of oral syringes to be dispensed for the prescribed day 1 dosage (15 mg).

Set up a ratio-proportion equation (see Example 5.12 in Chapter 5 for an example of how to use the ratio-proportion method to calculate liquid dosages):

$$strength\ on\ hand = amount\ to\ be\ dispensed$$

$$\frac{15\ mg}{5ml} = \frac{1\ mg}{y\ mL}$$

Cross-multiply:

$$15\ mg \times y\ mL = 5\ mL \times 15\ mg$$

Divide both sides of the equation by 15 mg to isolate the unknown variable (y), cancel like units, and solve for y:

$$\frac{15\ mg \times y\ mL}{15\ mg} = \frac{5\ mL \times 15\ mg}{15\ mg}, \quad so\ y\ mL = 5mL$$

$y = 5$ mL; the prescription calls for 5 mL per dose.

Step 2 Now, repeat what was done in Step 1 for the remainder of the days. You should come up with the following totals:

Day 1 - 10 mL
+ Day 2 - 6.6 mL
+ Day 3 - 5 mL
+ Day 4 - 3.4 mL
+ Day 5 - 3.4 mL
28.4 mL needed in total

Answer: The total amount of Orapred required to fill the prescription is 28.4 mL

4.6 Online Claims Submission

All medications have a National Drug Code (NDC) to identify them, and this code is a key component in the online claims submission process. When entering and submitting prescriptions into the pharmacy software for the DUR, the software or technician transmits the prescription online to the pharmacy benefit manager (PBM) to complete the crucial online insurance **adjudication**. Online adjudication electronically submits the prescription billing claims to the appropriate PBM to determine if reimbursement will be provided. The PBM's online response then states the proportion of the pharmacy reimbursement as compared to the average wholesale price (AWP) and the patient's out-of-pocket costs. It usually takes less than 30 seconds to receive a reply from the PBM.

Accepted Claims

The message from the PBM usually confirms payment of a claim, also known as **claim capturing**. The adjudication usually includes information on preferred formulary products that will lower the copay or adjusted copay for certain choices. Pharmacy technicians and pharmacists should look at the claim capture screen and make sure the pharmacy is not losing money on the transaction. If this is the case, alert the pharmacist so another product or generic can be suggested or substituted based on the patient's policy.

Rejected Claims

Study Idea

It is important to know the different ways to handle rejected claims based on the specific reasons for rejection.

While adjudication usually results in claim capturing, sometimes it results in a rejected claim, often accompanied by a reject code. Claims get rejected for many reasons, including problems with missing or mistyped information, wrong birth date, wrong name, wrong dosages, or special medications requiring prior authorization. Each rejection message requires its own response action to resolve the problem. If questions about coverage arise, the technician should use the appropriate toll-free insurance or PBM contact phone number.

Formulary Issues

A common message for any brand-name or high-cost medication is *NDC Not Covered*. When this message or *Not an Option* appears on the screen in adjudication, it means that this drug is not covered by the PBM formulary. A technician can then present the following options to the patient: (1) the patient can pay the out-of-pocket costs (2) the pharmacy can keep the prescription on file for a later date; (3) the patient can call the prescriber and request a cheaper alternative, if available; (4) the pharmacist can consult with the patient and then call the prescriber to recommend alternative options or prior authorization if needed.

Prior Authorization

The alert *Requires Prior Authorization* may pop up as a reason for rejection. In this case, the pharmacy technician may need to notify the prescriber's office of the rejected claim to allow the prescriber to seek prior authorization (PA) from the insurance company or PBM for a nonformulary medication. For example, a prescriber might request prior authorization for the brand-name drug, Lipitor, because the patient had an allergic reaction to the generic atorvastatin. In this situation, the prescriber would contact the insurance provider by phone, email, or in writing to request coverage of the more expensive brand-name drug. The PBM has physician, nurse, and pharmacist consultants on staff who review each case to determine the merits and approve or deny payment.

Practice Tip

Be aware that some prior authorization or approval issues can take hours and days to resolve. Warn the patient of this, so they do not wait at the pharmacy.

Cases exist in which the medication selected by the physician is not covered by the insurance under any circumstances—not even with a PA. This lack of coverage often applies to new, innovative drugs that are extremely expensive, drugs that promote weight loss or sleep, certain medications for anxiety or nervous disorders, certain cough syrups for adults, and drugs that have cheaper alternatives or are available as OTC drugs. If the insurer denies coverage, the patient has the right to appeal by calling the appropriate toll-free insurance contact phone number. This is not done by the technician or pharmacist but by the patient (it takes time and much paperwork). However, the technician generally must break this news to the patient.

Prescribers' National Provider Identifier Issues

The correct **NPI number** is required for each prescription to be processed. (NPs or physician assistants may use the NPI number of their supervising physicians with their knowledge and approval.) These NPI numbers must always be carefully checked to ensure that they match up with the prescribers' names. In the case of controlled substances, the prescriber must also have a DEA number on file in order for the claim to be processed and billed.

Out-of-Network Prescriber

In rare cases, a claim can be rejected because the prescriber is not contracted with the patient's insurance plan (as with Medicaid). In this case, another prescriber or supervising physician in the network must be contacted by phone, and that prescriber must agree to put their name on the prescription to process the claim. If the pharmacist or pharmacy technician can identify no alternative prescriber, the patient must pay cash for the prescriptions.

Drug Interactions and Combination Rejections

There are also the DUR rejections where the PBM software compares the prescriptions with the patient's PBM medication profile and finds that the patient is receiving more than one similar medication, such as two antibiotics at the same time. Or it could be that the drug may interfere with another prescribed drug (a drug interaction) or produce an allergic reaction. In these cases, the technician must alert the pharmacist to carefully review the rejection. The pharmacist may choose to override the rejection with the pharmacy's software, but if not, the PBM and/or prescriber must be notified.

Refill Too Soon

Refills with most insurers can be processed within five to seven days of the end date of the current medication (based on days supply), but some plans are more restrictive. In this case, a technician may get the message *Refill Too Soon* with information on when the refill can be processed. Communicate with the patient the exact date the insurance claim can be processed.

Incorrect Days Supply

A rejection may also be due to an incorrect amount for **days supply**—the amount of medication required to last for the duration of the prescription according to the physician's instructions. If you make a mistake in calculating or inputting the days supply, or if the PBM only permits a limited portion at a time, the claim will be rejected.

4.7 Filling a Prescription or Medication Order

For all prescriptions, medication orders, and for specialty compounding, DURs must be performed. The DUR will provide alerts for any problems from drug/drug, drug/allergy, drug/medical condition, or drug/supplement interactions. All issues must be resolved by the pharmacist (often with assistance from the technician by contacting the prescriber's office for more information). For many prescriptions, the technician will have to calculate dosage conversion and days supply. In the community pharmacy, the technician will also run the insurance and third-party claim processing. In the hospital, the billing department will handle these claims.

For both prescriptions and medication orders, a patient label or fill list is generated. The technician uses the drug name and strength to select the correct medication, scanning the NDC bar code to aid in identifying the exact drug, dose, and package size. The NDC number and bar code are on the stock drug label and unit dose packaging (see Figure 4.4).

The first number set, or *labeler*, designates the manufacturer; the second number set indicates the strength, dosage form, and formula; and the last number set, or product code, or package code, indicates the size and types (see Figure 4.5).

Each drug product is also assigned a **lot number**, or control number, by the manufacturer that identifies its manufacturing batch and date. The date of manufacturing determines the expiration date. That is why the lot number is listed on the label in Figure 4.4 as "Expiration Date/Control No." This lot number allows the product to be traced if there needs to be a product recall because of some contamination to this specific batch.

Also generated with the medication label or list are the auxiliary labels—the small, colorful labels about warnings and side effects that may be added to supplement the directions on the medication container label (see Chapter 1 for examples). The pharmacist or pharmacy software will choose which auxiliary labels to use.

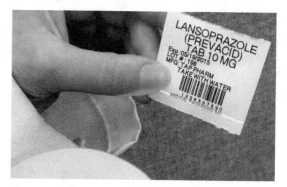

Commercially available unit dose labels contain the drug, dose, and NDC barcode.

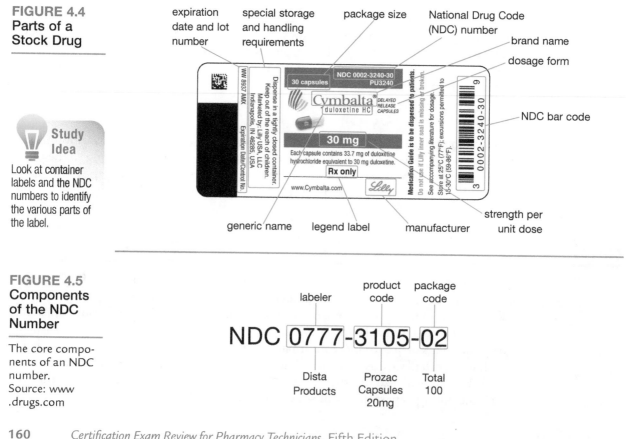

FIGURE 4.4 Parts of a Stock Drug — labels: expiration date and lot number; special storage and handling requirements; package size; National Drug Code (NDC) number; brand name; dosage form; NDC bar code; strength per unit dose; manufacturer; legend label; generic name

FIGURE 4.5
Components of the NDC Number

The core components of an NDC number. Source: www.drugs.com

NDC 0777-3105-02

labeler — 0777 — Dista Products
product code — 3105 — Prozac Capsules 20mg
package code — 02 — Total 100

Prescription Filling

Study Idea

Review the PPPA for the definition of a child-resistant container.

Study Idea

Review various types of containers used to dispense medications, including vials, bottles, and ointment jars.

After confirming the NDC on the stock bottle, the technician may have to reconstitute a product according to manufacturer instructions and then make a notation of the expiration date on the label. (Flavorings may also need to be added.) The expiration dates are determined by the manufacturer's guidelines. Medications must be dispensed in the proper containers. Most pharmacy containers used for tablets, capsules, and liquids are amber-colored plastic or glass to prevent ultraviolet (UV) light exposure that can cause degradation of the medication. Any product packaging from the manufacturer ensures stability and potency until the listed expiration date.

To comply with the Poison Prevention Packaging Act (PPPA) of 1970, all medications should be dispensed in child-resistant containers unless specifically requested by the patient. The caps on these containers are designed to be difficult for children to open. Certain drugs in original packaging are exempt from this requirement, for example, nitroglycerin sublingual tablets.

Patient Education Materials

Patient information about use, warnings, side effects, and storage are very important. There are five distinct ways of communicating necessary medication information to the patient: (1) medication container label, (2) auxiliary labels, (3) medication information sheet, (4) an FDA-mandated Medication Guide for select medications, and (5) counseling by the pharmacist.

Medication Container Labels

After medication review and verification by the pharmacist, the medication container label is affixed to the bottle, box, or other container of prescribed medication and includes the following: the date dispensed; name, address, and phone number of the pharmacy; ℞ number; patient name; number of refills; prescriber name; drug name; dose; directions; and manufacturer. The label's instructions must read as indicated in the signa on the original prescription. Some pharmacy labels also include a description of the medication.

Study Idea

Review auxiliary labels in Chapter 1. Study the common labels used and examples of drugs requiring the label. Also study the types of drugs needing Medication Guide and/or REMS in Chapter 3.

The storage information on the labels is significant to maintain medication stability and potency. For example, most reconstituted antibiotics require refrigeration and expire after 14 days. Vials of insulin at room temperature often have an expiration of 28 days before they lose some potency. Other insulins and many eye drops, suppositories, and injectable medications require refrigeration in the pharmacy and at home. At a pharmacy, the shingles vaccine (Zostavax) is stored in a freezer and is stable for only 30 minutes after it is reconstituted.

Medication container labels for Schedule II–V drugs must contain a transfer warning that reads, "Caution: Federal law prohibits the transfer of this drug to any person other than the patient for whom it was prescribed."

Medication Information Sheets and Medication Guides

After the pharmacist conducts a final check of the prescription and medication, they print the information sheet. It is attached to the prescription bag, which then is ready for patient pickup. Some prescriptions require a Medication Guide, which advises consumers about potential adverse reactions or the proper use of selected high-risk medications. Medication Guides are required for all high-risk drugs with a Risk Evaluation and Mitigation Strategy (REMS). Birth control pills must also be packaged with a Medication Guide.

Pharmacist Counseling

Finally, by law, at the time of prescription pickup, the technician must offer the patient counseling by the pharmacist. Often the patient does not take advantage of this offer. In some cases, especially with first-time medications or potential drug interactions, the pharmacist will take the initiative to counsel the patient, whether the patient requests it or not. The pharmacy technician is never allowed to counsel a patient.

Patients must sign a document at pickup to verify they were offered counseling, and it will list the prescriptions being picked up by the patient. The document is usually on a computerized signature pad that will store the data in case of future insurance inquiries where proof is required that the patient received the filled medication.

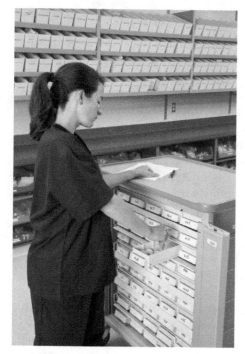

A technician fills a unit dose cart.

Medication Order Filling

Orders in the hospital are filled and delivered through daily unit dose carts, emergency carts, automated dispensing units on the nursing floor, or compounded parenteral medications that are delivered to the patients' rooms as needed. Table 4.5 lists the typical steps for filling a hospital order.

TABLE 4.5 Steps for Filling a Medication Order

The following list outlines the typical steps involved in filling a medication order in the hospital:

- The prescriber writes the medication order(s) on the patient chart or enters the order(s) in the computerized prescriber order entry (CPOE) system. Home medications, if confirmed for continued use in the hospital, must be added to the patient profile and medication orders.
- The order is transmitted via computer to the patient profile or transported to the pharmacy by a tube system, transportation department, in person, or by pharmacy personnel making regular rounds. The technician or pharmacist transcribes it into the profile.
- The medication order is reviewed for accuracy and safety by the pharmacist.
- A cart unit fill list per nursing floor or station is generated from the medication orders for the next 24-72 hours for patients in that unit. The medication order list is checked by the pharmacist for accuracy.
- The technician fills each patient medication drawer in a unit dose cart by selecting the correct medications at a pick station. (Technicians may also manage the robotic pick stations in the pharmacy for filling unit dose carts.) Each unit dose of a medication is labeled by the manufacturer with the generic or brand name of the drug, dosage and strength, administration instructions, manufacturer's name, lot number, expiration date, NDC, and bar code. This information must be matched to the medication cart list.
- The pharmacist reviews the unit dose cart according to the generated list or patient profile.
- Pharmacy technicians are then responsible for delivering the medication cart to the nursing unit. This is usually done once a day in a large acute care hospital, though the cart may carry medications for more than one day in a smaller hospital or long-term care facility.
- Stat orders are processed separately from the unit dose carts. They are given top priority by technicians and delivered quickly for the nurse or doctor to administer immediately.
- Emergency crash carts are checked and refilled by technicians with all the most commonly used emergency medications, so they are always available. In a Pyxis automated dispensing system, some emergency medications, like nitroglycerin sublingual tablets, can be accessed by the nurse before the pharmacist checks the order.
- A Pyxis or other automated dispensing system may also be used to fill a medication order, especially on nursing floors, with the technicians also checking for and replacing expired medications. The technicians fill the automated dispensing units using the drug names and NDCs, removing expired drugs and reordering those that are low. Once the pharmacist approves a medication order, the nurse may retrieve it from the dispensing station to administer it. Some institutions use a combination of cart-fill and automated dispensing technology.

Large hospital pharmacies use a variety of time- and cost-saving devices to assist technicians in medication preparation and repackaging, such as automated pill counting machines and high-speed packaging and dispensing machines for oral medications (for example, PACMED by McKesson). Such automation reduces cart fill times, lowers inventory costs, and improves patient safety. Automated systems can also interface with robotic systems to further increase efficiency and safety in hospital pharmacy operations.

Repackaging Drugs for Unit Doses

Practice Tip

A BUD and lot number must be included on all repackaged medications, which is different from the stock expiration date.

Not all drugs are commercially available in unit dose packaging, so the pharmacy technician often needs to repackage medications from bulk containers into unit doses and give them a bar-coded label.

For solid oral medications, technicians use heat-sealed bags, adhesive-sealed bottles, blister packs, and heat-sealed strip packages. For oral liquids, the medications are measured and sealed into airtight plastic or glass cups, heat-sealable aluminum cups, and plastic syringes labeled "For Oral Use Only."

All repackaged unit doses are placed in an envelope or a plastic bag and labeled with the patient's name, the drug name and dose, the medication administration time, lot number, beyond-use date (BUD), and an identifying bar code.

After repackaging, the essential information must be documented in a digital **repackaging control log** (or handwritten repackaging logbook as in Figure 4.6). It must be initialed by the repackaging technician as well as by the pharmacist who checked the medication. Automated repackaging machines can be used that generate and affix the labels.

Any home medications that are to be delivered in the daily dose carts also need to be repackaged as unit doses, affixed with a bar-coded label, and portioned out in correct scheduled doses for the cart fill. At discharge, any remaining stock of the home medications will be returned to the patient.

FIGURE 4.6
Repackaging Control Log Information

This information must be entered and filed in the computer or logbook to document and track repackaging.

Repackaging Control Log
Department of Pharmaceutical Services

Date Repackaged	Pharmacy Lot Number	Drug Name, Strength, and Dosage Form	Manufacturer and Lot Number	Expiration Date	Quantity Packaged	Initials	
						Prep. By	Approved By

Parenteral Medication Orders

Study Idea

Review parenteral fluids in the Chapter 7 on sterile and hazardous compounding.

A patient's survival often depends on swift administration of an individualized sterile drug product, or **compounded sterile preparation (CSP)**. See Chapter 7 for more information on types of parenteral preparations.

Large volume parenteral (LVP) solutions usually consist of water with salt (saline, or NaCl) and/or glucose (dextrose). It is not unusual for an LVP to have additional additives, such as potassium chloride (KCl) or multivitamins, depending on the patient's requirements. LVPs may be sent to the nursing unit or may be available at the nursing unit via a Pyxis workstation. Table 4.6 lists the most common IV fluid products and their typical abbreviations.

Pharm Fact

IV solutions are also known as IV infusions and admixtures.

TABLE 4.6 IV Fluids and Abbreviations

IV Fluid	Abbreviation
Normal saline (0.9% NaCl)	NS
1/2 Normal saline (0.45% NaCl)	1/2 NS
5% Dextrose	D_5W
10% Dextrose	$D_{10}W$
5% Dextrose and normal saline	D_5NS
Lactated Ringer's solution	LR or RL

IV medication orders include additional information including fluid and amount, infusion period (e.g., "infuse over 30 minutes"), flow rate (e.g., 100 mL/ hour), BUD, and time of administration. (See Figure 4.7 for examples.)

FIGURE 4.7 Common Physician's Orders for Parenteral Solutions

These are medication orders with sterile compounding sigs and abbreviations. To translate, see Table 4.6.

℞ cefoxitin 1 g IV every 6 h × 24 hours

℞ nafcillin 1 g IV every 4 h

℞ penicillin 2 million units IV every 4 h

℞ add 100 units Humulin R regular insulin to 500 mL NS @ 20 mL/hour (label ℞ concentration 0.2 units/mL)

℞ begin magnesium sulfate 5 g in 500 mL NS to run over 5 hours × 1 dose only

℞ change IV fluids to 1/2 NS with 20 mEq KCl 125 mL/hour

4.8 Final Check by the Pharmacist

It is extremely important—and required by law—that the pharmacist checks every prescription and medication order to verify its accuracy before it is dispensed to the patient or sent to the nursing unit. Typically, in a community pharmacy, the pharmacy technician will present the prescription printout or original hard-copy prescription, the medication information sheet, and the labeled container with the prescribed medication to the pharmacist for a final check. The pharmacist reviews the original prescription, compares it with the patient profile, confirms that the medication information sheet has been printed, verifies that the drug selected by the technician (from the stock bottle) is correct, and checks the accuracy of the medication container label.

In the hospital, the medication order, label, compounding procedure, preparation records, and all materials used to prepare or make a CSP must be inspected by the pharmacist before the medication is sent to the nursing unit. The inspection should include verification of the identity and amount of ingredients, technique for aseptic mixing and sterilization, packaging, labeling, and physical appearance. A pharmacist will also perform a physical check to look for incompatibilities between the additives and an IV solution.

In the case of states and facilities that allow **tech-check-tech**, the TCT personnel can do the main checking of specific medications that have been verified and dispensed before. For instance, the University of Wisconsin Hospital and Clinics assigned TCT personnel to check the filling of unit-dose medication cassettes, and TCT personnel achieved a >99.8% accuracy rate. The TCT personnel must have advanced training for this responsibility.

4.9 Equipment and Supplies Required for Drug Administration

When dispensing medications, it is important to provide the proper dosage delivery devices for use by the patient, parent, or caregiver. These devices are calibrated and marked to proper measurement of the intended dose. This section will discuss various dosage delivery devices.

Devices for oral administration include cups, droppers, calibrated spoons, and oral syringes. They are typically marked to measure in teaspoons, tablespoons, or milliliters. One teaspoon equals 5 mL and one tablespoon equals 15 mL. Cups are used for volumes such as 5 mL or 10 mL. Medication is poured into the cup and measured at the bottom of the meniscus for accuracy. Droppers are usually used to measure small amounts of liquid to the eyes, ears, or mouth. Droppers are usually calibrated by the manufacturer for use with a specific product and should not be interchanged. Calibrated spoons are used for volumes up to 5 mL. The medication is poured into the hollowed portion of the spoon using the proper measurement and then administered to the patient orally. Oral syringes are the most used oral administration device. They typically come in 1, 3, 5, and 10 mL sizes and are chosen based on the intended volume of the dose. Sometimes an oral syringe is used with a bottle adapter, which is a small insert that fits into the top of a bottle and allows the user to draw out liquid from the inverted bottle.

Syringes for injection should not be confused with oral syringes. Injectable syringes allow administration of a medication by IV, IM, or another injected route using a needle. Syringes and needles come in various sizes. Both are disposable and should not be reused. Always dispose of used needles in a sharps container.

Many patients with diabetes administer their insulin using syringes and needles, but others use pen systems to deliver precise doses of insulin. When using insulin pens, patients with diabetes will need pen needles, which are thin, short needles for subcutaneous injection. The higher the number, or gauge, of the needle, the smaller the size of the needle. Other supplies for patients with diabetes include blood glucose test strips, lancets (for pricking the finger to obtain a blood sample), and quick-acting sources of glucose (typically tablets or gel) to treat low blood sugar.

Unit-use items are usually dispensed in their original packaging and can include items like medicated shampoos, creams, or lotions. These may be difficult to label due to the size and configuration of their packaging, so consult with your pharmacist if you have doubts about label placement. Unit-dose items are most often used in the hospital where medications are prepackaged for single administration.

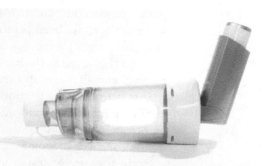

Patients can use a spacer with their inhaler to help with the distribution of their medication.

Patients with respiratory conditions who receive medications via inhalers often receive spacers with their devices. Spacers attached to certain inhalers hold the medication in a chamber until it is breathed in by the patient.

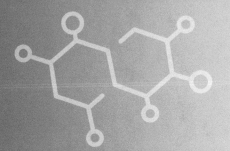

Review and Assessment

STUDY SUMMARY

A major portion of pharmacy technicians' work is the processing of prescriptions and medication orders. To allow the pharmacist more time for clinical activities and counseling, it is crucial for a technician to understand the steps involved from prescription or medication order intake to dispensing. The technician must have great attention to detail and accuracy. For the exam, focus on the following:

- the steps in the ordering and filling process
- being able to interpret orders
- reviewing calculations necessary for dosage and quantities to be dispensed
- knowing the labeling requirements for prescriptions and unit-dose packaging
- studying the legality of the order process as it relates to HIPAA
- preventing forgeries
- knowing the pharmacist's role in the final dispensing to the patient or nurse for administration.

ADDITIONAL RESOURCES

For more in-depth explanations, check out *Pharmacy Practice for Technicians, Seventh Edition* from Paradigm Education Solutions. To master and extend the material presented in this chapter, take advantage of the resources available through the eBook resources links. These include digital supplements, study resources, and a practice exam generator with 1,000+ exam-style questions. End-of-chapter tests are accessible through the eBook for individuals using the self-study course and through Cirrus for individuals enrolled in the instructor-guided course.

5

Pharmacy Conversions and Calculations

Learning Objectives

1 Adopt consistent methods for answering calculations questions for a certification exam. (Introduction)

2 Convert temperatures between the Fahrenheit and Celsius systems. (Section 5.1)

3 Convert standard time into military time. (Section 5.1)

4 Convert common systems of measurement into the metric system. (Section 5.1)

5 Understand the concepts for solving problems using ratio-proportion techniques. (Section 5.1)

6 Apply dimensional analysis in solving pharmacy dosage calculations that also include conversions. (Section 5.1)

7 Calculate oral drug dosages using proportions. (Section 5.2)

8 Calculate the dose of a drug based on the patient's weight. (Section 5.2)

9 Compute concentration percentages and the amounts of diluents needed to make desired prescribed concentrations. (Section 5.3)

10 Calculate days' supply accurately for tablets, capsules, liquids, and otic or opthalmic solutions or suspensions. (Section 5.4)

Access eBook links for resources and an exam generator, with 1,000+ questions.

Pharmacy conversions and dosage calculations are a major component of any pharmacy technician certification exam. Although some students express apprehension about this part of the exam, with the right preparation and sufficient study, this challenge can become a source of confidence and satisfaction. Conversions and pharmacy calculations are covered in all domains of the PTCE and in domain 3 of the ExCPT. This chapter and its examples—as well as the end-of-chapter practice problems and the exam generator accessed through the eBook or Cirrus—provide excellent preparation for your certification exam and career as a pharmacy technician.

Although there are often numerous ways to approach a pharmacy calculation problem, adopting consistent approaches to the different types of problems will help you develop confidence in finding accurate solutions. Being precise in conversions and calculations as a pharmacy technician will mean safety for patients and trust from pharmacists. That is why math questions are such a significant part of the PTCE and ExCPT. Table 5.1 offers helpful tips for answering calculation questions on a certification exam.

5.1 Reviewing Conversion Formulas and Measurements

To help answer calculation questions in a timely manner on a certification exam, memorize common conversion formulas and amounts, and practice using them.

Temperature Conversions

Practice Tip

Refrigerators should be maintained between 2°C and 8°C and freezers between -25°C and -10°C.

When converting temperatures between Celsius and Fahrenheit, you have to apply formulaic equations. Table 5.2 lists conversion formulas, which are important for pharmacy technicians to know. For instance, technicians are often asked to monitor refrigerator and freezer temperatures to ensure that pharmaceuticals are properly stored. If a frozen nafcillin IV solution needs to be kept at $-15°$ C, what would that be on the freezer's Fahrenheit thermometer? You would calculate $(-15 \times 1.8) + 32 = 5°$ F. Example 5.1 shows the process to convert Fahrenheit to Celsius.

Study Idea

Memorize your favorite temperature conversion equations.

TABLE 5.2 Conversion Formulas for Temperature

From Celsius to Fahrenheit	$(°C \times \frac{9}{5}) + 32 = °F$
	$(°C \times 1.8) + 32 = °F$
From Fahrenheit to Celsius	$(°F - 32) \div \frac{9}{5} = °C$
	$(°F - 32) \times \frac{5}{9} = °C$
	$(°F - 32) \div 1.8 = °C$

Example 5.1

NuvaRing vaginal contraceptive rings must be refrigerated at a temperature between 36° F and 45° F before dispensing. Calculate the equivalent temperatures in degrees Celsius. (Two different but equivalent formulas will be applied.)

Calculate the Celsius equivalents of 36° F and 45° F.

$$°C = (36 - 32) \times \frac{5}{9}; \quad °C = 2.2$$

$$°C = (45 - 32) \div 1.8; \quad °C = 7.2°$$

Answer: The refrigerator must be kept between 2.2° C and 7.2° C for NuvaRing contraceptives.

Time Conversions

While the 12-hour clock works for most everyday activities, it has become common internationally in health care to use the 24-hour clock, also called **military time**. The military system counts from midnight continuously until 2359 (written in international time as 23:59), to start again at 0000, the next midnight as shown on the clock on the left. The designations a.m. and p.m. do not exist in military time. Instead, hours escalate from midnight (0000) to noon (1200) up to 2359, the time just before midnight. See Table 5.3 for some examples of time conversions from a 12-hour clock to a 24-hour clock.

Pharmacy technicians must be able to convert between the two time systems for the correct administration time to be labeled on the medication in a hospital. Review Example 5.2.

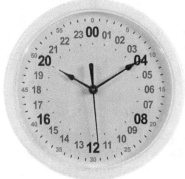

24-hour clocks begin at midnight (0000) each day, and the first 12 hours until noon (1200) are similar to the 12-hour clock. From noon to midnight, the counting after continues after noon up to 2359 instead of starting to count from 1 again.

Study Idea

Some hospitals use international time notation, which uses the 24-hour clock, but inserts a colon between the hours and the minutes, as in 23:59 (11:59 p.m.).

TABLE 5.3 Time Conversions

12-Hour Clock	24-Hour Clock
midnight	0000
12:30 a.m.	0030
1:00 a.m.	0100 (the 1st hour)
2:30 a.m.	0230
6:00 a.m.	0600 (the 6th hour)
8:45 a.m.	0845
noon	1200 (the 12th hour)
4:45 p.m.	1645
6:00 p.m.	1800 (the 18th hour)
9:30 p.m.	2130
11:00 p.m.	2300 (the 23rd hour)

A patient is to receive the intravenous antibiotic penicillin every 6 hours around the clock. If the first dose is taken at 8:00 a.m., when will the next dose be taken in military time?

Step 1 Calculate what time it would be for the next dose using the familiar 12-hour clock.

$$8{:}00 \text{ a.m.} + 6 \text{ hours} = 2{:}00 \text{ p.m.}$$

Step 2 Since 2:00 p.m. is 2 hours after 12 noon, think of the military clock count continuing for the 2 hours (0200) after 12 noon as 1200:

$$0200\,1200 = 1400 \text{ hours (fourteen hundred hours or}$$
$$14{:}00 \text{ international time).}$$

Answer: The next dose will be taken at 1400 hours.

Earlier Measurement Systems and Conversions

Throughout history, pharmacy practices have utilized three different measurement systems: avoirdupois, apothecary, and household systems. In health care today, most products are dosed in metric units, such as milligrams (mg) or milliliters (mL). Memorize the common conversion values in Table 5.4 before taking the exam.

TABLE 5.4 Common Conversion Values from Earlier Systems

Volume	Weight
1 grain (gr) = 60–65 milligrams (mg)*	1 ounce (oz) = 30 grams (g)
1 teaspoons (tsp) = 5 milliliters (mL)	1 pound (lb) = 454 grams (g)
1 tablespoons (tbsp) = 15 milliliters (mL)	2.2 pounds (lb) = 1 kilograms (kg)
1 fluid ounce (fl oz) = 30 milliliters (mL)	
1 cup = 240 milliliters (mL)	
1 pint (pt) = 480 milliliters (mL)	
1 quart (qt) = 960 milliliters (mL)	
1 gallon (gal) = 3,840 milliliters (mL)	

*=Grain measurements can vary; see explanation on following page.

The avoirdupois, apothecary, and household systems have survived. However, with very few exceptions, these measurements are not used in general pharmacy practice today and can lead to medication errors if put into practice. The only apothecary unit still sometimes used in prescription stock labels is the grain (gr), a dry weight measure. A common example can be seen in aspirin, acetaminophen, and ferrous sulfate products, which are sometimes labeled as 5 gr, an amount approximately equivalent to 325 mg (since 1 gr equals 65 mg).

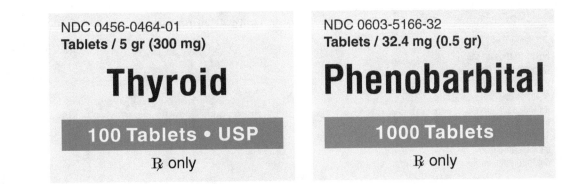

NDC 0456-0464-01
Tablets / 5 gr (300 mg)

Thyroid

100 Tablets • USP

℞ only

NDC 0603-5166-32
Tablets / 32.4 mg (0.5 gr)

Phenobarbital

1000 Tablets

℞ only

Practice Tip

Remind patients that when measuring OTC dosages with teaspoons and tablespoons, they need to use measuring spoons, not those from their silverware drawer.

Pharm Fact

The most commonly used metric units for pharmacy are liquid volumes in liters and mass and weight in grams. Meters are not commonly used, but the centimeter is used to measure a patient's height.

However, using the grain can be problematic: 1 gr can also be equal to 60 mg (as in thyroid) and 64.8 mg (as in phenobarbital). Some drug stock labels reflect both units of measurement (see thyroid and phenobarbital images above). Often the differences in grain conversions to other measurements depend on whether the drug is synthetic, semisynthetic, or naturally sourced. Because of the lack of standardized conversion, the grain is not a safe measurement to use and is being phased out.

The household system is based on the apothecary system and was used for cooking and helping patients take their medications at home. Because some over-the-counter (OTC) medications still use the household system of teaspoons (tsp) and tablespoons (tbsp) for dosages, it is essential to memorize how they compare to the metric system.

Knowing the Metric System

The metric system is based on multiples of 10. The advantages of the metric system include the following:

- consistent measurement values across the world and fields of use, especially science
- consistent decimal notation in which units are based on multiples of 10
- consistent escalation and de-escalation in value for ease of memory and use
- same correlations of value proportion in units of measurement across the dimensions of length, volume, and weight.

The metric system of measurements is considered universal, so it is necessary to memorize the units of measurement in Table 5.5.

TABLE 5.5 Common Metric Units

Measurement Unit	Equivalent
Length: Meter	
1 meter (m)	100 centimeters (cm)
1 centimeter (cm)	0.01 meter (m); 10 millimeters (mm)
1 millimeter (mm)	0.001 meter (m); 1,000 micrometers or microns (mcm)

continues

TABLE 5.5 Common Metric Units—*Continued*

Measurement Unit	Equivalent
Volume: Liter	
1 liter (L)	1,000 milliliters (mL); 1,000 cubic centimeters (cc)*
1 milliliter (mL)	0.001 liter (L); 1,000 microliters (mcL)
Weight: Gram	
1 gram (g)	1,000 milligrams (mg)
1 milligram (mg)	0.001 grams (g); 1,000 micrograms (mcg)
1 kilogram (kg)	1,000 grams (g)

*=Milliliters is the preferred measurement. Sometimes cubic centimeters is used but it's being phased out due to being the source of many medical errors.

Prefixes, or syllables placed at the beginnings of words, are added to the names of the basic metric units to specify a particular size of unit measure, such that *milli-* (meaning $1/1,000$) can be added to liter to form a new unit **milliliter**, or one-thousandth of a liter (L). The set of standardized metric prefixes based on powers of 10 is called the Système International (SI)—for examples, see Table 5.6.

TABLE 5.6 Système International Prefixes

Prefix	Symbol	Meaning
kilo-	k	one thousand times (basic unit $\times 10^3$, or unit $\times$ 1,000)
hecto-*	h	one hundred times (basic unit $\times 10^2$, or unit $\times$ 100)
deca-*	da	ten times (basic unit $\times$ 10)
deci-*	d	one-tenth (basic unit $\times 10^{-1}$, or unit $\times$ 0.1)
centi-*	c	one-hundredth (basic unit $\times 10^{-2}$, or unit $\times$ 0.01)
milli-	m	one-thousandth (basic unit $\times 10^{-3}$, or unit $\times$ 0.001)
micro-	mc or µ	one-millionth (basic unit $\times 10^{-6}$, or unit $\times$ 0.000001)

* These units are generally not used in pharmacy.
Note: Liters (L), grams (g), and meters (m) are base units and, therefore, do not have prefixes.

Converting to Proportionally Larger or Smaller Metric Units

The most common calculations in pharmacy involve conversions up to higher metric proportional amounts and down to lower amounts using milligrams, grams (g), and kilograms (kg), or milliliters and liters. Multiplying or dividing by 1,000 moves up and down the unit steps. In proper calculations, the decimal point will move to the left when converting to larger units, and to the right when converting to smaller units. Table 5.7 and Figure 5.1 show how these conversions work.

TABLE 5.7 Common Metric Conversions

Conversion	Instruction	Example
kilograms (kg) to grams (g)	multiply by 1,000 (*move decimal point three places to the right*)	6.25 kg = 6,250 g
grams (g) to milligrams (mg)	multiply by 1,000 (*move decimal point three places to the right*)	3.56 g = 3,560 mg
milligrams (mg) to grams (g)	multiply by 0.001 (*move decimal point three places to the left*)	120 mg = 0.120 g
liters (L) to milliliters (mL)	multiply by 1,000 (*move decimal point three places to the right*)	2.5 L = 2,500 mL
milliliters (mL) to liters (L)	multiply by 0.001 (*move decimal point three places to the left*)	238 mL = 0.238 L
microliters (mcL) to milliliters (mL)	multiply by .001 (move decimal point three places to the left)	1,000 mcL = 1 mL

FIGURE 5.1
Steps Worth a Thousand

Common metric units of measurement used in pharmacy calculations go up and down by steps of 1,000. Each step is separated by three decimal places (by a power of 1,000). To go to smaller measurements, move from left to right. For larger measurements, move from right to left.

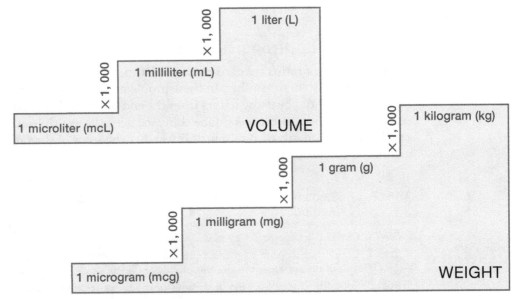

Reviewing Ratio-Proportion Equations

Perhaps no mathematical technique is used more frequently in pharmacy practice than that of ratios and proportions. Ratios and proportion equations are used in converting measurement units, determining dosages, and in compounding formulas.

Proportions with Means and Extremes

Study Idea

Pharmacy technicians should always double-check the units in a proportion, the set up of their ratio equations, and their calculations. The pharmacist must also check them.

Two ratios that have the same value when simplified are different ways of saying the same ratio, such as 1:2 and 4:8. They are called *equivalent ratios*. A pair of equivalent ratios together is called a *proportion*. The first and fourth numbers, or outside numbers, are called the *extremes*, and the second and third numbers, or inside numbers, are called the *means*.

For instance, $\frac{3}{4} = \frac{15}{20}$ is the same as:

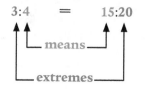

$3 \times 20 = 60$, and $4 \times 15 = 60$; or $3 \times 20 = 4 \times 15$

When you see it with the colors above, you can see why some people call this cross multiplication the *butterfly technique* or *butterfly multiplying*. This cross multiplying can be stated as a rule:

If $a:b = c:d$,

then $a \times d = b \times c$;

extremes = means

Applying Ratio-Proportion Equations

Pairs of equivalent ratios are used often in pharmacy to make conversions from one measurement system to another. In these problems, it is common to express the unknown quantities by using letters from the end of the alphabet to represent them, especially x, y, and z. Because x can be confused with the multiplication sign $\times$, y and z will be used primarily throughout this text. See the steps of the ratio-proportion method in Table 5.8.

TABLE 5.8 Steps for Solving for the Unknown Number in the Ratio-Proportion Method

Step 1 Create the proportion by placing the ratios in fraction form.

Step 2 Check that the unit of measurement in the numerators is the same and the unit of measurement in the denominators is the same.

Step 3 Solve for y by multiplying both sides of the proportion by the denominator of the ratio containing the unknown, and cancel.

Step 4 Check your answer by determining if the product of the means equals the product of the extremes.

Pharm Fact

When calculating with rounded conversion measurements, the margin of error becomes much larger when larger volumes are multiplied. More precise measurements should be used in larger calculations (e.g., IVs) and measurements should be rounded down in pediatric calculations.

Using Ratio-Proportion Equations to Convert Non-Metric Measurements to Metric Measurements

To convert any non-metric measurements to metric measurements, first convert the units into decimals and then apply the conversion amount ratios listed on Table 5.4 in ratio-proportion equations. Most conversion amounts have been rounded to whole numbers for ease of use. For example, when converting from fluid ounces to milliliters, it is common practice to round 29.57 mL to 30 mL.

However, rounding introduces a margin of error that increases for larger volumes or weights. Consider converting a household pint (pt), or 16 fluid ounces (fl oz), which is a common bottle size for bulk solutions, to metric units. When the rounded off 30 mL is multiplied by 16, it equals 480 mL. Yet when calculating with the more exact 29.57 mL, the answer is only 473.12 mL—a difference of almost 7 mL! However, pharmacy solutions bottled in 8 fl oz or 16 fl oz containers are usually dosed out in 30 mL increments. The rounded 30 mL value can be used for a fluid ounce and the rounded 480 mL for a pint when performing pharmacy calculations for this chapter, but it is important to be aware of this issue of precision.

Practice the ratio-proportion method for calculating conversions, going through the steps outlined in Example 5.3.

Example 5.3

A patient weighs 66 pounds (lb). What is their weight in kilograms (kg)?

Use the ratio-proportion method to solve the problem:

$$66 \text{ lb} = y \text{ kg}$$

The conversion rate is:

$$1 \text{ kg} = 2.2 \text{ lb}$$

Step 1 Create a proportion by writing the ratios in fractional form:

$$\frac{y \text{ kg}}{66 \text{ lb}} = \frac{1 \text{ kg}}{2.2 \text{ lb}}$$

Step 2 Set up the ratio-proportion equation, and use the means–extremes property of proportions to solve for y:

$$y \text{ kg} \times 2.2 \text{ lb} = 66 \text{ lb} \times 1 \text{ kg}$$

Next, divide each side of the equation by 2.2 lb to isolate the unknown variable (y), cancel like units, and solve for y:

$$\frac{y \text{ kg} \times 2.2 \, \cancel{\text{lb}}}{2.2 \, \cancel{\text{lb}}} = \frac{66 \, \cancel{\text{lb}} \times 1 \text{ kg}}{2.2 \, \cancel{\text{lb}}}$$

$$y \text{ kg} = \frac{66 \times 1 \text{ kg}}{2.2} = 30 \text{ kg}$$

Answer: The patient weighs 30 kg

Check the math by verifying that the product of the means equals the product of the extremes:

$$\frac{30 \text{ kg}}{66 \text{ lb}} = \frac{1 \text{ kg}}{2.2 \text{ lb}}$$

$$30{:}66 = 1{:}2.2$$

$$30 \times 2.2 = 66 \times 1$$

$$66 = 66$$

Using Dimensional Analysis to Calculate Conversions

Many conversions can also be done using process known as *dimensional analysis calculation*. This is an intimidating term for a simple process that uses techniques technicians should already know: multiplying by fractions that equal 1 and canceling out elements that balance each other out. In fact, dimensional analysis is often considered an accurate shortcut, cutting out extra steps to get to the same end by combining multiple steps into one equation.

When any number is multiplied by 1, that number stays the same. So, when converting pounds to kilograms, the pounds can be multiplied by a fraction of different measurements that equal the value of 1, as in 1 kg/2.2 lb.

When working out the equation, the known units on the top and bottom of the multiplication equation cancel, or balance, each other out, leaving a clean equation with the answer in the new unit of measurement (see Example 5.4). This is why dimensional analysis is also called *unit cancellation* or calculation by cancellation. Review the steps in Example 5.4.

Study Idea

Any time there is an element that is equally proportioned on the top or bottom of a fraction, they can be crossed out to simplify the equation or fraction because they cancel each other out.

Example 5.4

The pharmacy receives a prescription for:

℞   Acetaminophen 400 mg tablets

However, the stock bottle only measures the drug in grains (gr). How many grains of acetaminophen are prescribed?

Step 1 Look up the conversion rate for grains to milligrams (see Table 5.4). The conversion rate is:

$$1 \text{ gr} = 65 \text{ mg}, \quad \text{so } \frac{1 \text{ gr}}{65 \text{ mg}} = 1$$

Set up the equation with the unknown factor (y) on one side, and the known factors multiplied by the conversion rate on the other side (the unit of measurement needed should be on the top of the conversion fraction). Use the dimensional analysis method to solve for y:

$$y \text{ gr} = 400 \text{ mg} \times \frac{1 \text{ gr}}{65 \text{ mg}}$$
$$y \text{ gr} = \frac{400 \text{ gr}}{65} = 6.153846\ldots \text{ gr}$$

Step 2 Round the answer to the nearest whole number or to an amount that can be measured with the pharmacy balance. In this case, the nearest whole number is 6, so 6 gr should be measured and used in the prescription. If the tablets are 3 gr each, 2 tablets will be needed for each dose.

Study Idea

In conversions, the ratio-proportion method can be used to check the dimensional analysis answer and vice versa.

Check the math with a ratio-proportion equation: To double-check, this conversion can also be done as a ratio-proportion equation. Using the butterfly technique, multiply the ends and means, and then cancel like units to get the same end equation and answer. Because the ratio-proportion method has more steps, dimensional analysis is sometimes seen as a shortcut.

$$\frac{y \text{ gr}}{400 \text{ mg}} = \frac{1 \text{ gr}}{65 \text{ mg}}$$

$$y \text{ gr} \times 65 \text{ mg} = 400 \text{ mg} \times 1 \text{ gr}$$

$$\frac{y \text{ gr} \times 65 \text{ mg}}{65 \text{ mg}} = \frac{400 \text{ mg} \times 1 \text{ gr}}{65 \text{ mg}}$$

$$y \text{ gr} = \frac{400 \text{ gr}}{65} = 6.153846\ldots \text{ gr}$$

Answer: 6.153846 . . . gr can be rounded to 6 gr; 6 gr of acetaminophen are prescribed

5.2 Calculating Dosages

Ratios are commonly used in dosage calculations to express the number of parts of one substance contained in another substance of known parts. For example, suppose that there are 3 mL of an ophthalmic solution dissolved in a total of 60 mL sterile saline solution. This can be expressed as the ratio 3:60 or $\frac{3}{60}$, which reduces to $\frac{1}{20}$. In other words, the ratio of the active ingredient to the sterile saline solution is 1 to 20, or 1 part in 20 parts.

Drug Ratio Strengths

Drug stock is generally labeled with the concentration ratio of an active ingredient in the carrying vehicle: weight/volume (w/v) and volume/volume (v/v) for solutions and suspensions, and weight/weight (w/w) for solid formulations. In pharmacy, the term **ratio strength** refers to the ratio of concentration level of active ingredient to the final product or substance that holds the active ingredient. The first number (numerator) is the number of parts of active ingredient in a solution, suspension, or solid formulation, and the second number (denominator) is the total number of parts.

$$\frac{active\ ingredient\ (by\ weight\ or\ volume)}{final\ product\ (weight\ or\ volume)}$$

Ratio strengths of stock medications versus prescribed/ordered medications are used in ratio-proportion equations to determine the missing information—both in practice and on a certification exam.

A crucial step is arranging the equation properly with y for the missing information. Because a proportion is a mathematical comparison of similar things, it is essential that the units of measurement are the same in the numerators and are the same in denominators. On one side of the equation, write out the strength or concentration of the available drug, and on the other, write the prescribed strength or concentration (or vice versa, with the prescription on one side and the available drug on the other). Review this process in Example 5.5.

Example 5.5

A technician needs to make 35 mL of a distilled water solution with a concentration of 2 g sodium chloride (NaCl) to each 7 mL of distilled water (or 2 g:7 mL). How many grams of sodium chloride are needed?

Step 1 Write the variables as ratios, then write the ratios in fractional form:

$$y\ g{:}35\ mL = 2\ g{:}7\ mL$$

$$\frac{y\ g}{35\ mL} = \frac{2\ g}{7\ mL}$$

Step 2 Use the ratio-proportion method to set up an equation:

$$y\ g \times 7\ mL = 35\ mL \times 2\ g$$

Step 3 Divide both sides of the equation by 7 mL to isolate the unknown variable (y), cancel like units, and solve for y:

$$\frac{y\ g \times 7\ mL}{7\ mL} = \frac{35\ mL \times 2g}{7\ mL}$$

$$y \, g = \frac{70 \, g}{7} = 10 \, g$$

Answer: 10 g of NaCl are needed

Study Idea

When ratio strengths are given, it is often easiest to convert them into percentages for calculation: liquid v/v percents are % mL/100 mL as in 70% isopropyl alcohol (IPA); solid w/w percents are % g/100 g.

Converting a Strength Ratio to a Percent

Prescription strengths can also be expressed in a ratio, not between specific measurements, but as percentages of a whole. For instance, the percent strength of a v/v ratio would be $y \, mL/100 mL$ and a w/w ratio would be $z \, g/100 \, g$.

To express a strength ratio as a percent, designate the first number of the ratio as the numerator and the second number as the denominator. Multiply the fraction by 100 ($^{100}/_1$) and add a percent sign after the product.

To turn 1:20 into a percent, take: $\frac{1}{20} \times \frac{100}{1} = \frac{100}{20}$;   then $100 \div 20 = 5\%$

For 5:1, take: $\frac{5}{1} \times \frac{100}{1} = 5 \times 100 = 500\%$

For 1:2.5, take: $\frac{1}{2.5} \times \frac{100}{1} = \frac{100}{2.5}$;   then $100 \div 2.5 = 40\%$

To see how this is applied, see Example 5.6.

Example 5.6

If the ratio of dexamethasone in a 100 mL oral suspension is 1:3, what is the percent of dexamethasone in the suspension?

$$\frac{1}{3} \times \frac{100}{1} = \frac{100}{3}; \quad \text{then } 100 \div 3 = 33\%.$$

Answer: The oral suspension contains 33% dexamethasone.

Concentrations with Weight/Volume Percentage Strength

When the strength or concentration of a solution is expressed as a w/v percentage, the notation is grams/milliliter. For example, the intravenous fluid D_5W is a shorthand notation for a solution of 5% dextrose in water, or 5% of the 100 mL volume of final solution of dextrose dissolved in water. Therefore, a D_5W solution can be expressed mathematically as:

$$\frac{5 \text{ g dextrose}}{100 \text{ mL solution}}$$

This fractional form can be used to solve a problem with w/v (g/mL) solution concentrations, as in Example 5.7.

Example 5.7

How many milligrams of dextrose are in 75 mL of D_5W? Express D_5W as a percentage fraction, and then determine the amount of dextrose in grams required to create this concentration in 75 mL. Convert that amount to milligrams in the final answer.

Step 1 Set up a ratio-proportion equation to determine the amount of dextrose in 75 mL of D_5W:

$$\frac{5 \text{ g dextrose}}{100 \text{ mL solution}}$$

$$\frac{5 \text{ g}}{100 \text{ mL}} = \frac{y \text{ g}}{75 \text{ mL}}$$

$$100 \text{ mL} \times y \text{ g} = 5 \text{ g} \times 75 \text{ mL}$$

$$\frac{\cancel{100 \text{ mL}} \times y \text{ g}}{\cancel{100 \text{ mL}}} = \frac{5 \text{ g} \times 75 \cancel{\text{mL}}}{100 \cancel{\text{mL}}}$$

$$y \text{ g} = \frac{375 \text{ g}}{100} = 3.75 \text{ g}$$

Step 2 Convert grams to milligrams:

$$3.75 \cancel{\text{ g}} \times \frac{1,000 \text{ mg}}{1 \cancel{\text{ g}}} = 3,750 \text{ mg}$$

Answer: There are 3,750 mg of dextrose in 75 mL of D_5W

Check the math with dimensional analysis: To double-check and simplify, this problem can be solved using a single dimensional analysis equation.

$$y \text{ mg} = \frac{5 \cancel{\text{ g}}}{100 \cancel{\text{ mL}}} \times 75 \cancel{\text{ mL}} \times \frac{1,000 \text{ mg}}{1 \cancel{\text{ g}}} = 3,750 \text{ mg}$$

Converting a Percent to a Strength Ratio

Study Idea

If decimal places are moved to change a decimal to a percent, always double-check by multiplying by 100.

To convert a percent to a ratio, the percent is divided by 100 and the fraction expressed as a ratio with the numerator as the first number and the denominator the second number.

$$2\% = 2 \div 100 = \frac{2}{100}; \quad \text{then } 2:100$$

This ratio can be simplified by reducing the original fraction—dividing both the numerator and denominator by 2 to get:

$$\frac{1}{50} = 1:50$$

To see how this is applied, see Example 5.8.

Example 5.8

The pharmacy receives a prescription for:

> ℞   100 mL IV bag of 4% lidocaine to treat arrhythmia

The active ingredient in the lidocaine solution is measured in grams. What is the ratio of grams to milliliters of sterile water solution?

$$4\% = 4 \text{ g} \div 100 \text{ mL} = \frac{4 \text{ g}}{100 \text{ mL}}$$

4 g/100 mL   simplifies to 1 g/25 mL,   or 1 g:25 mL

Answer: The strength ratio of grams to milliliters of sterile water solution is 1 g:25 mL

Calculating Tablet Dosages

For solid oral formulations, the drug strength of the medication stock supply is displayed on the container's label as drug weight per tablet or capsule. Pharmacy technicians need to know how to use an equal proportion equation to calculate the proper dosage amount to fulfill the prescription strength per dosage form. You can see these steps laid out in Example 5.9.

Example 5.9

The pharmacy receives a prescription for:

> ℞ Lamotrigine 87.5 mg PO BID, q12H

On hand, the pharmacist has a drug stock of lamotrigine 25 mg scored tablets. How many tablets should be dispensed?

Step 1 Using the ratio-proportion method, determine how many tablets should be dispensed:

$$strength\ on\ hand = amount\ to\ be\ dispensed$$

$$\frac{25\ mg}{1\ tablet} = \frac{87.5\ mg}{y\ tablets}$$

$$25\ mg \times y\ tablets = 1\ tablet \times 87.5\ mg$$

$$\frac{25\ mg \times y\ tablets}{25\ mg} = \frac{1\ tablet \times 87.5\ mg}{25\ mg}$$

$$y\ tablets = \frac{1\ tablet \times 87.5}{25} = 3.5\ tablets$$

Answer: 3.5 tablets should be dispensed

Not all tablets are scored, so technicians may have to split tablets before dispensing. Scored tablets usually have a line down the middle with an equivalent amount of drug distributed on each side of the line. This scoring will help the patient cut the tablet in half as is needed for the dosage.

Calculating Dosages Using Body Weight Ratios

The prescribed or ordered dosage for a specific patient may be calculated based on the patient's body weight in kilograms rather than pounds. So, these dosage calculations have to include converting pounds to kilograms. During a certification exam, be careful to remember this step and that 1 kg equals 2.2 lb. Example 5.10 shows this process.

Example 5.10

Sally S., a 50-year-old patient who weighs 140 pounds, has a seizure disorder. She has been prescribed the following:

> ℞ Levetiracetam 15 mg/kg PO BID

What dosage has Sally S. been prescribed per day?

Step 1 Using the ratio-proportion method, calculate Sally's weight in kilograms (kg):

$$\frac{y \text{ kg}}{140 \text{ lb}} = \frac{1 \text{ kg}}{2.2 \text{ lb}}$$

$$y \text{ kg} \times 2.2 \text{ lb} = 140 \text{ lb} \times 1 \text{ kg}$$

$$\frac{y \text{ kg} \times 2.2 \text{ lb}}{2.2 \text{ lb}} = \frac{140 \text{ lb} \times 1 \text{ kg}}{2.2 \text{ lb}}$$

$$y \text{ kg} = \frac{140 \times 1 \text{ kg}}{2.2} = 63.636363\ldots \text{ kg}$$

$63.636363\ldots$ kg can be rounded to the nearest hundredth: 63.64 kg; Sally S. weighs 63.64 kg

Step 2 Using the ratio-proportion method, calculate the dosage that Sally S. has been prescribed per day:

$$\frac{z \text{ mg}}{63.64 \text{ kg}} = \frac{15 \text{ mg}}{1 \text{ kg}}$$

$$z \text{ mg} \times 1 \text{ kg} = 63.64 \text{ kg} \times 15 \text{ mg}$$

$$\frac{z \text{ mg} \times 1 \text{ kg}}{1 \text{ kg}} = \frac{63.64 \text{ kg} \times 15 \text{ mg}}{1 \text{ kg}}$$

$$z \text{ mg} = 63.64 \times 15 \text{ mg} = 954.6 \text{ mg}$$

Sally has been prescribed 954.6 mg twice a day. To find the dosage she has been prescribed per day, multiply the answer by 2:

$$954.6 \text{ mg} \times 2 = 1{,}909.2 \text{ mg}$$

Then, convert to grams (1,000 mg = 1 g):

$$\frac{1{,}909.2 \text{ mg} \times 1 \text{ g}}{1{,}000 \text{ mg}} = \frac{1{,}909.2 \text{ g}}{1{,}000} = 1.9092 \text{ g}$$

Answer: 1.9092 g can be rounded to the nearest tenth: 1.9 g; Sally S. has been prescribed a dosage of 1.9 g per day

Calculating Dosages for Children

Safety Alert

Always remember to round down the dosage for pediatric and neonatal patients down rather than up for safety reasons.

Many medications have a wide range of recommended dosages. Patients' body shapes, sizes, bodily responses, and adverse reactions vary widely, even among adults. Children are particularly vulnerable to problems in dosing because they vary even more than adults as they go through their developmental stages. Since their cells, systems, and bodies are still forming, incorrect doses—particularly higher doses than are healthy for them—can do even more harm to them than to an adult.

Most pediatric prescribers favor medications that have been specifically formulated by the manufacturer for pediatric doses rather than strict body weight ratios. However, there are times when a medical order comes in for a child's portion of an adult-use drug. The prescriber or pharmacist will determine the proper calculation approach, which is often based on body surface area.

Applying Body Surface Area for Dosages

A dosing formula that considers both metric height and weight is called **body surface area (BSA)**. This formulation is calculated in square meters. Dosage prescriptions are then written as mg/m^2. The prescriber's or pharmacist's software determines this number and then technicians apply it. Physicians prescribing cancer chemotherapy drugs in particular use BSA dosing formulas, so their dosages of these toxic drugs can be more precise. See Table 5.9 for US averages for BSA. Note that these are very general averages since adults assigned female at birth of different ages would have different subcategory averages, as would males of different ages. Each of these categories could have very different averages for subcategories within them, so it is best to use the patient's BSA formula for dosages.

TABLE 5.9 Average US Pharmacy BSAs

General Body Type	Average BSA
Male adult	1.9 m^2
Female adult	1.6 m^2
12–13-year-olds	1.33 m^2
10 years	1.14 m^2
9 years	1.07 m^2
2 years	0.5 m^2
newborn	0.25 m2

After the patient's BSA in m^2 has been determined, the technician uses the BSA dosing prescription in an equal proportion equation, which is something that may be tested in the certification exam. The process is shown step by step in Example 5.11:

$$\frac{y \text{ mg}}{patient's \text{ m}^2} = \frac{average\ adult\ dose \text{ mg}}{1 \text{ m}^2}$$

Example 5.11

Jenny, a 20 year-old patient with a BSA of 1.6 m^2, has breast cancer. To treat her cancer, the oncologist writes a prescription for

> ℞ Doxorubicin at a dose of 40 mg/1 m^2

Doxorubicin is toxic to the blood cells and heart in excessive doses. What is the proper dosage for Jenny?

Using the ratio-proportion method, calculate the proper dosage for Jenny:

$$\frac{y \text{ mg}}{patient's \text{ BSA } (m^2)} = \frac{average\ adult\ dose\ (mg)}{1\ m^2}$$

$$\frac{y \text{ mg}}{1.6 \text{ m}^2} = \frac{40 \text{ mg}}{1 \text{ m}^2}$$

$$y \text{ mg} \times 1 \text{ m}^2 = 1.6 \text{ m}^2 \times 40 \text{ mg}$$

$$\frac{y \text{ mg} \times 1 \text{ m}^2}{1 \text{ m}^2} = \frac{1.6 \text{ m}^2 \times 40 \text{ mg}}{1 \text{ m}^2}$$

$$y \text{ mg} = 1.6 \times 40 \text{ mg} = 64 \text{ mg}$$

Answer: The proper dosage of doxorubicin for Jenny is 64 mg

Calculating Liquid Dosage Amounts

When a drug is put into a solution or suspension, whether for oral use or a parenteral injection, the drug generally loses its properties as a solid and merges with the liquid. Even so, it is important to know how much of a given drug is contained in the liquid drug solution. For example, an amoxicillin oral suspension is manufactured in different strengths expressed as follows:

$$\frac{200 \text{ mg}}{5 \text{ mL}}, \quad \frac{400 \text{ mg}}{5 \text{ mL}}$$

Practice Tip

The first rule of thumb when substituting one drug concentration for another to fulfill a prescribed drug strength: follow the drug's directions for use, and set up ratios based on the recommended ratios and prescribed strength.

These show two different milligram amounts of amoxicillin, both contained in 5 mL of oral drug solution. This information is essential when setting up equations properly for determining the correct dosage amounts for a prescribed drug strength using an available stock of a different concentration.

If the amount of active drug prescribed is larger or smaller than in the stock concentration, the medication volume dispensed of the stock medication must be proportionally larger or smaller. By setting up a proportion or using dimensional analysis, technicians can easily solve problems of calculating the right dosage using a stock concentration. Follow the steps shown in Example 5.12. Example 5.13 provides more practice for calculating dosage amounts.

Example 5.12

A prescriber orders:

> ℞ **Amoxicillin 350 mg PO q12H**

Study Idea

Remember to simplify the numbers in your equations when you can. For instance, when you have equal numbers of ten at the top and bottom of an equation, you can cancel an equal number of zeros from the numerator and the denominator.

On hand, the pharmacy has amoxicillin 400 mg/5 mL. What is the prescribed dosage in milliliters?

Using the ratio-proportion method, calculate the prescribed dosage:

$$strength\ on\ hand = amount\ to\ be\ dispensed$$

$$\frac{400 \text{ mg}}{5 \text{ mL}} = \frac{350 \text{ mg}}{y \text{ mL}}$$

$$400 \text{ mg} \times y \text{ mL} = 5 \text{ mL} \times 350 \text{ mg}$$

$$\frac{400 \text{ mg} \times y \text{ mL}}{400 \text{ mg}} = \frac{5 \text{ mL} \times 350 \text{ mg}}{400 \text{ mg}}$$

$$y \text{ mL} = 5 \text{ mL} \times 350/400 = 4.375 \text{ mL}$$

Answer: 4.375 mL can be rounded to the nearest tenth: 4.4 mL; the prescribed dosage is 4.4 mL

Example 5.13

A prescription for a sick child is received from the emergency department on Saturday night for:

> **℞**   Cephalexin 125 mg/5 mL sig: 4 mL PO BID

Study Idea

Remember that when solving word problems, understanding the words may be more difficult than the mathematical computation. Phrases such as "can be made from" will usually refer to an initial solution or a stock solution that is literally taken off the shelf.

No other pharmacies are open in town. The pharmacy technician discovers that the prescribed 125 mg/5 mL concentration of the cephalexin suspension is out of stock. The child needs the medication the same night, and the prescribed concentration will not be available until Monday at noon. However, the pharmacy has the 250 mg/5 mL concentration in stock. Since the child needs 4 mL of a 125 mg/5 mL concentration, what is the amount of cephalexin per dose? How much of the 250 mg/5 mL concentration is needed for the prescribed dose?

Step 1 Using the ratio-proportion method, calculate the original prescribed dose in milligrams:

$$\frac{y \text{ mg}}{4 \text{ mL}} = \frac{125 \text{ mg}}{5 \text{ mL}}$$

$$y \text{ mg} \times 5 \text{ mL} = 4 \text{ mL} \times 125 \text{ mg}$$

$$\frac{y \text{ mg} \times 5 \text{ mL}}{5 \text{ mL}} = \frac{4 \text{ mL} \times 125 \text{ mg}}{5 \text{ mL}}$$

$$y \text{ mg} = \frac{4 \times 125 \text{ mg}}{5} = 100 \text{ mg}$$

According to the original prescription, the child should take 100 mg of cephalexin twice a day

Step 2 Now, determine the volume in milliliters (mL) of the available 250 mg/5 mL concentration required for a single dose of the prescription:

$$\frac{250 \text{ mg (in stock)}}{5 \text{ mL}} = \frac{100 \text{ mg (prescribed)}}{y \text{ mL}}$$

$$250 \text{ mg} \times y \text{ mL} = 5 \text{ mL} \times 100 \text{ mg}$$

$$\frac{250 \text{ mg} \times y \text{ mL}}{250 \text{ mg}} = \frac{5 \text{ mL} \times 100 \text{ mg}}{250 \text{ mg}}$$

$$y = \frac{5 \text{ mL} \times 100}{250} = 2 \text{ mL}$$

Answer: A 2 mL dosage of the in-stock 250 mg/5 mL concentration of cephalexin suspension is equal to the 4 mL dosage of the prescribed 125 mg/5 mL concentration suspension; 2 mL of the 250 mg/5 mL concentration is needed for the prescribed dose

5.3 Calculating Dilution Amounts

Pharmacy technicians are often required to take a stock solution of a liquid and dilute it to a less concentrated solution. Though the pharmacist usually calculates the dilution amounts, technicians double-check the answers to ensure accuracy. If there is a discrepancy, the technician queries the pharmacist to recalculate. Dilution questions are common on certification exams.

Calculating Final Strength and Volume

The first step in calculating dilutions is to determine the sufficient volume needed to decrease the drug concentration to the prescribed or ordered percentage. The amount decreased in the concentration will be in inverse proportion to the amount that must be increased in volume for the diluted solution. The following formula can be used to determine final strength and volume:

initial strength (is) $\times$ initial volume (iv) = final strength (fs) $\times$ final volume (fv)

When solving a dilution problem, there are four variables—three from the problem statement and a fourth that needs to be determined. It is advisable to write down the basic formula, above, and plug in the terms from the word problem as shown in Example 5.14. There are two important things to remember about a dilution:

- The final volume will always be higher than the initial volume because water (or some other solvent) has been added.
- The final strength will always be lower than the initial strength because this is a dilution.

Example 5.14

You have 30 mL of a 20% *N*-acetylcysteine solution. How many milliliters of 10% solution can be made if sterile water is added?

Step 1 Begin by identifying the known values given in the problem statement and the value to be determined.

$$\text{initial strength (is)} = 20\% \text{ (or } 0.2 \text{)}$$
$$\text{initial volume (iv)} = 30 \text{ mL}$$
$$\text{final strength (fs)} = 10\% \text{ (or } 0.1 \text{)}$$
$$\text{final volume (fv)} = \text{to be determined}$$

Step 2 After identifying the known values, enter them into the equation:

$$0.2 \times 30 \text{ mL} = 0.1 \times fv$$

$$6 \text{ mL} = 0.1 \, fv$$

Step 3 Calculate the value for the final volume by dividing 6 mL by 0.1.

$$\frac{6 \text{ mL}}{0.1} = fv; \quad 60 \text{ mL} = fv$$

Answer: The final volume of 10% *N*-acetylcysteine solution is 60 mL, so 60 mL of 10% solution can be made from 30 mL of 20% solution

Calculating Amounts of Diluent to Add

Pharmacy technicians may also be asked to calculate the volume of diluent that must be added to reach the prescribed or ordered volume. To solve these problems, the following equation can be applied:

final volume (fv) − initial volume (iv) = diluent volume (dv)

Although this second step uses subtraction to determine the amount of diluent needed, the diluent will be added to the original concentration. Questions like this are also common on certification exams. Example 5.15 builds on Example 5.14, but requires one additional step.

Example 5.15

Now that the final volume of the 10% *N*-acetylcyteine solution has been determined to be 60 mL, how much sterile water must be added to the 20% solution to make the required product?

Step 1 Begin by identifying the known values given in the problem statement and the value to be determined.

$$\text{final volume} = 60 \text{ mL}$$
$$\text{initial volume} = 30 \text{ mL}$$

Step 2 Enter the known values into the equation:

$$60 \text{ mL} - 30 \text{ mL} = 30 \text{ mL}$$

Answer: The diluent volume is 30 mL, so 30 mL of sterile water must be added.

On a certification exam, always read the dilution questions very carefully. There could be a two-part question (such as Examples 5.14 and 5.15 together), the final volume must be calculated before the amount of liquid needed to reach the desired dilution is determined. An exam will likely offer the answer to the first part of the question as a distractor. So, technicians should watch out and make sure the question is asking for.

5.4 Calculating Days' Supply

Calculating the days' supply of a medication accurately is an important skill to prevent the rejection of insurance claims. Examples 5.16–5.20 show how to calculate medication amounts and days' supply for sample prescriptions.

Example 5.16

A prescription is received for:

> ℞ Ciprofloxacin 500 mg, #28
> Take one tablet twice daily.

What is the days' supply?

$$\frac{1 \text{ day}}{2 \text{ tablets}} \times 28 \text{ tablets} = 14 \text{ days}$$

Answer: The prescribed amount is 28 tablets with directions to take two tablets per day; so, the day supply for 28 tablets would be 2 weeks, or 14 days.

Example 5.17

How many days will the following medication last?

> ℞ Hydrocodone / APAP in a strength of 5 mg/325 mg #90.
> Take 1 tablet every 4 to 6 hours prn for pain.

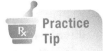

Practice Tip

When a # sign comes before a number in a prescription, it means that this is the total quantity to be prescribed or in the packaging. For instance, #90 means 90 units (such as tablets, capsules, patches, and other forms).

Step 1 Calculate the number of tablets the patient would take if the patient takes 1 tablet every 4 hours for 24 hours:

$$\frac{1 \text{ tablet}}{4 \text{ hr}} \times 24 \text{ hr} = 6 \text{ tablets}$$

The maximum number of tablets the patient could take per day is 6 tablets.

Step 2 Assuming the patient takes all 6 tablets per day, calculate the number of days the #90 supply will last:

$$90 \text{ tablets} \times \frac{1 \text{ day}}{6 \text{ tablets}} = 15 \text{ days}$$

Answer: If the patient takes the maximum dosage, the #90 supply of Hydrocodone/APAP will last for 15 days. Day supply calculations are always made based off the maximum use of the drug (in this case, every 4 hours).

Example 5.18

Study Idea

When a prescription is written as a range order, it means the patient has freedom within a prescription range of dosage and timing, as with some low-level pain medications. You always calculate the days supply using the maximum amount a patient could take per day.

A patient is prescribed to take 40 units of Humulin N NPH insulin in the morning and 25 units before dinner. This insulin is U-100 and is available in a 10 mL vial (1,000 units per 10 mL). The prescription is written to dispense 2 vials at a time. How many days will the prescribed medication last?

> ℞ Humulin N NPH insulin. Take 40 units in the morning and
> 25 units before dinner.

Step 1 Calculate the total daily dose of insulin.

$$40 \text{ units} + 25 \text{ units} = 65 \text{ units}$$

Step 2 Calculate the number of days that 2 vials will last using dimensional analysis:

$$2 \text{ vials} \times \frac{1,000 \text{ units}}{\text{vial}} \times \frac{1 \text{ day}}{65 \text{ units}} = 30.769230 \ldots \text{ days}$$

Answer: The prescribed medication will last 30.769230... days, which can be rounded to 31 days. The medication will last 31 days, or a 31 days supply.

Note: If a 56-day supply is mistakenly entered into the prescription (28 days for each vial instead of 2 vials for 30 days) for insurance processing, the initial claim will be processed; however, the patient will not be able to get a needed refill after 30 days without the pharmacist calling the insurance provider to change and correct the original prescription claim.

Example 5.19

A prescription is received for:

> ℞ Augmentin 250 mg/5 mL. Give 3/4 tsp 2 times a day for 10 days.

Augmentin is a brand suspension available as a generic suspension of amoxicillin and clavulanate potassium in quantities of 75 mL, 100 mL, and 150 mL. What is the days' supply? What size bottle should be used? How much dispensed product will be unused?

Step 1 Calculate volume taken in each dose by converting 3/4 teaspoon to milliliters.

$$1 \text{ tsp} = 5 \text{ mL} \quad \text{and} \quad \text{¾ tsp} = 0.75 \text{ tsp}$$

$$\frac{1 \text{ tsp}}{5 \text{ mL}} = \frac{0.75 \text{ tsp}}{y \text{ mL}}; \quad y \text{ mL} = 5 \text{ mL} \times 0.75; \quad y \text{ mL} = 3.75 \text{ mL}$$

Step 2 Calculate the amount of drug prescribed per day.

$$\frac{2 \text{ doses}}{\text{day}} \times \frac{3.75 \text{ mL}}{\text{dose}} = 7.5 \text{ mL/day}$$

Step 3 According to the prescription, the days' supply is 10 days. Calculate total volume needed for the days' supply.

$$\frac{7.5 \text{ mL}}{\text{day}} \times 10 \text{ days} = 75 \text{ mL}$$

Step 4 Select the bottle size from the available stock, and determine how much product will remain after the patient takes the prescribed amount. Because Augmentin comes in 75 mL, 100 mL, and 150 mL bottles, select the 75 mL bottle. Because the bottle amount equals the prescribed amount, none of the drug will be left over.

75 mL (dispensed amount) − 75 mL (prescribed amount) = 0 mL unused medication

Example 5.20

The pharmacy receives a prescription for:

> ℞ Augmentin 125 mg/5 mL. 1 tsp t.i.d. for 7 days.

The insurance will not cover this strength of 125 mg/5 mL but will cover Augmentin 250 mg/5 mL. Augmentin suspensions of 250 mg/5 mL concentration are available in 50 mL, 75 mL, and 100 mL bottles. If the substitution to the insured strength is made, which bottle size will be dispensed, what will the new signa (sig) be, and how much should remain after 7 days?

Step 1 Since 1 tsp equals 5 mL, one dose of the prescribed Augmentin would equal 125 mg. Calculate the volume of Augmentin 250 mg/5 mL needed to provide the prescribed 125 mg dose. Set up a dimensional analysis equation multiplying the prescribed strength by the number of milliliters of insured concentration:

$$y\ \text{mL} = 125\ \text{mg} \times \frac{5\ \text{mL}}{250\ \text{mg}} = 2.5\ \text{mL}$$

$$y\ \text{mL} = 2.5\ \text{mL}$$

The sig in the computer prescription must be changed to read, "Take 2.5 mL 3 times daily for 7 days."

Step 2 Calculate the volume needed per day for 7 days.

$$2.5\ \text{mL} \times \frac{3}{\text{day}} \times 7\ \text{days} = 52.5\ \text{mL}$$

Step 3 Select the 75 mL bottle of Augmentin and subtract the days, supply of 52.5 mL

$$75\ \text{mL} - 52.5\ \text{mL} = 22.5\ \text{mL}$$

So, 22.5 mL will remain. Some overage is allowed by insurance, so this bottle is appropriate. If the 50 mL size is incorrectly chosen, there would not be enough, and if the 100 mL was chosen, then 47.5 mL would be wasted, and the claim would likely not be processed. In the unlikely event it were approved, the claim could be reversed, so the pharmacy would not be reimbursed for dispensing more medication than necessary.

Practice Tip

A metric dosing spoon should be dispensed with oral solutions and suspensions.

Otic and Ophthalmic Calculation Challenges

Study Idea

Technicians can practice calculating the number of drops in different solutions and suspensions using 20 drops per mL of solution and 15 drops per mL of suspension.

Certain drug formulations, such as ear (otic) and ophthalmic solutions and suspensions, are particularly challenging to calculate when determining days' supply. Many are available in both a solution and a suspension formulation. When calculating drops for a solution, the standard measure is equivalent to 20 drops (gtt) per mL. For example, suppose that a prescription was written for Cortisporin otic solution, *4 drops into affected ear 3 times a day for 7 days*, or *12 gtt daily for 7 days*. That would equal 84 solution drops. The 5 mL package size (providing 100 gtt) would be dispensed.

However, suspension drops, because they are thicker in density, have fewer drops per mL than solutions. In the past, the measure was 16 gtt of suspension to 1 mL, but since IV drops go in rates of 10, 15, and 20 gtt per minute, there has been a movement toward standardization to round down the measurement to 15 gtt of suspension per mL rather than round up to 16. The suspension drop rate now depends on individual pharmacy and insurance reimbursement policies, but most often it is 15 gtt/mL.

Compounding-related dilution equations and examples will be covered in Chapter 6 on nonsterile compounding and Chapter 7 on sterile and hazardous compounding.

Calculations for inventory and other retail math will be covered in Chapter 8. In all calculations and conversions, the most important thing is practice, practice, practice to build up confidence!

Review and Assessment

STUDY SUMMARY

Calculations are an important component of certification exams. Technicians should memorize the formulas for converting temperatures between Fahrenheit and Celsius systems. It is important that they are confident converting times from the 12-hour clock to the 24-hour clock and back.

Technicians should also memorize the amounts for converting the most common apothecary, avoirdupois, and household measurements into the metric system. They can converting between proportionally larger or smaller units of metric measurement.

Most pharmacy calculations for dosages and concentrations can be easily set up in ratio-proportion or dimensional analysis equations. Technicians should practice both calculating techniques, and utilize them to solve and check your answers. Dilution and other complex calculations add some more steps of simple math. For practice, they can start with the end of chapter questions found on Cirrus. Technicians should carefully read each test question to identify what is being asked and in what units and be prepared to interpret concentration percentages and utilize them in calculations.

ADDITIONAL RESOURCES

For more in-depth explanations, check out *Pharmacy Calculations for Technicians*, Seventh Edition from Paradigm Education Solutions. To master and extend the material presented in this chapter, take advantage of the resources available through the eBook resources links. These include digital supplements, study resources, and a practice exam generator with 1,000+ exam-style questions. End-of-chapter tests are accessible through the eBook for individuals using the self-study course and through Cirrus for individuals enrolled in the instructor-guided course.

6

Nonsterile Compounding

Learning Objectives

1 Discuss guidelines for nonsterile compounding processes in *USP* Chapter <795>. (Section 6.1)

2 Know the documentation requirements for nonsterile compounding. (Section 6.1)

3 Understand the steps of preparing a nonsterile compounded product. (Section 6.1)

4 Know the commonly compounded nonsterile dosage forms and techniques used in nonsterile compounding. (Section 6.1)

5 Identify the equipment and supplies for nonsterile compounding. (Section 6.1)

6 Know how to use and maintain the balances used in nonsterile compounding. (Section 6.1)

7 Understand how to calculate concentrations for nonsterile compounding, including using the processes of geometric dilution and alligation. (Section 6.2)

8 Understand how to determine a product's stability, including beyond-use dates and signs of incompatibility. (Section 6.2)

9 Identify additional labeling requirements for nonsterile compounded products. (Section 6.2)

Access eBook links for resources and an exam generator, with 1,000+ questions.

The purpose of this chapter is to provide the pharmacy technician with knowledge of the basic skills involved in compounding simple and moderately complex nonsterile pharmaceuticals. Domain 4 of the PTCE includes nonsterile compounding. Nonsterile compounding is also included in domain 3 of the ExCPT. Complex nonsterile compounding is done by specialty pharmacies, and a pharmacy technician would need advanced training and may be required to have compounding certification to work in this environment.

Compounding is defined by the FDA as "the extemporaneous combining, mixing, or altering of ingredients by a pharmacist in response to a physician's prescription to create a medication tailored to the specialized medical needs of an individual patient." Nonsterile compounding may only legally be done to create a drug preparation that is not commercially available to meet a specific medication prescription or order.

A community pharmacy is not allowed to manufacture bulk quantities of product for sale, although the pharmacy can prepare an excess amount for refills and similar prescriptions in a short time period. This practice is called **anticipatory compounding**, and it is legal as long as the excess product is properly labeled with the assigned lot number, ingredients, and a short-term beyond-use date (BUD) which is usually six months or less.

6.1 Types of Nonsterile Compounding

For a high-grade, nonsterile compounded product, correct professional procedures and policies must be followed with quality control measures, documentation, and recordkeeping. To achieve this compounding technicians must follow *USP Chapter <795>* Pharmaceutical Compounding–Nonsterile Preparations for the preparation, dispensing, and administration of these products to humans and animals.

USP Chapter <795> classifies nonsterile compounding into three categories:

Study Idea

Categories of non sterile compounding are determined by *USP* <795> which takes into account the master formulation record, stability data, requirements for special calculations, and the need for advanced compounding training.

- **Simple nonsterile compounding** is for making a preparation from a *USP*-recommended formulation record or from a peer-reviewed journal article in which the components, procedure, equipment, and stability data are clearly specified. Simple nonsterile compounding also includes reconstituting or using commercial products that require adding one or more ingredients as directed by the manufacturer. Examples include captopril oral solution and benzoyl peroxide / erythromycin topical gel.
- **Moderate nonsterile compounding** requires special calculations or procedures for preparing the individual product or individual dosage units, or for determining the stability data. Examples include morphine sulfate suppositories, diphenhydramine troches, or two manufactured mixed creams together for which stability of the mixture must be determined.
- **Complex nonsterile compounding** requires special technician training, facilities, equipment, and procedures. Examples include transdermal dosage forms, modified-release preparations, and some inserts and suppositories for systemic effect.

In addition, technicians need to follow all the guidelines of the facility's policy and procedure (P&P) manual and Occupational Safety and Health Administration (OSHA) requirements. To compound nonsterile drug products with hazardous substances, technicians must have additional training on the storage, handling, and disposal of these chemicals as described in *USP* Chapter <800>. For animal-oriented preparations, technicians must also follow the rules of the American Veterinary Medical Association's (AVMA) *Guidelines for Veterinary Prescription Drugs*, at CertExam5e .ParadigmEducation.com/AVMA).

Basic Nonsterile Compounding Steps

It is important for the pharmacy to have a separate, designated compounding area that is removed from excessive traffic and air flow that might interfere with the accuracy of the balance and disturb stock powders. The dedicated area must be well-maintained, neat, clean, and uncluttered, with sufficient workspace and storage. If compounded pharmaceuticals are stored in a refrigerator or freezer, the temperature must be recorded at least daily to ensure proper storage conditions are maintained.

According to *USP <795>*, compounding pharmacy technicians must wear appropriate clean compounding garb, including hair covers, gowns, gloves, face masks, shoe covers, aprons, or other items depending upon what is necessary for protection from chemical exposure and for prevention of drug contamination. Additional personal protective equipment (PPE) can be identified from OSHA guidelines and the relevant Safety Data Sheet (SDS). Compounding garb should not be worn outside the compounding area.

Compounding technicians should wash their hands with soap and warm water, rubbing their hands together vigorously for a thorough cleaning before putting on gloves.

Compounding begins when the prescription is entered into the computer so that it can be checked against the patient profile for the Drug Utilization Review (DUR). The pharmacist then selects the proper **Master Formulation Record** (compounding recipe) to fit the prescription and patient needs. An overview of the full process is provided in Table 6.1, and

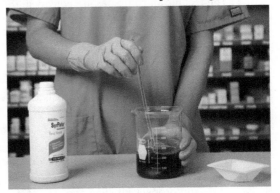

A pharmacy technicians often wear scrubs or a lab coat, gloves, and a hairnet when preparing nonsterile products.

the components of a Master Formulation Record are provided in Table 6.2. During compounding, only one product should be made at a time, and the equipment and compounding area should be cleaned before starting another preparation.

TABLE 6.1 Steps in the Compounding Process

1. The pharmacist judges the suitability of the prescription for appropriateness of dose, safety, and intended use, and accesses the results of the Drug Utilization Review (DUR), resolving issues.

2. The pharmacist reviews the technician's selection for the Master Formulation Record in the computer and approves or modifies the technician's selection. (See Table 6.2 for the components.)

3. The technician generates a Compounding Record (or log sheet) from the Master Formulation Record to make the nonsterile preparation. (See Table 6.3 for a description of requirements for a Compounding Record. Figure 6.1 is an example of a Compounding Record for Magic Mouthwash.)

4. The technician performs all necessary mathematical calculations for ingredient quantities and BUD and identifies the necessary equipment; the pharmacist double-checks all calculations.

5. The technician generates the medication label with computer software using information in the Compounding Record. The label includes the following:
   a. patient name
   b. prescriber name
   c. date of compounding
   d. name of preparation
   e. prescription and/or extemporaneous compounding ID or lot number
   f. BUD
   g. directions for use, including any special storage conditions
   h. any additional requirements of state or federal law
   i. initials of compounding technician and pharmacist.

6. The technician gathers all necessary active and inactive ingredients and prepares and calibrates any measuring equipment.

7. The pharmacy technician uses appropriate protective clothing and hand-washing technique.

continues

TABLE 6.1 Steps in the Compounding Process —Continued

8. The technician weighs all ingredients for the preparation, initials each step, and adds documentation (such as source, lot or batch number, expiration date, and National Drug Code [NDC] number) to the Compounding Record for the pharmacist to check before ingredients are combined.

9. The technician combines ingredients in the proper order and method according to the Master Formulation Record and stores the medication in a proper container for application, storage, and UV light protection.

10. The technician generates and affixes the medication label and pharmacist-recommended auxiliary labels to the proper container.

11. The pharmacist reviews the Compounding Record and labels, and assesses appropriate physical characteristics of the preparation, such as any weight variations, adequacy of mixing, clarity, odor, color, consistency, and pH.

12. The pharmacist signs and dates the Compounding Record and/or prescription, and files the records (computer entry and printed copy).

13. The technician places the compounded preparation in proper storage and notifies the patient for pickup.

14. The technician cleans all equipment thoroughly and promptly, reshelving all active and inactive ingredients, and properly labeling and storing any excess preparation.

15. The technician refers the patient to pharmacist counseling at the time of pickup.

TABLE 6.2 Components of the Master Formulation Record

1. Official or assigned product name, strength, and dosage form
2. Calculations needed to determine and verify quantities of components and doses of active pharmaceutical ingredients (APIs)
3. Description of all ingredients and their quantities
4. Compatibility and stability information, including references when available
5. Equipment needed to prepare the preparation, when appropriate
6. Mixing instructions, which include order of mixing, mixing temperature and other environmental controls, duration of mixing, and other factors relevant to replication of the product
7. Sample labeling information, that—in addition to legally required information—should contain: generic name and quantity or concentration of each active ingredient, assigned BUD, storage conditions, and prescription or control number, whichever is applicable
8. Container used in dispensing
9. Packaging and storage requirements
10. Description of the final preparation
11. Quality control procedures and expected results

Source: *USP* <795>

Study Idea

Know when a Master Formulation Record, SDS, and Compounding Record, are needed for nonsterile compounding.

Once the Master Formulation Record, or recipe, has been determined or approved by the pharmacist, the technician gathers the ingredients according to the record. The pharmacy must use high-grade chemicals and ingredients that meet US Pharmacopeia–National Formulary (USP–NF) guidelines for compounding. An SDS should be on file for every chemical stored in the pharmacy to facilitate the safe cleanup of any accidental spills or contamination. (More information on SDSs is in Chapter 7, Sterile and Hazardous Compounding.) An eyewash station should also be readily available.

Water used in compounding preparations must be purified. Sterile water is acceptable because it has been purified. To document the purified water, include the source, lot number, and BUD. Rinse equipment with purified water as required by *USP <795>*.

To ensure a high-quality product is produced each time, it is necessary to document the proper quantities and sequences were used to make the product. From the Master Formulation Record, the technician generates the **Compounding Record** (or log), which is filled in with the specific information from that instance of compounding. (See Table 6.3 for the required components of a Compounding Record.) This documentation is required each time a product is made, unique for each prescription. A specific prescription and/or extemporaneous compounding lot number must be assigned to each Compounding Record, so the compound can always be traced to its date and particular process. The Compounding Record contains the relevant calculations, notes on special equipment used, ingredient lot numbers and expiration dates, and the initials of the compounding technician and the pharmacist who checked the technician's work. For an example, see the Magic Mouthwash Compounding Record shown in Figure 6.1.

After the product is compounded, a beyond-use date (BUD) must be determined. The BUD is the date after which the compounded product should not be used, and it is calculated from the date the product was compounded and according to *USP <795>* guidelines.

TABLE 6.3 Components of a Compounding Record

1. Official or assigned product name, strength, and dosage form
2. Master Formulation Record reference for the preparation
3. Names and quantities of all components
4. Sources, lot numbers, and expiration dates of components
5. Total quantity compounded
6. The names of the person who prepared the preparation, the person who performed the quality control procedures, and the pharmacist who approved the preparation
7. Date of preparation
8. Assigned lot or prescription number
9. Assigned BUD
10. Duplicate label as described in the Master Formulation Record
11. Description of final preparation
12. Results of quality control procedures (e.g., weight range of filled capsules, pH of aqueous liquids)
13. Documentation of any quality control issues and any adverse reactions or preparation problems reported by the patient or caregiver

Source: *USP <795>*

FIGURE 6.1
Compounding Record for Magic Mouthwash

Patient Name _____   Date Prepared <u>12/2/20XX</u> _____

Rx # _____   Master Formulation Record # _____

Compounding Record for Magic Mouthwash

Ingredient Name	Amount Needed	Manufacturer	NDC #	Lot #	Expiration Date	Prepared By	Checked By
Lidocaine 2% viscous	60 mL	HiTech	50838-0775-04		12/10/20XX		
Diphenhydramine 12.5 mg/5 mL	60 mL	Walgreens	00363-0379-34		07/12/20XX		
Mylanta, generic	60 mL	Qualitest	00603-0712-57		03/12/20XX		
Nystatin suspension	60 mL	Qualitest	00603-1481-58		09/11/20XX		
Total quantity	240 mL						

Prepared by _____

Quality Control checked by _____

Approved by _____

Date and lot number _____

BUD_____

Directions _____

Auxiliary Labeling: SHAKE WELL

_____

Commonly Compounded Dosage Forms

A **tablet** is a solid dosage form made from dry powdered ingredients. The powdered ingredients are mixed together and then pressed together with a single punch tablet press. Compression tablets require expensive equipment and special expertise, and are labor intensive. They are not commonly made in the community pharmacy.

A **capsule** contains the active and inactive ingredients encased in a hard shell made of gelatin, sugar, and water. The capsule shell consists of two parts: (1) the body, which is the longer narrower part; and (2) the cap, which is the short part that fits over the body. Capsules come in standard sizes indicated by numbers: 5, 4, 3, 2, 1, 0, 00, and 000. The largest capsule size is 000, and it can contain up to 1,000 mg of medication. The smallest capsule size is 5, and it can contain up to 100 mg (depending on the substance).

Two methods for filling capsules are the manual punch method and the capsule machine. In either method, the capsule body is filled with the compounded powdered ingredients, and the cap is placed over the body and pressed down to seal the capsule.

A **solution** is a liquid dosage form in which an active ingredient, the *solute*, is dissolved in a liquid vehicle, the *solvent*. A solution may contain a liquid or powdered solute. The solvent can be aqueous (water based), alcoholic, or hydroalcoholic. Solutions can be for oral administration or topical administration, such as an otic solution for earwax softening. Simple syrup is a common aqueous solution in which 85 g of sucrose is dissolved in 100 mL of purified water.

Study Idea

Commonly used suspending agents include tragacanth, acacia, and carboxymethylcellulose.

A **suspension** is a liquid dosage form in which the solute is not dissolved in the solvent but dispersed throughout the liquid vehicle. Since the active ingredient may settle in a suspension, the pharmacy technician should always include a "Shake Well" auxiliary label on the compounded products label.

The order of mixing ingredients is important to prevent clumping, also known as **agglomeration** (or flocculation), of the active ingredients. Additionally, the tablet or powder must be vigorously triturated (see "Common Techniques for Ingredient Preparation and Blending," on page 201) before adding to the suspending agent and the final liquid vehicle.

A **troche**, which is also known as a lozenge, is used for buccal administration, or absorption by the mucous membranes into the blood vessels in the cheek. The active ingredients in powder form for troches gummies, and lollipops are slowly added to a liquid base with other formulated ingredients, which are heated and poured into a mold to cool into shape. They are used for pain relief, bioidentical hormones, and the antifungal drug clotrimazole, among other uses.

An **ointment** is a **water-in-oil (w/o) emulsion** that is usually greasy and not water washable. An occlusive ointment holds moisture in the skin for hydration. Emollient-based ointments, such as bath oils, are more softening to the skin. It is best to use water-repellant plastic equipment to compound an ointment.

A **cream** is generally an **oil-in-water (o/w) emulsion** that is nonocclusive, nongreasy, and water washable. A cream is best prepared using glass equipment. Creams may be made in a glass mortar and pestle.

A **lotion** is generally a liquid suspension or an oil-in-water emulsion used topically where lubrication is desired, such as on the skin or scalp. A lotion is similar to a cream but thinner in consistency. Calamine for poison ivy is an example of a commercially available suspension lotion.

Much like a suspension, a **gel** contains solid particles in a liquid, but the liquid is thickened with gelatin or another agent, and the particles are fine or ultrafine.

For ointments, creams, lotions and gels, the goal is not only an accurate, safe, and effective preparation, but also a **pharmaceutically elegant product**, which is smooth and without visible flaws. To create a pharmaceutically elegant ointment, add the active ingredients in small amounts and constantly work the mixture into the ointment base with a spatula on an ointment slab. Automated ointment mills are available that maximize the mixing of ingredients to improve the final preparation.

A **suppository** is a solid dosage form that has the active ingredient placed in a water-soluble base (like glycerinated gelatin or polyethylene glycol) or oleaginous base (like cocoa butter). Suppositories are inserted into body orifices, such as the rectum, vagina, or urethra, and they melt at body temperature to release the active ingredient. A suppository mold is used to shape the dosage form, or it is molded by hand. The suppository's shape and size is determined by the site of administration. Refrigeration of the final product is usually necessary to maintain shape and stability.

Nonsterile Compounding Equipment

Study Idea

Never touch the weights with your hands. Always use the forceps to transfer weights to and from the balance.

Before each compounding session, scales and measures should be checked and calibrated for accuracy. Many state boards of pharmacy (BOP) list the minimum equipment necessary for a licensed pharmacy, including a scale, spatulas, graduated cylinders, compounding slabs, storage containers, and mortar and pestle.

Measuring and Weighing Instruments

A **digital electronic analytical balance** is the easiest to use and most accurate scale, but it is expensive and may not be available in some community pharmacies. Most pharmacies have a **Class III prescription balance** (formerly called a Class A balance), which is a two-pan mechanical balance that uses pharmaceutical weights of various sizes to weigh small amounts of materials, as shown in Figure 6.2.

Typical weight sets include metric and apothecary weights, though the apothecary weights are rarely used. Metric weights vary in size, from 10 mg to 100 g. They should be stored in their original box and only handled with the forceps provided to prevent the transfer of hand oil that can result in inaccurate measurements. Pans should always be covered with weighing papers or boats to prevent damage that could cause inaccuracies.

A larger scale, called a **counterbalance**, is used to weigh heavier amounts up to 5 kg.

FIGURE 6.2
Weighing with a Class III Prescription Balance

(a) After the scale is level and locked, transfer weights with forceps to the right pan and ingredients to the left. (b) Make final measurement, and check with the cover down.

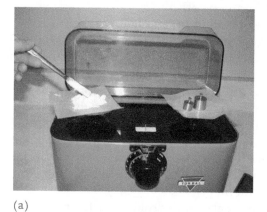
(a)

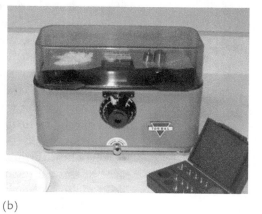
(b)

Mixing Instruments

A **spatula** is used to transfer solid dosage forms to weighing pans and for other tasks, such as preparing ointments and creams or loosening material from the surface of a mortar and transferring to a container. Spatulas may be made of plastic, rubber, or stainless steel. Hard rubber is used for corrosive materials like iodine or mercuric salts.

A **compounding slab**, or ointment slab, is a plate made of glass, which is smooth, hard, and nonabsorbent. The slab is used to evenly mix the ingredients of an ointment or cream by using a process called spatulation (see detailed definition below). Ointments and creams are stored in ointment jars that range in size from one ounce to one pound, or they are put into tubes. Ointment pads, made of parchment paper, are also used in preparing ointments and creams. The paper improves the ease of transferring the compounded product to its dispensing container.

A **mortar and pestle** is used for grinding and mixing pharmaceutical ingredients. Both the mortar and pestle can be made of glass or porcelain. The coarser the mortar surface, the finer the triturating (grinding) of the powder or crystal. The glass variety is used to mix liquids, and the porcelain type is used to grind crystals, granules, and powders. High-volume compounding pharmacies may have an electric mortar and pestle for grinding and mixing.

Cylinders, **pipettes**, and **beakers**, which are made of glass or polypropylene, are used to measure liquids. They are calibrated in metric and apothecary units. Out of all the volumetric equipment, graduated cylinders are considered to be the most accurate for measuring. Beakers are used for mixing, pipettes are used to measure volumes less than 1.5 mL, and cylinders are used for measuring larger volumes.

Miscellaneous Equipment

Depending on the amount of compounding done on site, the pharmacy may have other equipment, including a convection oven, single-punch tablet press, pellet press, or capsule machine. These facilitate making tablet, pellet, and capsule dosage forms.

Common Techniques for Ingredient Preparation and Blending

Comminution is the act of reducing the particle sizes of ingredients through various methods, including trituration, pulverization by intervention, levigation, and heating and dissolving for the purposes of integration.

- **Trituration** is the process of rubbing, grinding, or pulverizing a substance to create a finer particle. Minimal pressure and rotating of a pestle in a mortar grinds the ingredients into a powder. Trituration can also be used to combine two or more powders to standardize the powder blend.
- **Pulverization by intervention** reduces the particle size of a substance with the aid of an additional ingredient in which that substance is soluble. A volatile solvent like camphor, alcohol, iodine, or ether, is often used in the process. Only a small amount of the solvent is used, and then it is allowed to evaporate, so it is not part of the final product.
- **Levigation** is used to further reduce particle size of a solid during ointment preparation. A levigating agent, such as castor oil, glycerin, propylene glycol, or mineral oil, is slowly added to the large particles of dry ingredients in a glass mortar or on an ointment slab to wet (but not dissolve) the powder. The resulting paste is triturated with a mortar and pestle, and then added to the ointment base.
- **Heating and dissolving** involves applying gentle heat to dissolve a solid ingredient that is not easily dissolved. This allows for more uniformity and less precipitation.

Blending is the process of combining two substances, but it does not include any particle reduction. There are many methods of blending, including spatulation, sifting, tumbling, and geometric dilution.

Study Idea

Be able to identify each nonsterile preparation action in terms of the relative particle size being reduced or blended.

- **Spatulation** is the process of blending substances with a spatula. This is useful for fine powder mixing and mixing powders into an ointment base.
- **Sifting** is the mixing of powders using a fine wire mesh sieve. The powder is poured into an appropriate particle size sieve, and a rubber spatula is used to force the powder through the sieve and onto glassine paper.
- **Tumbling** is used to mix or blend powders with a container, such as a resealable plastic bag or glass bottle. After the powders are added, the container is rotated or tumbled to mix the powders.
- **Geometric dilution** is a method for combining two or more ingredients of differing strengths into an ointment or cream base. The ingredients are added a little at a time. The most potent ingredient (often the ingredient in the smallest quantity) is placed into the mortar first, then an equal amount of diluent is added before mixing well. The process is repeated by adding the second ingredient and an equal amount of diluent, and then mixing. This process occurs for each ingredient until all have been integrated effectively. Any small amount of leftover diluent should be added at the end and mixed well. This creates a smooth dispersion of drug(s) in the cream or ointment base.

Study Idea

Geometric dilution is used to prepare pharmaceutically elegant ointments, creams, and lotions.

To review how geometric dilution is calculated and combined, see Example 6.1.

Example 6.1

A prescription for 60 g of an ointment is to be compounded. It has three active ingredients: hydrocortisone powder, zinc oxide powder, and a hydrophilic ointment, in a ratio of 1:3:6. Calculate how many grams of each ingredient will be needed, and explain how to use the geometric dilution method for compounding these ingredients into a pharmaceutically elegant product.

Step 1 Find the total number of parts in the ointment, then find the weight per part.

$$\text{total parts} = 1 \text{ part} + 3 \text{ parts} + 6 \text{ parts} = 10 \text{ parts}$$

$$\text{weight per part} = \frac{60 \text{ g}}{10 \text{ parts}} = 6 \text{ g per part}$$

Step 2 Find the weight of each ingredient needed for the compounded ointment.

$$\text{grams of hydrocortisone powder needed} = 1 \text{ part} \times \frac{6 \text{ g}}{1 \text{ part}} = 6 \text{ g}$$

$$\text{grams of zinc oxide powder needed} = 3 \text{ parts} \times \frac{6 \text{ g}}{1 \text{ part}} = 18 \text{ g}$$

$$\text{grams of hydrophilic ointment needed} = 6 \text{ parts} \times \frac{6 \text{ g}}{1 \text{ part}} = 36 \text{ g}$$

Answer: To compound 60 g of prescribed ointment, 6 g of hydrocortisone powder, 18 g of zinc oxide powder, and 36 g of hydrophilic ointment are needed.

The method for geometric dilution for the prescribed ointment will be:

1. Put 6 g of hydrocortisone powder onto an ointment slab, add 6 g of hydrophilic ointment, and spatulate.

2. Put 18 g of zinc oxide powder on a different ointment slab, add 18 g of hydrophilic ointment, and spatulate.

3. Spatulate the hydrocortisone-ointment mixture and the zinc oxide-ointment mixture together.

4. Add the remaining 12 g of hydrophilic ointment to the mixture, and spatulate into the final product.

6.2 Compounding Calculations

Study Idea

Go back to Chapter 5 and review ratio and proportion calculations.

Pharmacy technicians need to do many calculations when creating nonsterile compounds. They need to convert dosages or ingredients from one measurement system to another, or calculate how to dilute medications or combine ingredients in the correct proportions. In the pharmacy profession, the term **ratio strength** refers to the concentration level of an active ingredient to a completed product. Solutions made of two or more liquids are described as **volume-in-volume** concentrations, such as mL/mL. (Compounding with solutions and using dilution and volume-in-volume calculations are often done in sterile compounding and will be addressed in Chapter 7.)

Solutions with powdered ingredients and suspensions are described as **weight-in-volume**, such as g/mL, and solids and gels are described as **weight-in-weight**, such as g/g. Proportion equations are often used for these calculations.

Calculating with Concentration Percentage Ratios

Ointments and creams use a percent concentration, which is defined as the percentage weight of the active ingredient per 100 g of the final drug formulation (cream or ointment). For example, a 2.5% hydrocortisone cream is equal to 2.5 g of active ingredient (hydrocortisone) per each 100 g of cream. Percentage concentrations are handled the same as for weight-in-volume percentages, except that the units of measure are all weights, either milligrams or grams (as reviewed in Chapter 5). To see how concentration percentages are applied in nonsterile compounding, study Example 6.2.

Example 6.2

A prescription for 4 oz of medicated lotion is to be compounded. The prescription is to contain 10% menthol and 2% camphor (active ingredients) in Lubriderm lotion (diluent). How many grams of each active ingredient and diluent are needed?

Step 1 Convert the prescribed weight from ounces to grams (1 oz = 30 g).

$$4 \text{ oz} \times \frac{30 \text{ g}}{1 \text{ oz}} = 120 \text{ g}$$

Step 2 Using the ratio-proportion method, determine the weight (in grams) of 10% menthol and 2% camphor needed.

10% menthol:

$$\frac{y \text{ g}}{120 \text{ g}} = \frac{10 \text{ g}}{100 \text{ g}}$$

$$y \text{ g} \times 10 = 120 \text{ g}$$

$$\frac{y \text{ g} \times 10}{10} = \frac{120 \text{ g}}{10}$$

$$y \text{ g} = 12 \text{ g}$$

2% camphor:

$$\frac{z \text{ g}}{120 \text{ g}} = \frac{2 \text{ g}}{100 \text{ g}}$$

$$z \text{ g} \times 100 = 240 \text{ g}$$

$$\frac{z \text{ g} \times 100}{100} = \frac{240 \text{ g}}{100}$$

$$z \text{ g} = 2.4 \text{ g}$$

Step 3 Determine the amount of Lubriderm lotion needed for the 120 g preparation.

12 g menthol + 2.4 g camphor = 14.4 g total active ingredients

120 g total preparation − 14.4 g active ingredients = 105.6 g Lubriderm lotion

Answer: To dispense 4 oz of the prescribed medicated lotion, 12 g of 10% menthol and 2.4 g of 2% camphor should be added to 105.6 g of Lubriderm lotion.

This preparation can be integrated using geometric dilution: (1) mix 12 g menthol with 12 g Lubriderm lotion; (2) mix 2.4 g camphor with 2.4 g Lubriderm lotion; (3) mix the menthol-Lubriderm mixture and the camphor-Lubriderm mixture together; (4) mix in the remaining Lubriderm lotion.

Using the Alligation Method to Combine More than One Concentration for a New Concentration

Physicians often prescribe concentrations of medications that are not commercially available, and these prescriptions must be prepared by integrating two different concentrations of the same active ingredient, one higher and one lower, for a midrange concentration. This process, called **alligation**, is used in nonsterile and sterile compounding for mixing varied concentrations of solutions, mixtures, creams, ointments, or other products. The resulting concentration will be greater than the weaker strength but less than the stronger strength.

The principles used to solve alligation problems remain the same regardless of the media combined (e.g., liquid, semisolid, or even solid). An alligation box is a useful tool to help visualize the process. By the end, the boxes look like a tic-tac-toe grid, which is why alligation is sometimes called *tic-tac-toe math*. See Example 6.3 for a step-by-step alligation problem.

Example 6.3

How many grams of a 10% urea cream and a 60% urea cream should be mixed to prepare 100 g of a 40% urea cream?

Step 1   To set up an alligation box, place the final concentration (40%) in the middle of the tic-tac-toe grid. Place the higher concentration (60%) in the upper left corner. Place the lower concentration (10%) in the lower left corner.

Step 2   Draw a diagonal line from the upper left higher concentration through the middle with the final concentration to the bottom right. Write the difference between 60% and 40% (20) in the bottom right corner.

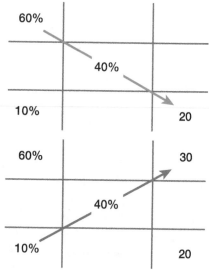

Step 3   Repeat the process for the lower concentration solution, subtracting the lower strength concentration (10%) from the final strength (40%). Write the difference in the top right corner.

Step 4   At this point, read across the lines from left to right to find the relative contributions of each concentration. You will note:

- The *30* at the top right represents how many parts are needed of the 60% urea cream to the final mixture.
- The *20* on the bottom right represents the parts of the 10% cream needed.

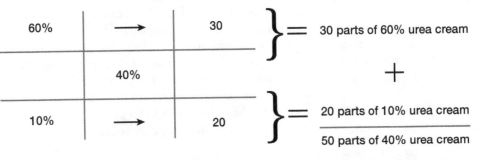

Study Idea

Always reread the question and see what it is really asking you to calculate.

- There will always be more parts of the ingredient that is closest to the final concentration than the other. Because 60% is closest to 40%, it will have more parts than that of the 10%. This has been demonstrated, with 30 parts of the 60% and 20 of the 10%.

Study Idea

Remember that in an alligation, the ingredient that is closest to the concentration of the final product will be added in the highest amount. Any answer that doesn't fit this guide can be eliminated.

You have worked out the alligation. Now return to the question. It asks to see how much of each concentration is needed for 100 g of the prescribed 40% lotion. Since grams are the measurement unit being used for urea cream, you can convert the parts into grams in the final equation.

Step 5 To calculate the contribution of the 60% concentration, put it in a dimensional analysis equation with the first ingredient.

$$y = \frac{30 \text{ parts}}{50 \text{ parts}} \times 100 \text{ g}$$

$$y = \frac{300 \text{ g}}{5}$$

$$y = 60 \text{ g}$$

Step 6 At this point, you can either do another dimensional analysis equation with the second ingredient, or you can subtract the first ingredient from the final weight to determine the amount.

final weight − first ingredient weight = remaining ingredient weight

100 g total − 60 g of 60% urea cream = 40 g of 10% urea cream

Answer: 60 g of 60% urea cream should be mixed with 40 g of 10% urea cream to create 100 g of the prescribed 40% urea cream.

On an exam, you could also have used logic and the process of elimination to cancel out any unlikely answer choices. Eliminating the distractor answers is a helpful way to narrow the choices and improve the likelihood of correctly answering the question. Look at the prescribed concentration (40%). Is 40% closer to the higher concentration (60%) or the lower concentration (10%)? Since the 40% concentration is closer to the 60% prescribed, more of that will be used. Any answer in which the amount of 10% solution is equal to or greater than the amount of 60% solution used could not be correct.

Determining Beyond-Use Date

After the product is compounded, a BUD must be determined according to the stability of the compound as determined by *USP* guidelines and those of the manufacturer for each ingredient. Many compounded products have adequate stability information from the Master Formulation Record to allow for assignment of a BUD based on the expiration dates and stability of the manufactured ingredients.

In the absence of stability data, *USP* <795> has established maximum BUD recommendations for nonsterile compounded drug preparations that are packaged in tight, light-resistant containers and stored at controlled room temperatures. The BUD may never be later than the expiration date on the label of any component of the preparation. See Table 6.4 for *USP* <795> BUD guidelines. Example 6.4 shows how to determine the BUD for a nonsterile compounded preparation.

TABLE 6.4 Beyond-Use Dates by Type of Formulation

- **For nonaqueous formulations:** The BUD is not later than the time remaining until the earliest expiration date of the active ingredient or six months, whichever is earlier.
- **For water-based oral formulations:** The BUD is not later than 14 days when stored at controlled cold temperature.
- **For water-based topical/dermal, and mucosal liquid, and semisolid formulations:** The BUD is not later than 30 days.

Study Idea

Remember that, legally, the pharmacist must have a discussion with the patient on the use of the preparation for each compounded product dispensed.

Example 6.4

On March 24, 2021, the following ingredients are used to compound a topical analgesic. What would be the BUD for the final product?

Drug	Drug Source	Expiration Date
Ketoprofen powder	Bulk chemical	Dec. 2021
Lidocaine powder	Bulk chemical	Aug. 2021
Petrolatum	Bulk chemical	Mar. 2022

Answer: Since none of the ingredients are aqueous, we can calculate the BUD as not later than the time remaining on the earliest expiring ingredient or six months from the compounding date, whichever is earlier. Six months after the date of compounding is August 24, 2021. In this scenario six months from compounding and the earliest expiration of an ingredient are the same. The BUD is August 2021.

6.3 Completing Nonsterile Compounding

During the compounding process, the technician must have the pharmacist check the compounding process and preparation on at least three key material points:

- Beginning: prescription, DUR, and Master Formulation Record
- Middle: calculations and measurements before mixing
- End: Compounding Record, label, product integrity, and auxiliary labels.

The technician is responsible for accurate and thorough documentation of each step on the Compounding Record. The pharmacist also verifies that the final product looks, smells, and feels correct. If it is an ointment cream, lotion, or gel, it should be pharmaceutically elegant. If it is a solution, it must not have clumps or precipitation.

When the label is applied, it must include the necessary information (as listed in Table 6.5). The pharmacist will choose the proper auxiliary labels and approve of the patient education materials that the technician has printed out. After this, the technician handles the proper product storage and cleanup. At prescription pickup, the technician must also make sure the patient receives counseling on the drug's use and potential side effects and warnings from the pharmacist.

TABLE 6.5 Nonsterile Compounding Label

A nonsterile compounding label includes the following:

- patient's name
- physician's name
- date of compounding
- name of preparation
- prescription and/or extemporaneous compounding lot number
- BUD
- initials of compounding technician and pharmacist
- directions for use, including any special storage conditions
- additional requirements of state or federal law

Note: The pharmacist selects appropriate auxiliary labels.

Review and Assessment

STUDY SUMMARY

Nonsterile compounding is the extemporaneous combining, mixing, or altering of ingredients to create a medication tailored to the specialized medical needs of an individual patient. Pharmacy technicians must be knowledgeable about the requirements in *USP <795>* as it relates to nonsterile compounding.

As you study for the exam, review the guidelines for garbing in personal protective equipment (PPE), handwashing, correct use and maintenance of equipment, and how to calculate a preparation's BUD. Know the basic steps from prescription receipt to final packaging and storage to patient dispensing. Be able to differentiate between the Master Formulation Record and Compounding Record, and the importance of both. Master the calculations and steps necessary to integrate ingredients with appropriate methods for a pharmaceutically elegant product.

ADDITIONAL RESOURCES

For more in-depth explanations, check out *Pharmacy Practice for Technicians,* Seventh Edition and *Pharmacy Labs for Technicians,* Fourth Edition from Paradigm Education Solutions. To master and extend the material presented in this chapter, take advantage of the resources available through the eBook resources links. These include digital supplements, study resources, and a practice exam generator with 1,000+ exam-style questions. End-of-chapter tests are accessible through the eBook for individuals using the self-study course and through Cirrus for individuals enrolled in the instructor-guided course.

7

Sterile and Hazardous Compounding

Learning Objectives

1 Discuss *United States Pharmacopeial Convention* (USP) guidelines for sterile and hazardous drug compounding processes. (Section 7.1)

2 Differentiate between the different types of parenteral administration and common sterile and hazardous products. (Section 7.1)

3 Know the components of medication orders and the requirements for labeling and documentation of sterile and hazardous compounding. (Section 7.5)

4 Identify the equipment (including personal protective equipment) and supplies for sterile compounding. (Section 7.2)

5 Know the requirements of personal protective equipment and aseptic technique for sterile compounding. (Section 7.2)

6 Know how to clean, maintain, and use sterile compounding equipment. (Section 7.3)

7 Calculate overfill volume, dilution quantities, active ingredient weight, powder volume, flow rate and volume, drip rate, and the time for a replacement IV using the 24-hour clock. (Section 7.3)

8 Determine product stability including date and signs of incompatibility. (Section 7.4)

9 Define the role of the Occupational Health and Safety Administration, the National Institute for Occupational Safety and Health, and the US Nuclear Regulatory Commission in the protection of healthcare workers. (Section 7.4)

10 Describe some of the key safety requirements and personal protective equipment for hazardous and nuclear compounding. (Section 7.5)

11 Understand the basic requirements for handling and disposing of hazardous and nonhazardous pharmaceuticals. (Section 7.5)

Access eBook links for resources and an exam generator, with 1,000+ questions.

Though the practice of pharmacy uses mostly manufactured drug products, there are many medical conditions in the hospital and other healthcare facilities that require specially trained pharmacy personnel to prepare both sterile and hazardous products to fill medical orders.

Domain 3 of the ExCPT on the dispensing process includes questions on sterile and hazardous compounding.

7.1 Sterile Compounding for Parenteral Administration

Study Idea

Review hand-washing technique for sterile compounding.

Many drugs ordered for patients in hospitals and other healthcare settings are injected directly into the body, so they must be specially compounded in a strictly controlled environment that is as germfree as possible. Healthcare facilities are particularly concerned about **healthcare-associated infections (HAIs)**—infections that patients contract while receiving care at a medical facility. HAIs can result in the need for lengthy, multidrug therapies, extended and costly hospitalizations, permanent injuries, and sometimes death. Organisms that commonly cause HAIs include the **methicillin-resistant *Staphylococcus aureus* (MRSA)** bacteria that can cause serious bloodstream infections. MRSA is often passed by contaminated hands.

US Pharmacopeia–National Formulary Chapter <797>

To ensure the highest quality and safest possible sterile product, the United States Pharmacopeial Convention (USP) has set out guidelines for sterile compounding in the *United States Pharmacopoeia*, General Chapter <797> (rev. 2019), more commonly known as *USP Chapter <797>*. Sterile means the absence of *any* microorganisms, whereas *asepsis* is the absence of any destructive pathogens. Objects can be made sterile but people cannot. **Aseptic technique** is the set of special procedures used to ensure that harmful germs are not passed on, or introduced onto, surfaces and equipment, into the air, or into the compounded drug preparations.

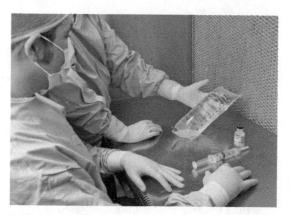

Technicians preparing IVs, injections, and other CSPs must be carefully trained to follow aseptic technique.

According to *USP <797>*, **compounded sterile preparations (CSPs)** must be prepared in a cleanroom with monitored air quality attained and maintained through primary and secondary engineering controls. Compounding technicians must use sterilized equipment and tools while following a strict aseptic technique that includes protocols for handwashing, donning **personal protective equipment (PPE)**, and careful manipulation of ingredients, containers, and CSPs during the preparation. See Table 7.1 for skills needed.

Pharmacy personnel are evaluated for competency in these skills as required by *USP <797>*. Based on the compounding risk level (low, medium, or high) of the products the facility prepares, competency evaluations must be completed annually or semiannually.

Study Idea

Parenteral solutions have the advantage of quicker action since they bypass the digestive system.

Types of Sterile Parenteral Drug Products

CSPs are generally administered through a **parenteral route of administration**, usually one that uses injection to reach its destination in the bloodstream either by direct administration (intravenous) or through intramuscular or subcutaneous injection. A sterile, or microbial-free, solution (with or without medication) is administered by means of a hollow needle or catheter inserted through one or more layers of the skin. Injectable parenteral dosage forms are administered through four paths:

- **intravenous (IV)**—into a vein via an IV line and catheter or syringe
- **intradermal (ID)**—between the layers of skin via a syringe
- **subcutaneous (SubQ)**—under the skin into the subcutaneous tissue via a syringe
- **intramuscular (IM)**—into a muscle vial a syringe or injection pen.

Study Idea

Two types of LVPs used for nutritional support are peripheral parenteral nutrition (PPN) and total parenteral nutrition (TPN). TPN must be administered through a central venous catheter.

Study Idea

Know that lactated Ringer's solution is a very common large-volume parenteral (LVP) used for fluid restoration after blood loss from injury, surgery, or burns. Lactated Ringer's solution includes sodium chloride (NaCl), sodium lactate, potassium chloride (KCl), and calcium chloride (CaCl), sometimes administered in combination with a dextrose solution.

TABLE 7.1 Sterile Compounding Skill Proficiencies

- hygiene, garbing, handwashing, gowning, and gloving
- aseptic manipulation
- proper cleanroom behavior
- measuring and mixing technique
- use of equipment and tools
- proper use of the primary engineering controls (PECs)
- understanding of the high-efficiency particulate air (HEPA) filtered unidirectional airflow within the rooms and equipment
- understanding of the potential impact of personnel activities, such as moving materials into and out of the compounding area
- documentation of the compounding process (e.g., Master Formulation Record and Compounding Record)
- cleaning and disinfection procedures
- methods of sterilization

There are three basic forms of parenteral IV solutions. Large- and small-volume parenteral solutions are the most commonly ordered. There are key distinguishing features that affect how each parenteral solution is compounded and administered.

- **Large-volume parenteral (LVP) solutions** are generally administered over a prolonged period that ranges from 8 to 24 hours, and are available in 250 mL, 500 mL, and 1,000 mL IV bag sizes. They may contain one or more electrolytes added to an IV solution of saline or dextrose.
- **Small-volume parenteral (SVP) solutions** are available in smaller bag sizes, 25 mL, 50 mL, 100 mL, and 150 mL, or 250 mL for rapid infusion. Many SVPs are administered as intravenous piggyback (IVPB) solutions. Their tubing is inserted into primary LVP lines to merge the solutions. SVPs are typically infused over 10 minutes to an hour and are made of a medication dissolved into a sterile **normal saline (NS)**—0.9% sodium chloride (NaCl)—or a dextrose in water (D_5W) solution.
- **IV bolus injections**, or **IV push (IVP) injections**, are small-volume medications inserted by syringe into the catheter or port near the catheter.

Study Idea

Additional CSPs include aqueous bronchial inhalations, baths and soaks for live organs and tissues, irrigations for internal body cavities, ophthalmic solutions, and implants.

Medication Orders for Compounded Sterile Preparations

Once the hospital pharmacy receives the compounded sterile preparation (CSP) order, a pharmacist (or in certain facilities, a senior technician) enters the order into the pharmacy's computer system, and the software runs the drug utilization review (DUR). This will check the order against the patient's medical history and medication profile to catch any allergies, cross-sensitivities, drug/drug or drug/food interactions, duplicate therapies, and/or contraindications.

The pharmacist resolves all computer-generated warnings and either modifies the order with the physician or approves it, and the sterile compounding labels are generated. Rather than just issuing a single label for the medication order, a separate label is issued for each individualized dose to be compounded. These are provided to the sterile compounding technician in the cleanroom.

The label formatting will differ among hospitals and software, but the CSP labels generally include the information in Figure 7.1 and in Table 7.2.

FIGURE 7.1
Small-Volume Parenteral Solution Label

IV Piggyback

Memorial Hospital

Pt. Name: Ogard, Christopher   **Room:** 560
Pt. ID#: 898372   **Rx#:** 03127

Ampicillin 500 mg
Sodium Chloride 0.9% (NS) 50 mL
Rate: over 20 min

Date prepared _____ Time prepared _____
RPh _____ BUD/Expiration Date _____
Tech _____ BUD/Expiration Time _____

Keep refrigerated – warm to room temperature
before use.

TABLE 7.2 Compounded Sterile Preparation Labeling Requirements

Each compounded sterile preparation (CSP) must have a label that encompasses most or all of the following information:

- medication order number or batch lot number
- name and identification (ID) number (bar code) of the patient for whom the medication is prescribed
- name, concentration, and amount of base solution (e.g., D5W 500 mL)
- brand or generic name and amount (or concentration) of each drug or additive in the compound (e.g., potassium chloride [KCl] 20 mEq)
- infusion rate (e.g., 100 mL/hr or infuse over 20 min), dosing interval, and/or administration time
- form and route of administration (e.g., for intravenous administration)
- beyond-use date (BUD) or manufacturer's expiration date
- storage requirements (e.g., keep refrigerated or protect from light)
- auxiliary labels or special instructions (e.g., Shake well before administering; Warm to room temperature before administering; For wound irrigation only)
- any device-specific instructions (e.g., MINI-BAG Plus must be activated and mixed prior to administering)
- preparer's and pharmacist's initials
- address and contact information of the infusion pharmacy or compounder if the CSP is to be sent outside of the facility in which it was compounded.

Note: Consult the hospital pharmacy's policy and procedure (P&P) manual for the institution's specific labeling requirements.

Each IV preparation requires a bag of a base solution to which additive(s) are injected. These additives may include active drug(s), electrolytes, or nutrients. The amount of drug or additive and the volume of the base solution must be listed on the label. See Table 7.3 for a list of common parenteral solutions and additives. The label may also contain the drug dosing interval or the time that the CSP is to be administered.

TABLE 7.3 Products Used in Sterile Compounding

large-volume parenteral (LVP) solutions	250 mL, 500 mL, 1,000 mL with medications in saline or dextrose solutions, or with lactated Ringer's solutions
small-volume parenteral (SVP) solutions	25 mL, 50 mL, 100 mL, 150 mL, 250 mL with medications in normal saline or D_5W
total parenteral nutrition (TPN) solutions	amino acid solutions, dextrose solutions, fat emulsions
TPN additives	electrolytes, trace elements, vitamins
diluents	sterile water for injection, lidocaine, sodium chloride (NaCl), bacteriostatic water for injection
pharmaceuticals	antibiotics, chemotherapy, proton pump inhibitors, H_2 blockers, and so on

Master Formulation and Compounding Records

Some pharmacy labeling programs provide sterile compounding instructions directly on the label. However, when the labels do not provide compounding instructions or when CSPs are prepared in a batch for multiple patients, *USP <797>* requires that a **Master Formulation Record** be followed. Generally, a Master Formulation Record for each type of ordered medication can be found in the hospital software, the *US Pharmacopeia -National Formulary* (USP-NF), in an approved peer-reviewed pharmacy-medical article, or at the website of the Professional Compounding Centers of America (PCCA). The Master Formulation Record lists the ingredients, specific procedures, equipment to be used, and testing required for each kind of CSP (see Table 7.4).

TABLE 7.4 Sterile Compounding Master Formulation Record Components

A Master Formulation Record for sterile compounding should include the following information:

- name, strength, and dosage form of the CSP
- physical description of the final preparation
- identities and amounts of all ingredients and appropriate container-closure systems
- complete instructions for preparing the CSP, including equipment, supplies, and a description of the compounding steps
- BUD and storage requirements
- quality control procedures (e.g., pH, filter integrity, and visual inspection)
- sterilization method, if applicable (e.g., filter, steam, or dry heat)
- any other information needed to describe the operation and ensure its repeatability (e.g., adjusting pH, tonicity, and temperature)

For every compounded product using a Master Formulation Record, a **Compounding Record**, with its specific medical order or batch lot number, must be established by the technician on the computer for each patient, as in nonsterile compounding. This record documents the ingredients, calculations, and compounding processes that were actually used for a particular preparation, allowing for traceability. It is critical that the record also describes in detail any deviations from the label directions or Master Formulation Record, any compounding problems or errors experienced, and the identities of the staff involved in its preparation and verification.

Each Compounding Record must be reviewed and approved, with the pharmacist's signature or initials and the date, before the CSP is released. For sterile products that are assembled according to manufacturer's directions, such as the standard reconstitution of powders for injectable medications, no Compounding Record is required.

Cleanroom and Air Quality Engineering Equipment

Name Exchange

Some manufacturers and pharmacy personnel use *cleanroom* to refer to both the ante-room and buffer room together. Others refer to the buffer room as the *cleanroom* or *IV room*.

The standard sterile compounding area required by *USP* <797> is separated into two rooms: a preparatory **ante-room** (or transition area) and a **buffer room** (also known as the **cleanroom**) that provides space for the sterile compounding workstations or benches. (The ante-room and buffer room together are sometimes referred to as the *cleanroom* or *cleanroom* suite.) A CSP workstation is called a ***primary engineering control* (PEC)** because it has **high-efficiency particulate air (HEPA)** filtered ventilation system to protect the CSPs from contamination. Within the PECs, the direct compounding area (DCA) must have an International Organization for Standardization (ISO) air quality classification of 5 (ISO Class 5). (Note that, for ISO air quality classifications, lower classification numbers correspond to cleaner air quality; so, ISO Class 1 air is the cleanest, and ISO Class 9 air is the least clean.)

The buffer room and ante-room have HEPA ventilation systems called **secondary engineering controls (SECs)**. The buffer room must have at least ISO Class 7 air, and the ante-room must have at least ISO Class 8 air. The common PEC for nonhazardous sterile compounding is called the ***horizontal laminar airflow workbench* (H-LAFW)**, also known as the *hood*. The ventilated airstream produced by the PEC and its hood create ISO Class 5 air quality in the DCA in the middle of the H-LAFW. Nonhazardous sterile compounding can also be done in a PEC called a **compounding aseptic isolator (CAI)**, which has an enclosed DCA inside a glove box. It offers even more protection for the compounding process.

Study Idea

An H-LAFW is used for sterile compounding of nonhazardous drugs. Hazardous drugs cannot be compounded in an H-LAFW.

The H-LAFW must be cleaned and sanitized according to *USP* standards at the beginning of each compounding shift and before each preparation (see Figure 7.2 for the order and process). The DCA must be cleaned after every 30 minutes of continuous compounding and after any spill or surface contamination. The PEC prefilters must be replaced every 30 days. The HEPA filters must be recertified every six months or any time the PEC is moved.

For sterile compounding, the air moves horizontally from the HEPA filter behind the grill over the CSP toward the compounder. The airflow must be unidirectional (going one way away from the CSP) with positive pressure, from filtered air pumped into the DCA toward the buffer room and outward to ever lessening air quality.

Study Idea

Cardboard boxes or material that may give off particulate matter should never be brought into the ante-room or buffer room.

According to *USP* <797>, the counters, work surfaces, and floors of the buffer room and ante-room must be cleaned daily. The buffer room and ante-room ceilings, walls, and shelving must be cleaned monthly. At specified intervals, the supervisor of the sterile compounding pharmacy will observe and document the cleaning and disinfecting techniques used by pharmacy staff.

FIGURE 7.2
Hood Cleaning Order for the H-LAFW

Wipe the bar and hooks first with a 70% isopropyl alcohol (IPA) wipe, followed by ceiling, both sides of the hood, and finally the work surface. The arrows show where to start in each section and the direction to wipe.

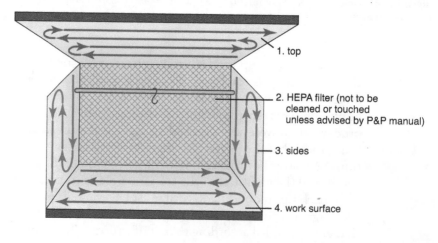

1. top
2. HEPA filter (not to be cleaned or touched unless advised by P&P manual)
3. sides
4. work surface

In addition, routine environmental monitoring is required for quality assurance. Nonviable and viable airborne particle testing must be conducted at least every six months. Regular surface sampling is done to ensure cleaning and disinfecting procedures meet the required standards. If any area is out of compliance, corrective action has to be taken and documented.

Aseptic Technique and Personal Protective Equipment

For aseptic technique, technicians must put away outerwear, jewelry, and electronic devices before entering the ante-room. In the ante-room, they must finish calculations, gather and wipe down supplies, and don PPE. The PPE garbing process for sterile compounding personnel follows a hospital or organizational policy. A sample garbing and hand-washing policy involves removing all unnecessary garments and jewelry in the ante-room. After removing prohibited garments and accessories, a technician will put on PPE, in the following order: shoe covers, hair cover, and face mask. Then comes handwashing and arm scrubbing. Sterile gowns (with sleeves) and gloves are put on last because they must be the cleanest items; the gown goes on in the ante-room, and the gloves are donned in the buffer room. The gown must be clean, disposable, and nonshedding, with arms that fit snugly around the wrists (see Table 7.5). Goggles, face shields, a nonpermeable gown, and two pairs of chemotherapy gloves are recommended when making hazardous CSPs.

TABLE 7.5 Compounded Sterile Preparation Garbing and Handwashing

In the Ante-Room

Remove all personal outer garments (e.g., sweaters, jackets).

Remove jewelry from hands, wrists, or other visible body parts.

No artificial nails, nail polish, cosmetics, or perfume are permitted.

Put on first layers of PPE, in the following order:
- shoe covers
- hair cover
- face mask (beard cover, if applicable).

Perform aseptic hand-washing procedures.

Put on a nonshedding gown.

In the Buffer Room

Apply foamed, sterile, 70% isopropyl alcohol (IPA) antiseptic hand cleanser.

Don sterile, powder-free gloves.

7.2 Sterile Compounding Calculations

Study Idea

Review ratio and proportions and dimensional analysis in Chapter 5.

In the ante-room, before preparing the CSPs with aseptic technique, technicians need to do or to double-check the calculations required by the medical order and/or the Master Formulation Record in order to fill in the Compounding Record. It is essential to memorize the equivalents and metric conversions provided in Chapter 5 to be confident in these calculations. You will also need to know conversions from standard time (12-hour clock time) to military time (24-hour clock time) to interpret the labels for drug administration times. Knowing how to translate temperatures in Fahrenheit to Celsius and back is essential for checking the refrigerator and freezer storage conditions for IVs.

Some important calculations needed for sterile compounding include dosage concentrations, alligations, dilutions, specific gravity, milliequivalents, base solution overfill, flow rates, and 24-hour supply for IVs. Some of these calculations are too complex and advanced for the ExCPT, such as specific gravity, and thus will not be covered in this text. Others are based on the knowledge already reviewed in Chapter 5 on calculations:

Safety Alert

Never rely solely on the directions on the CSP label or pharmacist's calculations, or on your own! The IV technician must always double-check the medication order, labels, and calculations, documenting them all in the Compounding Record.

- When doing conversions and a measurement is missing, the ratio-proportion calculation method is best (as reviewed on pages 79–80).
- For calculating dosages based on body weight or surface area, see pages 182–184.
- For multi step dosage questions using conversions and concentration calculations, dimensional analysis is favored (as reviewed on pages 80–81, 84, 86).
- For calculating dilutions, use the formula: $is \times iv = fs \times fv$ to determine the final volume; then use the equation: $fv - iv = volume\ of\ diluent$ (as reviewed on pages 91–93).

When combining two different concentrations of products for a midrange concentration, do an alligation calculation. One warning about alligation questions on the exam: it is common to see an incorrect answer choice that switches the concentrations. You can usually explore your answers to eliminate many of the distracter answer by logic, as demonstrated in Example 7.1.

Study Idea

Review alligation in Chapter 6 because it could be used in a problem like Example 7.1.

Example 7.1

How much D₅W (5% concentration) and D₅₀W (50% concentration) should be mixed to prepare 1,000 mL of D₄₀W (40% concentration)?

a. 700 mL of 5% and 300 mL of 50%
b. 777 mL of 5% and 222 mL of 50%
c. 222 mL of 5% and 777 mL of 50%
d. 222 mL of 40% and 777 mL of 50%

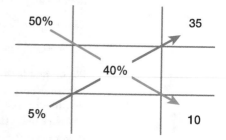

By process of elimination, the following can be determined:

- Answer *a* is incorrect because an equal split in volume would provide a concentration that is too low; there should be more of the 50% to offset the low 5%.
- Answer *b* has the correct numbers applied to the wrong solutions.
- Answer *d* uses 40% as part of the answer. The prescribed concentration cannot be part of a correct answer choice because it does not even exist until it is mixed. Any answer choice that contains the final-strength solution or mixture must be incorrect.
- Answer *c* must be correct.

If this were an actual test question, you could have arrived at the correct answer merely by inspecting your answer choices after setting up the alligation box (explained in depth on pages 204–205). Alligation problems take practice. Use the sample questions from the online end-of-chapter tests or exam generator to sharpen your skills.

Overfill of Base Solutions

Study Idea

The 10% rule for overfill requires that if the added volume with additives will be greater than 10% of the final volume, you should remove from the IV bag the amount equivalent to the volume of active ingredient(s) you will add.

Although manufactured base IV solutions are labeled to contain a set number of milliliters (e.g., 25, 50, 100, 250, 500, or 1,000 mL), the actual volume is greater because the containers include overfill. **Overfill** is the amount of solution manufacturers add to make up for the loss of water due to evaporation through plastic over time. This loss is somewhat dependent on conditions during transport and storage, the ratio of fluid volume to the surface area, and the time between manufacturing and use. The larger the IV bag base solution, the greater the potential loss, so the more overfill the manufacturers add to compensate.

Overfill Amounts

Manufacturers are not the same or consistent in their addition of overfill amounts, and they do not always label the overfill percentages they use. (See Table 7.6 for an example of possible overfill amounts.) Some overwrap their non-PVC (a type of plastic) IV solutions to reduce evaporation. These wraps should stay on until right before compounding or administration.

TABLE 7.6 Example of Possible Overfill in IV Bags

- 100 mL bags contain 7 mL overfill.
- 250 mL bags contain 25 mL overfill.
- 500 mL bags contain 30 mL overfill.
- 1,000 mL bags contain 50 mL overfill.

Note: The amount of overfill varies with the manufacturer.

Overfill Policies

Study Idea

Remember that the only way to accurately ensure a precise amount of medication is to prepare it in a new sterile empty IV bag or other container. This way there is no overfill to address. Make sure the label accurately indicates the percentage of drug solute to solvent.

Each hospital and home infusion pharmacy will have written protocols for dealing with overfill calculations for base solutions. SVPs and LVPs compose the majority of CSPs, and normally the overfill amount for these IVs does not appreciably affect the amount of fluids or drug dosages administered. However, in the case of IV premixed neonatal drugs or cancer chemotherapy drugs that must be reconstituted with a diluent before being transferred into an SVP or LVP solution, the combination of the overfill in the IV bag plus the diluent can cause an overdilution of the prescribed dose, especially if the entire contents of the IV solution are not administered. A diluted dose of a critical drug may adversely affect the disease outcome.

Many pharmacies implement the 10% rule for overfill that states that if the manufacturer's overfill plus any required additives equals 10% or more over the stock label amount for the base IV solution, then the overfill volume should be removed before adding the drug volume. To calculate if you might need to adjust for an overfill, see Example 7.2.

Example 7.2

Mitomycin 40 mg in a 0.5 mg/1 mL sterile water dilution must be added to 1,000 mL normal saline (NS) to be infused over six hours. The hospital has a policy that says the amount of overfill plus diluent should be withdrawn from an NS base solution. Will this CSP result in an overfill that needs an adjustment of the NS base solution? If so, how much NS will need to be withdrawn from the NS base solution?

Step 1 Convert 0.5 mg/1 mL to a whole number:

$$\frac{10}{10} \times \frac{0.5 \text{ mg}}{1 \text{ mL}} = \frac{5 \text{ mg}}{10 \text{ mL}}$$

Step 2 Using the ratio-proportion method, determine the amount of sterile water diluent to be added:

$$\frac{5 \text{ mg}}{10 \text{ mL}} = \frac{40 \text{ mg}}{y \text{ mL}},$$

$$5 \text{ mg} \times y \text{ mL} = 10 \text{ mL} \times 40 \text{ mg};$$

$$\frac{\cancel{5 \text{ mg}} \times y \text{ mL}}{\cancel{5 \text{ mg}}} = \frac{10 \text{ mL} \times 40 \cancel{\text{ mg}}}{5 \cancel{\text{ mg}}}$$

$$y \text{ mL} = \frac{10 \text{ mL} \times 40}{5} = 80 \text{ mL}$$

$$y \text{ mL} = 80 \text{ mL}$$

Step 3 Determine the final volume of the IV solution.

First, determine the initial volume of NS, accounting for overfill:

Using the overfill example in Table 7.6, it can be determined that a 1 L (1,000 mL) bag of NS will contain approximately 50 mL of overfill.

$$1,000 \text{ mL} + 50 \text{ mL} = 1,050 \text{ mL}; \quad \text{the initial volume of NS is 1,050 mL}$$

Then, determine the final volume of the IV solution:

final volume (fv) = initial volume (iv) + diluent volume (dv)

$$\text{fv} = 1,050 \text{ mL} + 80 \text{ mL} = 1,130 \text{ mL}$$

$$\text{fv} = 1,130 \text{ mL}$$

Step 4 Using the 10% rule, determine if the volume of the NS base solution must be adjusted.

Determine the stock label volume of NS plus 10% of the stock label amount of NS:

$$1,000 \text{ mL} + (\frac{1}{10} \times 1,000 \text{ mL}) = 1,100 \text{ mL}$$

The stock label amount of NS plus 10% of the stock label volume of NS equals 1,100 mL; since the final volume of the solution (1,130 mL) is greater than this volume, the volume of NS base solution must be adjusted.

Step 5 Determine the amount of NS to be withdrawn from the NS base solution before adding the medicated solution to the 1,000 mL IV bag.

Hospital protocol states that the amount of overfill plus diluent should be withdrawn from the NS base solution, so:

$$50 \text{ mL} + 80 \text{ mL} = 130 \text{ mL}$$

50 mL NS must be withdrawn from the NS base solution before adding the medicated solution to the 1,000 mL IV bag

Answer: This CSP results in an overfill that requires an adjustment to the NS base solution; 50 mL NS must be withdrawn from the NS base solution

General Medication Addition to an LVP Base Solution With a typical LVP continuously administered, the problem of overfill diluting a medication does occur, but the measurements do not need to be precise because another IV with the same drug will be following it.

Precise SVP Compounding For medications that need to be the most precise, as in SVP chemotherapy, sterile compounding technicians need to work with accurate medication amounts, so all ingredients including the base solution and any diluent must be precisely measured and injected into a new sterile container. This can be done manually or in an automated compounding device. Using a new container means that there will be no overfill to calculate or estimate.

An epidural pain medication must always be exact, with no overfill, so the base solution and the medication must be drawn into new syringes and then injected into a sterile medication reservoir cassette.

Calculating Sterile Compounding Doses and Dilutions

Study Idea

Return to Chapter 5 to study and apply conversion, dosage, and dilution calculation skills to parenteral solutions. Also, review and apply the compounding calculation skills in Chapter 5.

Injectable drugs and IV solutions use the same conversion, dosage, and dilution calculations explained in Chapter 5. Sterile compounding is particularly focused on working with liquids for IV solutions or sterile injections.

Calculating Weight/Volume (w/v) Percents

Many IV solutions are ordered as a percentage of active ingredient weight based on solution volume. Premade preservative-free lidocaine, for instance, is available in 1% and 2% concentrations for parenteral use. To calculate dilution levels, convert from percentages to fractions and sometimes from grams to milligrams of actual ingredient in a concentration (see Example 7.3).

Study Idea

Remember w/v percents are usually expressed as percentage of grams of the active ingredient per 100 mL of solution, as expressed in 1% = 1 g/100 mL.

Example 7.3

A technician is to prepare a 0.02% Nimotop solution administered in 1 liter of normal saline (NS) base solution. How many milligrams of Nimotop must they add to the NS base solution?

Step 1 Convert 0.02% Nimotop solution to w/v.

Using dimensional analysis, determine the amount of Nimotop solution in milligrams per 100 milliliters:

$$y \text{ mg}/100 \text{ mL} = \frac{0.02 \text{ g}}{100 \text{ mL}} \times \frac{1{,}000 \text{ mg}}{1 \text{ g}} = \frac{20 \text{ mg}}{100 \text{ mL}}$$

$$y \text{ mg}/100 \text{ mL} = 20 \text{ mg}/100 \text{ mL}$$

Determine how many milligrams of Nimotop must be added to the NS base solution.

Using dimensional analysis, determine the amount of Nimotop to be added:

$$y \text{ mg} = \cancel{1L} \; \frac{1{,}000 \; \cancel{mL}}{\cancel{1L}} \times \frac{20 \text{ mg}}{100 \; \cancel{mL}} = 200 \text{ mg}$$

$$y \text{ mg} = 200 \text{ mg}$$

Answer: The technician must add 200 mg Nimotop to the 1-liter bag of NS base solution

Calculating Dry Powder Volume and Dilutions

At times, you will need to do calculations with dry powdered forms of active ingredients. For example, parenteral products are often reconstituted by adding a diluent to a lyophilized or freeze-dried powder to prepare an IV solution. The product is commercially manufactured in powder form because of the instability of the drug in a solution over a long period. The active ingredient (the powder) is expressed in terms of weight, but it also occupies a certain amount of space, or volume. This space is referred to as **powder volume (pv)**. It is equal to the difference between the **total volume (tv)** of the final product and the volume of the diluting ingredient, or the **diluent volume (dv)**, as expressed in the following equations (see Example 7.4 for practice using these equations):

$$total \; volume \; (tv) - diluent \; volume \; (dv) = powder \; volume \; (pv)$$

$$total \; volume \; (tv) - powder \; volume \; (pv) = diluent \; volume \; (dv)$$

$$total \; volume \; (tv) = powder \; volume \; (pv) + diluent \; volume \; (dv)$$

For instance, a dry powder antibiotic must be reconstituted for use. The label states that the powder volume is 0.8 milliliters. When calculating amounts of powder and diluent, it helps to make a table of known and unknown information, as seen in Figure 7.3 and Example 7.4. Using the correct formula, determine the diluent volume for a total volume of 5 mL:

$$tv - pv = dv$$

FIGURE 7.3
Sample Reconstitution Table

Active Drug Weight	Concentration	Powder Volume	Diluent Volume	Total Volume of Final Drug Solution	How much to administer?
		0.8 mL	4.2 mL	5 mL	
		0.8 mL	5.5 mL	6.3 mL	

Total Volume		Powder Volume		Diluent Volume
5 mL	−	0.8 mL	=	4.2 mL

What is the total volume if you add 5.5 mL of diluent to 0.8 mL of powder volume?

Powder Volume		Diluent Volume		Total Volume
0.8 mL	+	5.5 mL	=	6.3 mL

Example 7.4

A technician is to reconstitute 1 g of a dry powder medication. The medication label states that 8.3 mL of diluent are to be added to a base solution to make a final medicated solution of 100 mg/1 mL. What is the powder volume of the medication? If the patient's medical order is for 60 mg of medication, how many milliliters of medicated solution must be drawn from the vial into the syringe?

FIGURE 7.3
Sample Reconstitution Table

Active Drug Weight	Concentration	Powder Volume	Diluent Volume	Total Volume of Final Drug Solution	How much to administer?
1 g (1,000 mg)	100 mg / 1 mL		8.3 mL		60 mg

Step 1 Convert the grams of active ingredient to milligrams:

$$1 \cancel{g} = \frac{1{,}000 \text{ mg}}{1 \cancel{g}} = 1{,}000 \text{ mg}$$

The medicated solution will have a strength of $\dfrac{1{,}000 \text{ mg}}{y \text{ mL}}$

Step 2 Use the ratio-proportion method to determine the total volume of 100 mg/1 mL medicated solution needed:

$$\frac{100 \text{ mg}}{1 \text{ mL}} = \frac{1{,}000 \text{ mg}}{y \text{ mL}}$$

$$100 \text{ mg} \times y \text{ mL} = 1 \text{ mL} \times 1{,}000 \text{ mg}$$

$$\frac{100 \cancel{\text{mg}} \times y \text{ mL}}{100 \cancel{\text{mg}}} = \frac{1 \text{ mL} \times 1{,}000 \cancel{\text{mg}}}{100 \cancel{\text{mg}}} \qquad \text{so } y \text{ mL} = 1 \text{ mL} \times 10 = 10 \text{ mL}$$

$$y \text{ mL} = 10 \text{ mL}$$

Step 3 Calculate the powder volume that must be added to the diluent:

$$tv - dv = pv$$

$$pv = 10 \text{ mL} - 8.3 \text{ mL} = 1.7 \text{ mL}$$

$$pv = 1.7 \text{ mL}$$

Step 4 Determine the milliliters of medicated solution to be drawn from the vial into the syringe for the ordered 60 mg dose of the 100 mg/1 mL medicated solution.

$$y \text{ mL} = 60 \text{ mg} \times \frac{1 \text{ mL}}{100 \text{ mg}} = 0.6 \text{ mL}$$

$$y \text{ mL} = 0.6 \text{ mL}$$

Answer: The powder volume of the medication is 1.7 mL; 0.6 mL of medicated solution must be drawn from the vial into the syringe

Measuring Electrolytes

Study Idea

Review the abbreviations for commonly ordered electrolytes like KCl and NaCl.

Many IV fluids used in hospital pharmacy practice contain dissolved mineral salts; such a fluid is known as an **electrolyte solution**, which provides needed electrical chemistry interactions for the body to rejuvenate.

Milliequivalents (mEq) are used to measure electrolytes in the bloodstream and/or in an IV preparation. The **equivalent (Eq)** weight is the number of grams of the substance that is able to fully dissolve in 1 mL of solution to react with another substance. The chemistry equation to determine the equivalent weight is based on each element's atomic structure. It is too complicated for this review and not needed for the ExCPT. Eq calculations are done by pharmacy software. However, you do need to know that the milliequivalents in a drug solution are measured by the number of milliequivalents per 1 mL. Then you can use a ratio-proportion equation to figure out the number of milliequivalents that should be dissolved in the IV solution to reach the prescribed concentration of electrolytes or other ingredients (see Example 7.5).

Example 7.5

A technician is to make a sterile preparation in the IV room by adding 88 mEq of sodium chloride (NaCl) to an IV bag. NaCl is available as a 4 mEq/ 1 mL solution. How many milliliters of NaCl must be added to the IV bag?

Determine the number of milliliters needed.

Use the ratio-proportion method to compare the available base solution concentration to the number of milliequivalents of NaCl:

$$\frac{4 \text{ mEq}}{1 \text{ mL}} = \frac{88 \text{ mEq}}{y \text{ mL}}$$

$$4 \text{ mEq} \times y \text{ mL} = 1 \text{ mL} \times 88 \text{ mEq}$$

$$\frac{4 \text{ mEq} \times y \text{ mL}}{4 \text{ mEq}} = \frac{1 \text{ mL} \times 88 \text{ mEq}}{4 \text{ mEq}} \quad \text{so } y \text{ mL} = \frac{1 \text{ mL} \times 88}{4} = 22 \text{ mL}$$

Answer: y mL = 22 mL; 22 mL of NaCl must be added to the IV bag

Calculating IV Administration Flow Rates and Volumes

The **infusion rate** (or dosing rate) is the prescribed rate at which an amount of fluid is infused into a patient over a given period of time. The actual **flow rate** (how fast a fluid is traveling) is determined by the size and nature of the tubing.

Calculating Volume Delivered with Ordered Flow Rate

By knowing the flow rate and the amount of time that an infusion has to run, it is possible to calculate the exact amount of fluid that will be delivered. Example 7.6 uses a ratio-proportion equation to solve a simple IV flow rate problem where you need to know how much fluid will be administered during a set amount of time based on its speed ratio of milliliters per hour.

Study Idea

When answering questions on the exam, pay close attention to the units of measure such as minutes versus hours or milliliters versus liters.

Example 7.6

A patient has an intravenous normal saline (NS) infusion running in at a rate of 125 mL/hr. How much fluid will the patient receive during an infusion that lasts 8 hours?

Determine the milliliters of fluid needed.

Use the ratio-proportion method to compare the rate of infusion to the number of hours the infusion will run:

$$\frac{1 \text{ hr}}{125 \text{ mL}} = \frac{8 \text{ hr}}{y \text{ mL}}$$

$$1 \text{ hr} \times y \text{ mL} = 125 \text{ mL} \times 8 \text{ hr}$$

$$\frac{1\cancel{\text{hr}} \times y \text{ mL}}{1 \cancel{\text{hr}}} = \frac{125 \text{ mL} \times 8 \cancel{\text{hr}}}{1 \cancel{\text{hr}}} \quad \text{so } y \text{ mL} = \text{mL} = 125 \text{ mL} \times 8 = 1{,}000 \text{ mL}$$

Answer: y mL = 1,000 mL; the patient will receive 1,000 mL of intravenous NS during an 8-hour infusion

Calculating Flow Rate Based on Volume Delivered

Often, pharmacies will have to calculate the IV flow rate for patients. The equation used to calculate IV flow rate is

volume/time = rate

The volume may be expressed in milliliters, liters, or drops (gtt). (Drop rates will be discussed later.) The time component of an IV flow rate may be expressed in terms of hours or minutes. (See Examples 7.7 and 7.8 for these types of calculations.)

Example 7.7

A patient receives 2.5 L of IV total parenteral nutrition (TPN) solution, infused over 12 hours. What is the flow rate in milliliters per hour if the flow rate is consistent throughout the entire 12-hour infusion?

Step 1 Convert liters of TPN to milliliters:

$$2.5 \text{ L} \times \frac{1{,}000 \text{ mL}}{1 \text{ L}} = 2{,}500 \text{ mL}$$

Step 2 Determine the flow rate.

Use the ratio-proportion method to compare the total volume of TPN administered over 12 hours to the milliliters of TPN received:

$$\frac{12 \text{ hr}}{2,500 \text{ mL}} = \frac{1 \text{ hr}}{y \text{ mL}}$$

$$12 \text{ hr} \times y \text{ mL} = 2,500 \text{ mL} \times 1 \text{ hr}$$

$$\frac{12 \text{ hr} \times y \text{ mL}}{12 \text{ hr}} = \frac{2,500 \text{ mL} \times 1 \text{ hr}}{12 \text{ hr}}, \quad \text{so } y \text{ mL} = \frac{2,500 \text{ mL}}{12} = 208.333333... \text{ mL}$$

y mL = 208.333333... mL, which can be rounded to the nearest whole number: 208 mL

Answer: The flow rate of TPN is 208 mL/1 hr

Example 7.8

A patient receives 2,640 mL of IV Lactated Ringer's solution over 24 hours. What is the flow rate in milliliters per minute?

Use a dimensional analysis equation to determine the flow rate in milliliters per minute:

$$y \text{ mL} = \frac{2,640 \text{ mL}}{24 \text{ hr}} \times \frac{1 \text{ hr}}{60 \text{ min}}, \quad \text{so } y \text{ mL} = \frac{2,640 \text{ mL}}{24 \times 60 \text{ min}} = 1.833333... \text{ mL/min}$$

Answer: y mL = 1.833333 ... mL/min, which can be rounded to the nearest hundredth: 1.83 mL/min; the flow rate of IV Lactated Ringer's solution is 1.83 mL/min

When taking the ExCPT, check that the answer you choose is in the correct unit of measure. For example, a likely distractor answer for this question would be 110 mL/hr, which would have the correct number, but the wrong unit of measure.

Calculating Time Duration for Infusion, Based on Flow Rate and 24-Hour Supply

To answer the question, *"How long will this IV bag last (or take to administer)?"* you divide the total milliliters by the infusion rate at milliliters per minute or milliliters per hour to find out how long it will take to empty. As you work through the problem, you may need to solve a time conversion at the end. If you need to finish your problem by doing a time conversion, you will find that setting up a dimensional analysis equation from the start is most efficient (see Example 7.9).

$$Time \text{ (hr or min)} = \frac{Volume \text{ (mL)}}{Rate \text{ (mL/hr)}}$$

When a time conversion is needed, the equation above can work into:

$$Time \text{ (min)} = volume \times \frac{hr}{mL} \times \frac{min}{hr}$$

Study Idea

When you work out the *Volume/Rate = Time* equation, you will note that, in order to divide the volume by a rate fraction, you have to flip the rate and multiply it by the volume. You end up with a dimensional analysis equation that can have the conversion rate of min/hr added to it, if needed.

Example 7.9

A 1,000-mL bag of solution containing 30 mEq of KCl is piggybacked into a continuous $D_{10}W$ solution. The flow rate of the infusion is 3 mL/min. How many hours will it take to complete the infusion of one bag? How many bags would be needed for a 24-hour supply?

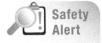

Safety Alert

When preparing IVs, remember tubing and bags made of PVC plastic can cause health problems because of PVC drug absorption or PVC leaching. Avoid using PVC IV sets for nitroglycerin, amiodarone, most biotechnology drugs, fat emulsions. as well as for any drugs for pregnant patients, neonates, children, and adolescent males.

Step 1 Use a dimensional analysis equation to determine the number of hours to complete the infusion of one bag:

$$y \text{ hr} = 1{,}000 \text{ mL} \times \frac{1 \text{ min}}{3 \text{ mL}} \times \frac{1 \text{ hr}}{60 \text{ min}}, \quad \text{so } y \text{ hr} = \frac{1{,}000 \times 1 \text{ hr}}{3 \times 60} = 5.555555... \text{ hr}$$

$y \text{ hr} = 5.555555... \text{ hr}$, which can be rounded to the nearest whole number: 6 hr

Step 2 Using the ratio-proportion method, determine how many bags of IV solution would be needed for a 24-hour supply:

$$\frac{6 \text{ hr}}{1 \text{ bag}} = \frac{24 \text{ hr}}{z \text{ bags}}$$

$$6 \text{ hr} \times z \text{ bags} = 1 \text{ bag} \times 25 \text{ hr}$$

$$\frac{6 \text{ hr} \times z \text{ bags}}{6 \text{ hr}} = \frac{1 \text{ bag} \times 24 \text{ hr}}{6 \text{ hr}}, \quad \text{so } z \text{ bags} = \frac{1 \text{ bag} \times 24}{6} = 4 \text{ bags}$$

$$z \text{ bags} = 4 \text{ bags}$$

Answer: It will take 6 hours to complete the infusion of one bag; 4 bags would be needed for a 24-hour supply

Calculating Flow Rate in Drops

For extremely concentrated solutions, as in chemotherapy, a pharmacy technician may be asked to calculate the IV flow rates per milliliter instead of per minute or per hour. Each IV infusion set has a particular drop factor based on the size of the tubing—the number of drops that will equal a volume of 1 mL, with **macrodrip tubing**, or **microdrip tubing** (often used for pediatric patients or chemotherapy)—as shown in Table 7.7. Infusion pumps can be set to regulate the infusion rate per drop (gtt).

TABLE 7.7 Common Drop Factors per Tubing Size

macrodrip tubing	10 gtt/1 mL
	15 gtt/1 mL
	20 gtt/1 mL
microdrip tubing	60 gtt/1 mL

The larger the drop factor, the smaller each individual drop is, so more drops are needed to make up a milliliter. A 10-drop set requires 10 gtt to add up to 1 mL volume, and a 60-drop set requires 60 gtt to add up to 1 mL volume. Example 7.10 calculates an IV infusion rate in drops using the ratio-proportion method and dimensional analysis.

Example 7.10

A patient is to receive 200 mL of IV 20% fat emulsion over 10 hours, using a 15-drop infusion (see Table 7.7 for the drop factor). What is the proper flow rate for this infusion pump in drops per minute?

Use a dimensional analysis equation to determine the flow rate in drops per minute:

$$y \text{ gtt/min} = \frac{200 \text{ mL}}{10 \text{ hr}} \times \frac{15 \text{ gtt}}{1 \text{ mL}} \times \frac{1 \text{ hr}}{60 \text{ min}},$$

$$y \text{ gtt/min} = \frac{200 \times 15 \text{ gtt}}{10 \times 60 \text{ hr}} = \frac{5 \text{ gtt}}{1 \text{ min}}$$

$$y \text{ gtt/min} = 5 \text{ gtt/min}$$

Answer: The proper flow rate for this infusion pump is 5 gtt/min

Calculating Time for the New Supply Based on Infusion Rate

If you have been given or have calculated the infusion rate per hour and you know what time the first bag will be administered, you can figure out when a new IV bag will be needed (see Example 7.11).

Example 7.11

The prescriber orders

> ℞ 20 mEq of medication in 2,000 mL of D_5W to be administered at 125 mL/hr

If each bag contains 1,000 mL of medication, and the first bag was hung at 9:00 a.m., what 12-hour clock time should the next bag be hung to complete the order?

Step 1 Use a dimensional analysis equation to determine the number of hours to complete the administration of one bag:

$$y \text{ hr} = 1,000 \text{ mL} \times \frac{1 \text{ hr}}{125 \text{ mL}}, \quad \text{so } y \text{ hr} = \frac{1,000 \text{ mL}}{125} = 8 \text{ hr}$$

$$y \text{ hr} = 8 \text{ hr}$$

Step 2 Determine what time the second bag will be needed.

First, convert the last administration time (9:00 a.m.) to 24-hour clock time:

$$0000 \text{ hours} + 900 = 0900 \text{ hours}$$

Then, add 8 hours to the last administration time (0900 hours):

$$0900 \text{ hours} + 800 = 1700 \text{ hours}$$

Since 1700 hours is 5 hours after 1200 hours (or noon on the 12-hour clock), the 12-hour clock time is 5:00 p.m.

Answer: The next bag should be hung at 5:00 p.m.

7.3 The Sterile Compounding Process

Study Idea

You must work six inches from the outside edge of the H-LAFW.

After performing several steps to ensure both the technician and the space are ready for sterile compounding, compounding can begin. (See Table 7.8 for an overview of the steps involved in the process.) The sterile compounding process involves handling needles and syringes, and adding ingredients from vials and ampules to base solutions, often in IV bags, in the protected space of the DCA.

The DCA is in the middle of the workbench, six inches from the edge of the counter. The clean air flows over the DCA, so the compounding technician's hands, tools, and ingredients must never be placed between the HEPA filter and the CSP.

TABLE 7.8 Overview of Steps in Sterile Compounding

This is a general outline of the process steps for sterile compounding in a two-room cleanroom area. Each facility is slightly different based on its layout and standard operating procedures. It is essential to take a sterile compounding course with practice labs to get a real sense of the detailed steps involved. *USP <797>* is the ultimate source for all sterile compounding guidelines.

1. In the main hospital pharmacy, receive medication orders and labels and run a drug utilization review (DUR). The pharmacist will do the initial calculations from the Master Formulation Record.
2. Receive the pharmacist's verifications, do any remaining calculations, and initiate a Compounding Record (may be done in pharmacy or ante-room, depending on procedures).
3. After removing outerwear and entering the ante-room, wipe down supplies and follow aseptic technique for garbing and handwashing.
4. Transport compounding supplies, ingredients, and primary engineering control (PEC) cleaning materials into the buffer room on a sanitized cart.
5. In the buffer room, sterilize hands and don sterile gloves.
6. Clean the PEC per manufacturer's directions and *USP <797>*.
7. Compound the CSPs in the PEC according to *USP <797>*; processes often include withdrawing medications from vials or ampules and then injecting them into IV base solutions or containers.
8. Complete a quality check of each CSP by comparing the label(s) to the medication order and doing a visual check.
9. Pharmacist will verify final CSP, label, and ingredients in buffer room or ante-room before applying the label and any auxiliary labels.
10. The CSP will be delivered to nursing unit for administration.

Wherever the air is blocked or interrupted from having unidirectional airflow, **turbulence** is created. Turbulence occurs where the PEC airflow meets the buffer room air, behind the supplies, and wherever the body of the person compounding is moving or blocking the air. A **zone of turbulence** is created between the DCA and the compounding technician in the act of compounding. Compounding personnel must be careful not to let their hands or supplies be closer to the air vent than the CSP, or they will **shadow** (block) the CSP from the cleansing airflow.

In preparation for compounding, to avoid shadowing, ingredients and instruments to be used must be arranged in a logical order to the sides of the DCA on the workbench so as to not block other ingredients from the airflow from the HEPA filter.

Manipulating Needles and Syringes

Study Idea

Needlesticks during compounding will introduce contaminants into the CSP. Discard the product that may be contaminated.

Some of the main compounding instruments are needles and syringes. Needles come in gauge (or bore) sizes. Needles with the highest number have the smallest bore (opening), and needles with the lowest number have the largest bore. Pharmacy technicians need to be proficient in choosing the correct needle size and manipulating the syringe and needle properly. Technicians must never touch the critical sites of the needle, syringe tip, or syringe plunger, because doing so may transmit pathogens, such as bacteria, viruses, or fungi from fingers, hands, and work surfaces. (See Figure 7.4 for syringe and needle details, including the critical sites to avoid.)

FIGURE 7.4
Common Needle Lengths and Gauges Used in Sterile Compounding, and Critical Sites on a Needle and Syringe

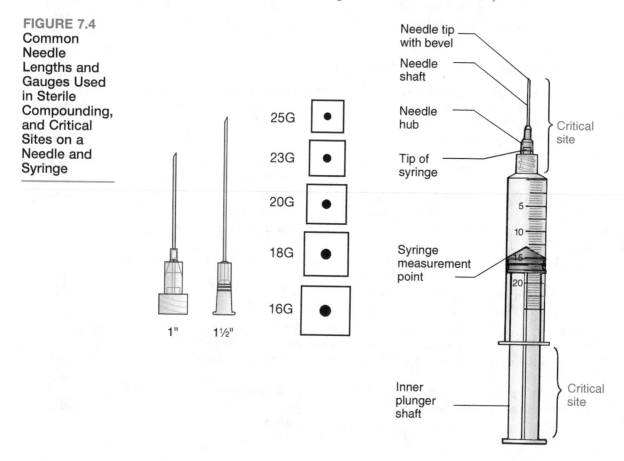

During compounding, universal precautions specify that needles used in patient care should not be recapped but should be placed uncapped into a puncture-proof sharps container. However, sterile compounding personnel are often required to perform compounding functions that require them to recap needles temporarily. So they use the *scoop* method with the needle to snag and scoop up the sterile cap without touching other surfaces.

Although there is no risk of exposure to patient blood or fluids during compounding, a needlestick could contaminate the final product with the compounding personnel's blood. If a needlestick occurs during compounding, the parenteral must be discarded, and the whole aseptic garbing and compounding processes must be started again once the wound is treated and covered. When multiple vials of pharmaceuticals are compounded for medium- to high-risk parenterals, a different needle and syringe should be used for each vial.

Adding Ingredients from a Vial

A **vial** is a sealed glass or plastic sterile container with a rubber seal and hard plastic cap. Vials contain sterile diluents or medications in either a liquid or powdered form and are available in sizes ranging from 1 mL to 100 mL (for batch CSPs). Two types of vials are the **single-dose vial (SDV)**, which does not contain preservatives, and the **multiple-dose vial (MDV)**, which does preservatives. (As an example, insulin often comes as a MDV.)

Information on the vial label includes the stock drug's concentration and the manufacturer's directions for reconstitution or use (see Figure 7.5).

The contents of the MDV are considered stable (with its preservatives) from its initial opening up to the manufacturer recommended BUD. (It is not generally longer than 28 days.) Once an MDV is opened, it must be marked with the BUD and stored under appropriate conditions (usually refrigeration) to alert other pharmacy personnel of the opening and the medication's change from an expiration date to a BUD.

FIGURE 7.5
Identifying the Components of an Injectable Medication Label

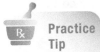
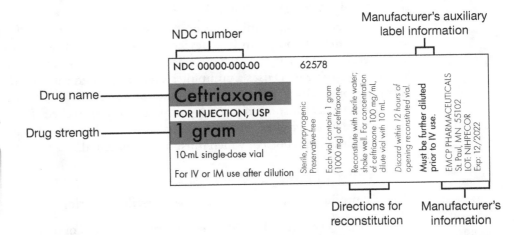

When preparing to remove contents from the vial, the plastic flip top must be removed, the rubber stopper wiped with 70% isopropyl alcohol (IPA), and the syringe needle inserted at a 45 degree angle to prevent **coring** (the accidental introduction of a microscopic piece of rubber into the solution). Remove the solution by using the **milking technique**. This is done by inserting a little air and removing some solution and repeating several times if you are not using a **vented needle**. Using a vented needle, which has an opening in it, prevents air pressure buildup and makes it so the technician doesn't have to use the milking technique to remove solution from the vial.

Adding Ingredients from an Ampule

An **ampule** is a small, hermetically sealed sterile glass container. An ampule stores a single dose of sterile medication in either a liquid (most common) or a powder form. Ampules contain no preservatives, and some drugs are available only in an ampule because they are incompatible with the rubber top or any plastic sealing components of the vials.

Because an ampule is a glass container without an opening, it is designed with a **break ring**, or scoring on its neck. Before breaking, the neck must be wiped with a sterile 70% IPA swab to remove any contaminants. Some technicians wrap a sterile 70% IPA wipe around the neck of the ampule before breaking it, but gauze may not be used, per *USP <797>*. To break open an ampule, grasp the ampule body in your nondominant hand with thumb and fingers below the ampule neck away from the HEPA filter, exert gentle but firm pressure, and snap the ampule's neck cleanly towards the side wall of the hood.

Study Idea

A filter needle or straw should only be used to remove medication from the ampule and then be removed to attach a sterile needle to the syringe.

Because there may be broken glass in the medication, a blunt, **filter needle** or a **filter straw** must be used to withdraw the medication, according to *USP <797>*, to catch any microscopic glass shards and impurities to prevent them from entering the CSP. The filter needle or straw must have a 5-micron (or finer) filter within its core and should be attached to the syringe just like a regular needle.

Filter needles are for one-directional use only, meaning that the needle may be used only to withdraw fluid from an ampule or inject fluid into an IV or IVPB. The same needle may not be used to do both. Before injecting the syringe contents into an IV, change to a regular needle in front of the HEPA filter to prevent introducing glass or particles into the IV admixture. When delivering the final IV, an inline filter should accompany the IV tubing to screen out any microscopic glass shards that might still be in the admixture. This is particularly necessary for neonatal and pediatric patients.

Using Automated Compounding Devices

Large hospitals and many infusion compounding pharmacies for home health care use an **automated compounding device (ACD)**. The ACD generally comes with 12 to 24 sterile fluid ports, and each dispenses a commonly needed nutritional additive for TPN bags. The ACD uses a pumping system calibrated with metric measurements of volume or gravity to fill the bags with the correct elements. The technician who oversees the ACD must measure each compounded bag to check that it is of the desired volume or weight. The ACD must also be checked for accuracy and correct calibration each day, both of which must be documented.

Preparing Premade IV Solutions

Study Idea

Docked vial-and-bag drugs may be returned to the pharmacy, if they are not activated, to be relabeled and used on another patient with a similar order.

Other IV products come premixed but need sterile activation.

Vial-and-Bag IVs A **vial-and-bag system** provides a vial of powdered medication that will be attached with an adaptor to a specified IV bag solution. Though the technician does not compound the vial-and-bag product, it must be assembled, or **docked** (the vial linked to the bag with the connector device) in a DCA with aseptic technique. These products do not require sterile compounding, so they are not considered CSPs. Labels must be generated for the bag-and-vial products with similar information as the CSPs, but they will come with manufacturer expiration dates rather than BUDs.

After scanning the product's labeled bar code, the nurse will use aseptic technique to break the seal of the attached powder vial, releasing the medication into the IVPB bag. This action activates the medication, which, once fully dissolved, is administered in short order to the patient via the secondary line tubing.

Premixed Frozen Solutions Manufactured frozen IV solutions, such as particular antibiotic solutions, are premixed products that are also not considered CSPs. When a frozen IV is ordered, it is thawed at room temperature or in the refrigerator (if there is sufficient time). After thawing, the technician prepares a patient-specific label. Once thawed, these frozen preparations cannot be refrozen.

Practice Tip

Manufacturers' recommendations for thawing frozen IVs vary between products, so be sure to check each product's label or package insert. The use of a warming bath or microwave to expedite the thawing process (*forced thaw*) is not recommended.

Determining Compounded Sterile Preparation Stability and Beyond-Use Date

After the various types of CSPs and other IVs are prepared and labeled, they must be inspected once more by the technician and pharmacist and assigned a BUD or the manufacturer's expiration date on the label (if not preprinted), and signed off by both the preparer and pharmacist. As noted, *USP <797>* guidelines specify the procedures for the dating, labeling, storage, handling, packaging, and transporting of CSPs in the hospital or infusion pharmacy. Improper procedures could adversely impact the sterility or stability of the products.

BUD Guidelines

BUD guidelines are based on the contamination risk or specific sterility testing provided by the hospital or manufacturer, as well as storage conditions and stability ratings. *USP <797>* provides guidelines for risk levels depending on the number and sterility of ingredients, the presence or absence of preservatives, the number of transfers from vials or ampules, and the use of automated compounding devices. Since CSPs may be compounded in anticipation of use, the longer a compound is stored, the greater the risk of microbial and pyrogen formation. Information about the chemical stability of a CSP is found in the Master Formulation Record, the manufacturer's literature, or specific product testing.

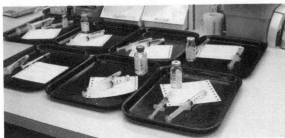

Medications compounded by the technician must await approval by the pharmacist.

Final Checks by Technician and Pharmacist

The technician checks to make sure there are no leaks in any of the IVs, precipitates, or incompatibilities, then lays out all the CSPs and all the components used in the compounding for the pharmacist's approval. The pharmacist's final CSP inspection will include checking the appearance and the accuracy in the proper selection and quantities of ingredients, technique for aseptic mixing and sterilization, packaging, and labeling that includes the BUD or expiration date. The pharmacist's inspection often includes rechecking the syringes used.

There should never be visible particles floating in the final parenteral solution. CSPs with precipitates must be discarded, not filtered. A *precipitate* is a nonsoluble particle or salt. A precipitate may clog an IV site or vein. A common cause of TPN precipitation is calcium gluconate and potassium phosphate added in too high of concentrations, in the wrong order, or without adequate mixing. To verify ingredient compatibility, use a compatibilities handbook, such as *Trissel's Stability of Compounded Formulations.*

7.4 Hazardous Compounding

Any drug that is known to have a risk of at least one of the following six criteria is considered a **hazardous drug (HD)**:

1. carcinogenicity (causes cancer)
2. teratogenicity (causes developmental damage/problems)
3. reproductive toxicity (causes reproductive damage/problems)
4. organ toxicity (causes organ damage/problems)
5. genotoxicity (causes genetic damage)
6. drugs that mimic HDs in structure or toxicity.

Safety Alert

A technician who is pregnant or may become pregnant should not count (or prepare) cancer chemotherapy drugs, including methotrexate (also used for rheumatoid arthritis), or drugs such as isotretinoin or finasteride (Proscar), due to the potential risk to the fetus.

Because of the special dangers involved in hazardous compounding, the Centers for Disease Control and Prevention (CDC) and Occupational Health and Safety Administration (OSHA) worked together to create the **National Institute for Occupational Safety and Health (NIOSH)**, which has published the "NIOSH Alert: Preventing Occupational Exposures to Antineoplastic and Other Hazardous Drugs in Health Care Settings." A **Safety Data Sheet (SDS)**, for each hazardous agent or investigational drug must be readily accessible in a compounding facility, so employees can see what they are handling and know what to do in the case of an accidental exposure or spill. The American Society of Health-System Pharmacists (ASHP) has also established HD guidelines.

According to *USP* Chapter <800> *Hazardous Drugs Handling in Healthcare Settings*, personnel in a hospital or compounding facility who come into any level of contact with HDs require specialized equipment, training, protective clothing, and procedures for handling, preparing, and disposing of these substances. Hospitals are required to develop written policies and procedures for each aspect of HD use to be in compliance with the USP and The Joint Commission (TJC), as well as state and federal regulations. Hospitals and compounding facilities must have intensive personnel training, protective PECs and SECs, personal protective clothing and gear, and specific techniques and supplemental engineering equipment. Routes of potential exposure are outlined on Table 7.9.

TABLE 7.9 Routes of Exposure to Hazardous Drugs

- receiving and unpacking hazardous drug (HD) orders
- counting individual oral doses and tablets from bulk containers
- crushing tablets or opening capsules to make oral solutions, suspensions, or syrups
- pouring oral or topical liquids from one container to another
- mixing topical dosage forms
- weighing or mixing components
- constituting or reconstituting powdered or lyophilized (freeze-dried) HDs
- withdrawing or diluting injectable HDs from parenteral containers
- expelling air from syringes filled with HDs

continues

TABLE 7.9 Routes of Exposure to Hazardous Drugs—*Continued*

- expelling HDs from a syringe
- coming into contact with HD residue present on drug container exteriors, work surfaces, floors, and final drug preparations (e.g., bottles, bags, cassettes, and syringes)
- inhaling HD residue or vapors
- handling contaminated waste generated at any step of the preparation or dispensing
- deactivating, decontaminating, cleaning, and disinfecting areas contaminated or suspected of being contaminated with HDs
- undergoing maintenance activities for contaminated equipment and devices
- spilling substances, cleaning up a spill, and disposing of cleanup materials

Medical Surveillance

Study Idea

HDs are not only given intravenously; they may be a **tablet** or topical preparation. Finasteride tablets are HDs because of the risk to pregnant individuals.

With exposure to HDs, workers can suffer acute, chronic, and long-term health consequences if proper precautions, procedures, and training are not followed. To prevent health issues, *USP* <800> requires a medical surveillance program by the hospital or compounding facility to collect and interpret data on HD workers to detect any changes in their health status due to potential exposure.

Any individual who can become pregnant and routinely works with HDs must confirm in writing an understanding of the risks and the importance of taking additional precautions to prevent pregnancy. A pharmacy technician who is pregnant, breast-feeding, or trying to conceive must notify their supervisor, so they can be reassigned to a different department position, take extra precautions, or have different work responsibilities to minimize contact with any HDs.

Hazardous Compounding Engineering Controls

Safety Alert

HDs must be compounded in a shielded vertical airflow hood or isolation box that has the proper biological safety rating.

HDs and sterile HDs must be compounded away from sterile products in a **containment secondary engineering control (C-SEC)** area with an exterior venting system. With this airflow control, the trace hazardous substances do not flow into other CSP compounding areas, the hospital, or the rest of the compounding facility. C-SEC rooms come in two kinds: one for the nonsterile and lower-risk nonsterile HDs, and one that has a buffer room with ISO Class 7 air for preparing sterile toxic HDs. Both C-SECs have to follow the appropriate *USP* <800> standards.

Hazardous compounding airflow goes in the reverse pattern of that in the sterile compounding cleanroom. C-SEC areas must provide **negative pressure**, with the ventilation system causing unidirectional airflow that is suctioned out of the buffer room and away from the compounding technicians and outer rooms. A sink must also be available for handwashing and for emergency access to water. An eyewash station within the contained HD compounding area is necessary for removal of HDs from the eyes and skin.

Containment Primary Engineering Controls

Per *USP* <800> standards, all HD compounding must be done in a **containment primary engineering control (C-PEC)**, which provides some level of shielding or isolation of the DCA, to contain the HDs and protect the compounding personnel. The C-PEC should be a Class II-B biological safety cabinet (BSC) or compounding aseptic containment isolator (CACI)—see Table 7.10 for the various types and levels of protection. These C-PECs still provide ISO Class 5 air quality in the DCA but have **vertical airflow**, or downward moving air that is suctioned away from the compounding technician to prevent exposure.

TABLE 7.10 General Types of Containment Primary Engineering Controls for Sterile Hazardous Compounding

Each containment primary engineering Control (C-PEC) unit has vertical HEPA-filtered airflow, air exchanges, and some level of HEPA-exhausted air according to USP Chapter <800> standards.

Containment Primary Engineering Controls
Class II Biological Safety Cabinets
• **Class II-A Biological Safety Cabinet (BSC):** partially shielded unit with downward filtered airflow onto the direct compounding area (DCA), with high amounts of recirculated air (including the vertical laminar airflow workbench [V-LAF]) • **Class II-B BSC:** similar unit to Class II-A (with barriers and vertical airflow) though with exterior filtered venting and little to no recirculated air
Aseptic Isolators
• **Compounding Aseptic Containment Isolator (CACI):** a unit with enclosed DCA in glovebox with external venting for sterile, hazardous compounding (for Class I or II hazardous substances)
Sealed Sterile Compounding Isolators
• **Class III BSC:** sealed unit for high-risk hazardous compounding; vented and filtered to outdoors with no recirculated air • **Radiopharmacy Isolator:** a lead-shielded, sealed unit designed specifically for compounding nuclear diagnostic and therapeutic agents

Supplemental Protections

Study Idea

Closed-system transfer devices and chemotherapy dispensing pins help protect the compounding technician from exposure to HDs during the transfer of drugs from vial to syringe to IV bag.

As mentioned when discussing aseptic garbing, extra PPE must be worn during hazardous compounding: goggles, a face shield with a respirator, a gown made of impervious material, and double chemotherapy gloves. Upon completion of compounding activities, garb must be disposed of in a special hazardous waste container.

Supplemental Engineering Controls In addition to those already mentioned, a few more protective supplies are needed: a **chemotherapy compounding mat**, **closed-system transfer devices**, and **chemotherapy dispensing pins**. The devices and pins supply additional containment when transferring HD ingredients. These three types of protective supplies are called **supplemental engineering controls**.

Labeling All CSPs containing hazardous agents must be properly labeled. These CSP labels must contain the patient's name and room number, the solution name and volume, the drug name(s) and dosage, CSP administration information, and storage requirements. Hazardous agents also require additional labeling that clearly identifies the CSP as a hazardous agent, with a colored caution label.

Study Idea

To ensure staff know how to properly clean a HD spill, mock HD spill drills are held for safety and quality assurance.

HD Cleaning and Spill Kit A **spill kit** must be readily accessible in any area where HDs are handled, compounded, or administered. A spill kit is a container of supplies,

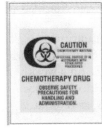

warning signage, and related materials used to contain an HD spill. Table 7.11 lists the contents of a typical spill kit.

In general, the standard HD PPE, including eye and face protection and chemotherapy gloves, should always be worn for cleaning, disinfecting, decontaminating the C-PECs and CACIs, and deactivating HDs in the compounding area, using appropriate products. Chemical **deactivation** of a nonnuclear HD should be done with 2% sodium hypochlorite (chlorine bleach). Alcohol is not an effective deactivating or HD cleaning agent.

HD spills, however, must be contained and cleaned immediately. Only trained workers with appropriate PPE should manage an HD spill, and they must post warning signs to restrict access to the spill area. The goal is to ensure that the staff, patients, and visitors are not exposed and that the healthcare environment (both inside and outside the medical facility) is not contaminated.

Safety Alert

When cleaning spills, trained personnel must wear proper PPE—including a gown, double chemotherapy gloves, goggles, and a mask or a NIOSH-certified respirator.

TABLE 7.11 Typical Contents of a Spill Kit

A commercially available spill kit may be purchased, or one may be assembled with the following contents:

- absorbent chemotherapy pads and towels
- 2 disposable chemotherapy-resistant gowns (with back closure)
- 2 pairs of chemotherapy-resistant shoe covers
- 4 pairs of chemotherapy gloves
- 2 pairs of chemical splash goggles
- 2 respirator masks approved by NIOSH
- 1 disposable dustpan
- 1 plastic scraper
- 1 puncture-proof container for glass
- 2 large, heavy-duty, sealable waste-disposal bags
- 1 hazardous waste label (if bags are unlabeled)

Source: American Society of Health-System Pharmacists (ASHP).

Nuclear Compounding

Study Idea

Nuclear hazardous waste is handled completely differently from other hazardous waste or pharmaceuticals, and it is regulated by the NRC

A specific kind of hazardous compounding occurs in a **nuclear pharmacy**, which prepares radioactive materials to diagnose and treat specific diseases. Nuclear medicine scans record radiation emitted from elements injected into the body, rather than from external elements like x-rays. **Radiopharmaceuticals** are irradiated HDs.

Unlike hazardous CSPs, these preparations are not prepared in a hospital pharmacy. They are most commonly prepared off-site in a nuclear pharmacy by specially trained and certified nuclear pharmacists and pharmacy technicians. The US Nuclear Regulatory Commission (NRC) regulates the medical use of radioactive materials to minimize radiation exposure to patients and healthcare staff.

A **nuclear pharmacy technician (NPT)** prepares radiopharmaceuticals. Working knowledge of radiopharmaceuticals and their risks and benefits is essential, as these technicians often advise healthcare providers regarding their toxicity and dangers. NPTs work under the direct supervision of nuclear pharmacists and receive special training and education on radiation safety. They must wear PPE to reduce radiation exposure, and follow strict guidelines with regard to the receipt, handling, disposition, disposal, and transfer of radioactive materials. Radiopharmaceutical compounders must use leaded glass or tungsten syringe shields, transfer devices, and containers in the nuclear pharmacy isolator.

Worker protection and medical surveillance programs for nuclear pharmacy personnel are even stricter than those for chemical HDs. Pharmacists, technicians, and other nuclear pharmacy personnel wear badges to monitor their exposure on a weekly, monthly, quarterly, annual, and lifetime basis. In addition, nuclear hazardous wastes are handled differently from other hazardous wastes or pharmaceuticals, as regulated by the NRC.

7.5 Waste Handling and Disposal

Sterile and hazardous compounding produce waste that must be disposed properly. Traces of hazardous wastes and residual pharmaceuticals have been found in surface water, groundwater, and drinking water in the United States, which has raised concern about the environmental contamination from waste from sterile and hazardous compounding as well as from general pharmaceuticals.

Hazardous Waste Disposal

During the admixture and administration of chemotherapy, any unadministered medication left in the IV bags and tubing, bottles, and vials must be disposed of in a hazardous waste container with a yellow label identifying it as hazardous waste. The US Environmental Protection Agency (EPA) defines *hazardous waste* as waste that causes or contributes to an increase in mortality or an increase in irreversible or incapacitating reversible illness. The definition also includes waste that poses a threat to human health when improperly treated, stored, transported, disposed of, or otherwise mismanaged. Table 7.12 lists examples of hazardous pharmaceutical waste based on the EPA's waste determinations. Further information about hazardous waste is available on the EPA's website at https://www.epa.gov and from state environmental protection agencies.

Nuclear hazardous wastes are handled differently from other hazardous wastes or pharmaceuticals, and are regulated by the NRC.

TABLE 7.12 Examples of Hazardous Pharmaceutical Waste

Waste Determination	Example
ignitable	flammable liquid or gas/aerosol or oxidizer, ethanol, ethyl chloride spray, silver nitrate swabs
reactive	nitroglycerin
heavy metals	products with thimerosal preservatives, burn ointments with silver compounds, *m*-cresol preservatives, selenium, mercury, silver sulfadiazine, and barium
corrosive	acids (e.g., acetic acid) and bases
specifically listed drugs	highly hazardous unused pharmaceuticals and chemicals, nicotine, physostigmine, chlorambucil, and warfarin

Sterile Compounding and General Pharmaceutical Wastes

Even small concentrations of certain drugs can have detrimental effects on aquatic and terrestrial wildlife species and on human health and development. A pharmacy technician must be aware of disposal requirements for sterile compounding and individual pharmaceuticals based on the employer's policies and procedures. The EPA and state governments monitor pharmaceutical waste disposal. There are significant fines for inappropriate disposal of any waste. Black waste containers are used for pharmaceutical waste, which must be labeled by contents. Storage and removal of filled containers must be handled in accordance with federal hazardous waste regulations.

Unused medications at healthcare facilities, pharmacies, and patient homes should not be flushed down the toilet or sink, because they flow into the wastewater system and work their way into rivers, groundwater, reservoirs, and oceans. This results in unintentionally medicating any person or animal drinking water with trace elements. These substances often accumulate in bodily tissues and fat and in aquatic plants, having unintended and often damaging effects. That is why the EPA now requires careful disposal of pharmaceutical waste.

Certain types of pharmaceutical waste are more dangerous than others, such as used fentanyl transdermal patches and other controlled substances. Because of their danger to children and pets, these patches should be folded in half and put into a sealed container with unappealing food waste like coffee grounds or cat litter and then put into a sealed trash container, away from child access.

For patients with pharmaceutical remainders, many pharmacies have established their own safe medication return containers. The National Community Pharmacists Association (NCPA) offers the Dispose My Meds program that allows patients to use their zip codes to find a disposal site at the closest participating community pharmacy. The National Association of Boards of Pharmacy (NABP) Foundation has worked with police departments and sheriff offices to set up permanent medication disposal dropboxes through its AWARxE program.

For pharmacies, outdated stock that can be returned to the manufacturer for credit is exempt from waste disposal regulations. If credit is not available, the pharmacy must dispose of outdated pharmaceuticals in accordance with hazardous waste regulations.

Review
and Assessment

STUDY SUMMARY

The ExCPT exam will require you to have a basic knowledge of the guidelines set up by the USP, OSHA, NIOSH, and NRC for safe compounding. Each hospital will also have its own P&P manual that includes these and additional guidelines. PPE, hand-washing, and aseptic technique should be reviewed.

Pharmacies compound many different types of parenteral products. Be aware of the procedures for compounding, calculations you will need to be able to compute, determining BUDs based on level of risk of contamination of the sterile product, documentation of the compounding process, and maintenance of equipment. You should be versed in the appropriate procedures for waste disposal from sterile and hazardous compounding and drug dispensing.

ADDITIONAL RESOURCES

For more in-depth explanations, check out *Sterile Compounding and Aseptic Technique* from Paradigm Education Solutions. To master and extend the material presented in this chapter, take advantage of the resources available through the eBook resources links. These include digital supplements, study resources, and a practice exam generator with 1,000+ exam-style questions. End-of-chapter tests are accessible through the eBook for individuals using the self-study course and through Cirrus for individuals enrolled in the instructor-guided course.

8

Pharmacy Inventory Management

Learning Objectives

1 Identify components in profitable inventory management, including average wholesale price and acquisition cost, reimbursement, markup, and profit. (Section 8.1)

2 Calculate inventory turnover rates and identify how these calculations relate to good inventory management. (Section 8.1)

3 Understand the different systems of reordering: periodic automatic replenishment level versus maximum/minimum levels. (Section 8.2)

4 Explain stock rotation using expiration dates. (Section 8.2)

5 Become familiar with purchasing concepts. (Section 8.2)

6 Discuss the advantages and disadvantages of a closed or open formulary. (Section 8.4)

7 Understand the receiving process and the Drug Quality and Security Act requirements. (Section 8.2)

8 Discuss storage requirements for refrigerated and frozen products, and for look-alike packages. (Section 8.2)

9 Discuss beyond-use dates for insulin. (Section 8.2)

10 Understand the handling of controlled substances, including the special US Drug Enforcement Administration forms for purchasing, recording diversions, and documenting destruction. (Section 8.2)

11 Identify product removal requirements related to overstock, outdated drugs, and medications returned by patients. (Section 8.2)

 Access eBook links for resources and an exam generator, with 1,000+ questions.

One of the responsibilities of a pharmacy technician is inventory management. Drug inventory is one of a pharmacy's largest investments, and a busy retail pharmacy may have $400,000 or more in inventory on the shelves. Proper ordering, receiving, posting, pricing, documenting, rotating, and other aspects of managing pharmaceutical and over-the-counter (OTC) inventory are important to a pharmacy's bottom line. Pharmacies must keep sufficient drug stock on hand to meet customer needs while minimizing costs, including the cost of stock sitting on the shelves and waste generated from expiring pharmaceuticals. At the same time, insufficient inventory can cost a community pharmacy sales if the pharmacy is not able to fill customers' prescriptions. In an institutional pharmacy, stock shortages may force the pharmacy to purchase products at higher prices.

The pharmacy technician is often responsible for ordering and receiving medications, durable medical equipment, and OTC products. Knowledge of inventory management is included in domain 1 of the ExCPT.

8.1 Inventory Accounting

A community pharmacy operates under the same principles as any other business—it must make a **profit** to survive. In other words, it must have more income than expenses to continue to provide services.

A **profit and loss (P&L) statement**, or report, is the financial statement that summarizes the revenues, costs, and expenses incurred for a specific period of time.

Acquisition Cost versus Pharmacy Reimbursement

Study Idea

AWP is the highest price or upper limit of what a pharmacy would pay to buy a drug from a wholesaler. Acquisition cost is what the pharmacy actually pays for the drug.

Pharmacies purchase their products from a wholesaler or supplier at a generally lower-than-retail price, called the **acquisition cost**.

In contrast, the **average wholesale price (AWP)** of a drug is the benchmark price or "*sticker price*" that wholesalers list for each drug, dose, and package size. There is a difference between the AWP and the actual acquisition cost because the AWP does not include the discounts pharmacies receive for bulk purchasing, prompt payment, or rebates from manufacturers for brand-name drugs.

Estimating Third-Party Reimbursements

Usually, insurance companies and other third parties reimburse pharmacies at a brand-name drug's AWP minus the third-party discount agreed upon in a negotiated contract, plus a pharmacy dispensing fee (in the range of $2.50 to $6.00 per prescription). The dispensing fee is a sum of all the pharmacy's personnel costs in providing services divided by the number of prescriptions, on average. This amount is added to each prescription that passes through the pharmacy so that they may attempt to cover their cost of operations.

Insurance companies and their pharmacy benefits managers (PBMs) calculate the prescription reimbursement amount paid to the pharmacy with the following formula:

$$AWP - (AWP \text{ x reimbursement percentage rate}) + dispensing\ fee = reimbursement\ amount$$

To maximize the pharmacy's income, it is essential to purchase a stock quantity from a wholesaler at less than AWP to make up for low reimbursement percentages. Consider Examples 8.1 and 8.2.

Example 8.1

You receive a prescription for 30 tabs of a cholesterol-lowering drug. The drug comes in a stock bottle that contains 90 tablets. The AWP for the bottle is $300.00. The insurance PBM has contracted with the pharmacy to pay the AWP minus 4% (converted to 0.04) plus a $6.00 dispensing fee. What is the reimbursement amount the pharmacy will receive?

Step 1 Determine the AWP for 30 tablets with a ratio-proportion equation:

$$\frac{90\ tablets}{285\ dollars} = \frac{30\ tablets}{y\ dollars}$$

$$90 \text{ tablets} \times y \text{ dollars} = 285 \text{ dollars} \times 30 \text{ tablets}$$

$$\frac{90 \text{ tablets} \times y \text{ dollars}}{90 \text{ tablets}} = \frac{285 \text{ dollars} \times 30 \text{ tablets}}{90 \text{ tablets}},$$

$$\text{so } y \text{ dollars} = \frac{285 \text{ dollars} \times 3}{9} = 95 \text{ dollars}$$

$$y \text{ dollars} = 95 \text{ dollars}, \quad \text{or } \$95.00$$

Step 2 Determine the reimbursement amount the pharmacy will receive:

AWP − (AWP reimbursement percentage rate) + dispensing fee = reimbursement amount

$$\$100.00 - (\$100.00 \times 0.04) + \$6.00 = \$102.00$$

Answer: The reimbursement amount that the pharmacy will receive is $102.00

Example 8.2

Using the AWP of $300.00 for a stock bottle of 90 tablets, determine the potential profit when considering a product purchase for a prescription of 30 tablets. Calculate the pharmacy's profit for a prescription for 30 tablets if the pharmacy has contracted with the supplier to pay AWP minus 5% (converted to 0.05).

Step 1 Determine the discount amount for the stock bottle:

AWP × reimbursement percentage rate = discount amount

$$\$300.00 \times 0.05 = \$15.00$$

Step 2 Determine the acquisition cost of the stock bottle:

AWP − discount amount = acquisition cost

$$\$300.00 - \$15.00 = \$285.00$$

Step 3 Using the ratio-proportion method, determine the cost of the prescribed quantity (30 tabs):

$$\frac{90 \text{ tablets}}{285 \text{ dollars}} = \frac{30 \text{ tablets}}{y \text{ dollars}}$$

$$90 \text{ tablets} \times y \text{ dollars} = 285 \text{ dollars} \times 30 \text{ tablets}$$

$$\frac{90 \text{ tablets} \times y \text{ dollars}}{90 \text{ tablets}} = \frac{285 \text{ dollars} \times 30 \text{ tablets}}{90 \text{ tablets}},$$

$$y \text{ dollars} = \frac{285 \text{ dollars} \times 3}{9} = 95 \text{ dollars}$$

$$y \text{ dollars} = 95 \text{ dollars}, \quad \text{or } \$95.00$$

Step 4 Determine the profit by subtracting the acquisition cost from the reimbursement amount. Use the reimbursement amount from Example 8.1 ($102.00):

$$\$102.00 - \$95.00 = \$7.00$$

Answer: The pharmacy's profit is $7.00. As you can see, the lower the pharmacy's acquisition cost, the more money will be available to cover operating costs and, hopefully, to generate a profit.

Markup and Profits

Pharmacies also buy their OTC products from wholesalers and sell them at higher prices. The pricing of OTC items is primarily determined by competition in the marketplace and customer expectations.

The difference between the retail selling price and the store acquisition cost is called the **markup**. It is determined by the pharmacy and used in the following formulas:

$$pharmacy\ acquisition\ cost + markup = retail\ selling\ price$$

$$retail\ selling\ price - acquisition\ cost = markup$$

Pharm Fact

The markup percentage affects the P&L statements. Too much markup will chase customers away and bring down profits. Too little markup will not cover expenses or create a profit.

The total profits from retail sales, patient pharmaceutical sales, and third-party reimbursements add up to the business's **gross profit**. The gross profit must cover a pharmacy's **overhead**, or operating costs, including personnel and benefits, facility costs, technology, utilities, marketing, and other expenses. What is left after all the expenses are paid is the **net profit**. A **loss**, or negative profit, occurs when the total retail sales plus claims reimbursement is lower than the total of the acquisition prices plus overhead. Having the right retail markup can help balance the bottom line toward profitability. Too high a markup drives customers away. Too low a markup means the pharmacy cannot meet its expenses and generate enough profit to stay in business.

Each independent pharmacy or pharmacy chain determines the percentage of each sale that must go toward the operation costs and profit. This percentage is called the **markup percentage**. To determine the exact **markup amount** to charge per item, whether prescription or retail, start with the acquisition cost from the wholesaler (supplier price) and multiply it by the pharmacy's markup percentage. (Pharmacies may set different retail markup percentages than prescription drug markup percentages.)

To calculate this markup amount, turn the markup percentage into a decimal by dividing it by 100, which is your **markup rate**. To get the markup amount, multiply the acquisition cost by the markup rate. Add the markup amount to the acquisition cost to get the customer price. The formula steps are as follows:

$$markup\ percent \div 100 = markup\ rate$$

$$markup\ rate \times acquisition\ cost = markup\ amount$$

$$acquisition\ cost + markup\ amount = customer\ price$$

You can see these formulas applied in Examples 8.3 and 8.4.

Example 8.3

The pharmacy acquires one case (12 bottles) of ABC All-Natural Fish Oil 1,200 milligram (mg) capsules for $180.00. To determine the customer price, a 34% markup must be applied to the acquisition cost. What is the customer price for one bottle of ABC All-Natural Fish Oil?

Step 1 Determine the markup rate:

$$\frac{markup\ percent}{100} = markup\ rate$$

$$\frac{34}{100} = 0.34$$

Step 2 Determine the markup amount for the case:

$$markup\ rate \times acquisition\ cost = markup\ amount$$

$$0.34 \times \$180.00 = \$61.20$$

Step 3 Determine the customer price for one bottle.

$$acquisition\ cost + markup\ amount = customer\ price\ (per\ case)$$

$$\$180.00 + \$61.20 = \$241.20;$$

The customer price for one case is $241.20

Divide by 12 bottles to determine the customer price for one bottle:

$$\frac{\$241.21}{12\ bottles} = \frac{\$20.10}{1\ bottle}$$

Answer: The cash price for one bottle of ABC All-Natural Fish Oil is $20.10

Pharm Fact

Markup for OTC items may seem high, but the profit on these front-end items helps make up for the small profit realized on prescription drugs, due to insurance contract pricing agreements.

Example 8.4

The customer price of one bottle of Senna with stool softener #100 is $34.95. The pharmacy's acquisition cost for this product is $22.45. What is the markup amount? What is the markup rate?

Step 1 Determine the markup amount:

$$customer\ price - acquisition\ cost = markup\ amount$$

$$\$34.95 - \$22.45 = \$12.50$$

Step 2 Determine the markup rate:

$$\frac{markup\ amount}{acquisition\ cost} = markup\ rate$$

$$\frac{\$12.50}{\$22.45} = 0.556792\ldots$$

Round $0.556792\ldots$ to the nearest hundredth: 0.56

Step 3 Convert the markup rate to a percent:

$$0.56 \times 100 = 56\%$$

Answer: The markup amount is $12.50; the markup rate is 56%

Managing Inventory Value and Turnover

Inventory value is the total value, or cost to acquire, the entire stock. The inventory includes prescription and OTC drugs, dietary supplements, medical and home health care supplies and equipment, front-end retail, and impulse merchandise. To determine inventory value, a pharmacy must keep a careful count of each product. This can be done manually or through technology.

Maintaining a Perpetual Inventory

As each drug prescription is filled, the pharmacy operations software and the point-of-sale (POS) system (which is connected electronically to the product barcode scanner and pharmacy inventory software) automatically deduct the product unit from the inventory count. This provides a **perpetual inventory**, or a continually up-to-date inventory count.

Each item in stock must also be counted once a year, and the manual counts compared to the software's perpetual inventory to reconcile them. For example, pharmacy software may indicate that there are 120 tablets of 20 mg famotidine remaining in stock. If the minimum reorder level is 100 tablets, famotidine will not be on the generated reorder list. However, if the drug is retrieved from the shelf and only 25 tablets remain, the inventory count should be updated in the system so that the drug can be ordered for the next business day. The technician, along with the pharmacist, must then try to figure out what caused the stock discrepancy.

One of the responsibilities of the pharmacy technician is to help keep track of the inventory and manage the inventory by making wise purchasing orders. To do this, it is important to know the inventory **turnover**—the number of times the whole inventory sells out per year—to make any necessary adjustments in stock ordering levels and ranges for more profitability. A high turnover rate without any shortage gaps is good. It means the pharmacy has closely estimated the individual stock movement needed to meet patient needs, and has ordered enough stock that it does not run out of the medications and loses sales or customers. A low turnover rate indicates that the inventory has been sitting on the shelves too long. If the inventory turns over every other month, the turnover rate is 6 (or 6 turns a year). If the inventory turns over every month the rate is 12. Pharmacies generally aim for a turnover rate of approximately 10 to 12 times a year, though most pharmacies do not usually exceed 10 turns. Most pharmacies average between 8 to 10 turnovers a year.

Calculating Inventory Turnover Ratios and Rates

To calculate the annual inventory turnover, you will use a **turnover ratio**, which compares the total annual cost of acquisition to the value of the current inventory. Divided out, the turnover ratio gives you the number of turnovers in a year, or **turnover rate**, as seen in the formula below.

$$\textit{turnover rate} = \frac{\text{annual acquisition cost}}{\text{current inventory value}}$$

You can see how to apply this formula in Example 8.5.

Example 8.5

The pharmacy has a monthly acquisition cost of $60,000.00. They have $140,000.00 invested in the inventory on hand. What is the inventory turnover rate?

$$\frac{\textit{annual acquisition cost}}{\textit{current inventory value}} = \textit{turnover rate}$$

Step 1 Determine the annual acquisition cost:

$$\frac{\$60,000}{1 \text{ month}} \times \frac{23 \text{ months}}{1 \text{ year}} = \frac{\$720,000.00}{1 \text{ year}}$$

Step 2 Determine the turnover rate:

$$y \text{ times a year} = \frac{\$720,000.00}{\$140,000.00} = 5.142857\ldots \text{ times a year}$$

Answer: y times a year $= 5.142857\ldots$ times a year, which can be rounded to the nearest whole number: 5 times a year; the inventory turnover rate is 5 times a year.

As Example 8.5 shows, this pharmacy is not controlling its inventory well, because a turnover rate of 5 is low. Pharmacy personnel will have to ask several important inventory questions:

1. Which products are the move the fastest, and which move the slowest?
2. Which products that require the most investment to maintain, and to what extent are they needed by your patient population? Do these products have to be on the shelves, or could they be ordered as needed?
3. Which products are necessary for your patient population, and how much of each product should be kept on hand?
4. Where should each product be shelved or stored?
5. Is there sufficient room for new products, or should other items counts be adjusted to make room?

In addition to these questions (which will be addressed in-depth in this chapter), other factors to be considered for inventory management include a knowledge of new products scheduled for release that the pharmacy will stock, floor space allocation, design and arrangement of shelves, and available refrigerator or freezer space. Inventory adjustments may include returning a portion of the current drug stock to a wholesaler, selling or transferring stock to another pharmacy, and/or lowering automatic restock levels.

8.2 Inventory Levels and Ordering Strategies

Practice Tip

For expensive refillable drugs, patients should be asked to alert the pharmacy when their drugs are at half to three-fourths level, so the pharmacy can do JIT ordering.

With the exception of Schedule II (C-II) controlled substances, ordering and purchasing are often initiated by the pharmacy technician. In addition to pharmaceuticals, the technician is also responsible for ordering pharmacy supplies, prescription vials, bottles, labels, information sheets, measuring devices, syringes, needles, and other items. In hospital settings, the technician is responsible for ordering supplies—including personal protective equipment (PPE) and intravenous base solutions for compounding—from the materials management department, which is in charge of ordering supplies for the entire institution.

In community pharmacies, medications are often ordered daily to minimize inventory costs and promote stock turnover. Most of the time, drugs are ordered from a wholesaler or corporate warehouse to be delivered to the pharmacy the following day. This is known as **just-in-time (JIT) ordering**—receiving medications just in time to sell. JIT ordering can also refer to waiting to order an expensive, rarely prescribed drug until someone needs it to avoid the cost of carrying it on the shelf until it is needed.

Chain pharmacies generally receive warehouse deliveries only once a few times per week and they rely heavily on JIT ordering to cover potential shortages during the week.

Investigational Drugs

Institutional pharmacies that work with research institutions acquire investigational drugs directly from the lead investigator or manufacturer, instead of the wholesaler. A **drug accountability record** must be maintained to account for the receiving and dispensing of the investigational drugs. This is generally done by a dedicated technician who also assists in dispensing. The drugs in the investigational study must be labeled and stored separately from the rest of the institution's pharmacy stock.

Periodic Automatic Replenishment Levels and Reorder Ranges

Put Down Roots

The inventory expression *PAR* in *PAR levels* comes from an acronym for periodic automatic replenishment levels.

Study Idea

A product with a PAR level of zero means it will not be reordered until it is out of stock. This could cause loss of sales.

In business, **economic order quantity** is the principle of ordering the optimal number of units to minimize the total cost associated with the purchase, delivery, and storage of a product. In pharmacy, this means ordering the highest amount of each drug that can be sold quickly enough to receive a quantity discount without wasting money and shelf space on units that sit on the shelves too long or drugs that expire.

On the one hand, buying in bulk is good, because it allows the pharmacy to acquire a drug at the lowest cost possible, but the pharmacy must be able to use the quantity purchased within a reasonable time frame. It may be cheaper per tablet to purchase a bottle of 1,000 tablets, but if the pharmacy only sells 50 tablets a month, it could take 20 months to use up the bottle. This is money sitting on the shelf.

Unlike some businesses, pharmacies often keep some slow-moving products on their shelves as a service to the few customers who will need them medically. If the pharmacy frequently runs out of needed supplies and medications, inconveniences patients, who will often just go to a different pharmacy. So, pharmacies set a **periodic automatic replenishment (PAR)** level in their software for each item, or the minimum level at which each stock item will generate automatic reordering. To accommodate fluctuations in demand, seasonal adjustments are made to the PAR levels for certain products, such as stocking more allergy products in the spring, sun protection products in the summer, flu vaccines in the fall, and antibiotics in the winter. If a new medication is increasingly prescribed in your geographical area, its PAR level will need to be increased.

Pharmacies that do not have an automated inventory ordering system must track drug stock by hand. These pharmacies usually have inventory ranges for each item—a minimum and maximum number of units to have on hand. The maximum number is the **safety point**, which allows a level of **safety stock** for higher than average sales. Orders are calculated using these levels. The minimum level marks the point when the stock must be ordered to avoid an interruption of stock availability, as with a PAR level. When inventory falls below the minimum level (or PAR level), the pharmacy makes an order. The order is for product that will take the inventory closest to the maximum level without going over the maximum level.

Stickers on the stock shelves list the minimum and maximum quantities for each drug. To calculate the amount to order use the following equation:

maximum inventory level − present inventory = order amount

When quantities get low, the technician should note it on the inventory control sheet and calculate the quantity to order by using this formula, as shown in Examples 8.6 and 8.7.

Example 8.6

The pharmacy's maximum inventory of sertraline 100 mg tablets is 600 tablets and the minimum is 200 tablets. By the end of the day there are 100 tablets left on the shelf. How many bottles of sertraline 100 mg #100 per bottle should the pharmacy order to reach the maximum threshold?

$$maximum\ inventory\ level - present\ inventory = order\ amount$$

$$600\ tablets - 100\ tablets = 500\ tablets;$$

$$500\ tablets \times \frac{1\ bottle}{100\ tablets} = 5\ bottles$$

Answer: The pharmacy needs to order 5 bottles of 100 tablets

Example 8.7

The pharmacy buys sertraline in bottles of 30 tablets each that only need to be labeled before dispensing, saving the pharmacy the cost of a prescription vial. Using the calculated number of tablets the pharmacy should order from Example 8.6, how many bottles of 30 tablets should be ordered?

$$y\ bottles = 500\ tablets \times \frac{1\ bottle}{30\ tablets} = 16.666666\ldots\ bottles$$

Answer: y bottles = 16.666666... bottles, which can be rounded to the nearest hundredth: 16.67 bottles; however, since the maximum inventory level is 600 tablets, only 16 bottles should be ordered

Excessive inventory ties up capital and hinders the pharmacy's ability to invest in other areas, like marketing and staffing. It incurs waste due to product expiration and increases the likelihood of theft. Therefore, inventory levels must be kept adequate but not excessive, with a rapid turnover of drug stock on the shelf.

ABC Classification System and Stock Management

Pharm Fact

Most pharmacies work by the 80/20 rule: 80% of costs can be attributed to 20% of products—the prescription drugs.

PAR levels and ordering ranges should be set based on a thorough knowledge of pharmacy stock movement and costs. There is an 80/20 rule in business that can be applied to pharmacy inventory analysis, in which 80% of costs are attributed to 20% of products, and often 80% of a pharmacy's profit comes from abundant sales of lower-end, retail items. By classifying products into categories of cost, the pharmacy can more easily monitor the most expensive and high-use products and use JIT ordering for these products to keep inventory costs down.

Inventory can also be sorted by product type, as in Table 8.1, where 80% fits a pharmacy's core mission: to sell prescription drugs. The other two product types (the 20%) will have the most markup to make a profit.

Poor management of a few products in category A is more detrimental to the bottom line than inadequate attention to a large number of items in category C. That is why it is particularly important to track the movement of high-dollar drugs and order only when necessary, without making patients wait for medications. Many pharmacies dispense high-dollar drugs with auxiliary labels that read, "This item is special ordered for you; please call a few days prior to needing refills."

TABLE 8.1 ABC Classifications

Category	% of Resource $	Product Type
A	80%	prescription drugs
B	15%	OTC drugs and supplements
C	5%	retail items

Study Idea

Lead time is the amount of time necessary to special order or compound a drug for a patient's prescription.

Study Idea

A shortage cost may include the cost to deliver to the patient, loss of patient to another pharmacy, or increase in price because it is not ordered from the pharmacy's primary wholesaler.

When ordering inventory, it is important to know how soon the product will be available, which is the **lead time**—the time between ordering or compounding a product and its delivery or payment. A compounding pharmacy must also consider the time it takes to compound or mix as part of the lead time.

If the pharmacy runs out of a medication before more stock arrives and cannot fill prescriptions, the pharmacy experiences what is known as a **shortage cost**. Shortage cost is difficult to measure, because it is made up of differing elements. For instance, if medications are out of stock, the pharmacy may need to deliver medications to the patients at home, incurring extra costs. If medications are unavailable too often, the pharmacy may lose customers. These are a few examples of shortage costs.

To ensure the pharmacy does not run out of a specific product, pharmacies often keep a safety stock of supply on hand. This safety stock provides a cushion so that, if certain prescriptions exceed the daily average, the pharmacy can still fill these prescriptions in a timely manner. To calculate safety stock, the technician must know the maximum potential daily usage, the average daily usage, and the lead time. You can then use the required amount of safety stock to calculate the level at which the pharmacy should reorder. This is called the **reorder point** for the PAR or ordering range. Example 8.8 shows how to calculate the amount of safety stock and the reorder point needed for atenolol (a beta blocker used to treat high blood pressure and rapid heartbeats), by using the following formulas:

safety stock = (maximum potential daily usage – average daily usage) × lead time

reorder point = (average daily usage × lead time) + safety stock

---

Example 8.8

A chain pharmacy dispenses an average of 400 atenolol 50 mg tablets a day, but it has sold as many as 550 tablets in one day. How many bottles of atenolol 50 mg 100 tablets should the pharmacy keep as safety stock if it takes 2 days of lead time to receive a new supply? What is the reorder point?

Step 1 Determine the safety stock:

safety stock = (maximum potential daily usage − average daily usage) × lead time = safety stock

safety stock = (550 tablets – 400 tablets) × 2 = 300 tablets

Convert tablets to bottles:

$$300 \text{ tablets} \times \frac{1 \text{ bottle}}{100 \text{ tablets}} = 3 \text{ bottles}$$

safety stock = 300 tablets,   or 3 bottles

Step 2 Determine the reorder point:

$$reorder\ point = (average\ daily\ usage \times lead\ time) + safety\ stock$$

$$reorder\ point = (400\ tablets \times 2) + 300\ tablets = 1{,}100\ tablets$$

Convert tablets to bottles:

$$1{,}100\ \cancel{tablets} \times \frac{1\ bottle}{100\ \cancel{tablets}} = 11\ bottles$$

$$reorder\ point = 1{,}100\ tablets, \quad or\ 11\ bottles$$

Answer: The pharmacy should keep a safety stock of 3 bottles atenolol; the reorder point is 11 bottles

Study Idea

Highly automated pharmacy computer systems generate the daily reorder list based on PAR levels. Some pharmacies still use the paper order book system in which, if an item is used, it is reordered.

As a purchasing agent, you have to consider shortage costs in addition to counts of waste due to expired or almost expired medications. Once a month, or per store policy, technicians have to check and reposition the stock, placing the oldest items in front and the new stock behind—unless the new stock has an earlier expiration date than the packages on the shelf. This repositioning is known as **rotating the stock** to make sure that pharmaceuticals with the earliest expiration dates are used first. Products close to expiration dates need to be removed. Each pharmacy has a policy for an acceptable range of shelf dates. A typical requirement might be that products have expiration dates of at least 12 months from the date of wholesaler receipt, and products on the shelves must have a four- to six-month shelf life.

The goal is to have low waste and shortage costs while taking advantage of volume discounts and other good deals negotiated through established purchasing relationships.

Purchasing Relationships and Contracts

Before any ordering or purchasing can happen, a pharmacy must establish relationships with those who distribute, store, or manufacture specific drugs. Purchasing contracts can be negotiated by an individual pharmacy or with other pharmacies as part of a group purchase contract. This can help independent pharmacies obtain greater discounts to better compete with chain stores that can buy in far larger quantities as a group.

Every month, a **compliance report** is sent by each wholesaler to the pharmacy inventory manager. It lists all the purchases made that did not comply with the contract bid and notes cheaper alternatives. Reviewing these reports for strategic changes in purchasing can save the pharmacy money in the future and help them determine if they want to remain with their current wholesaler or forge new relationships.

Primary Wholesaler Purchasing

Study Idea

Many institutional and community pharmacies now belong to buying groups that help leverage lower acquisition costs based on the group's total purchases.

Independent pharmacies generally each secure a **primary wholesaler purchasing contract** with a local drug wholesaler to be its primary supplier, so it can receive the fastest moving products from a single source for the best negotiated price to be delivered on a daily basis. (Chain pharmacies negotiate as a group or have their own wholesalers.) The advantages of this include scheduled deliveries and ordering, automatic online ordering, reduced turnaround time for orders, lower inventory and lower associated costs, discounts, and reduced commitment of time and staff. The turnaround time for receipt of drug orders is usually the next business day, with the exception of weekends and holidays. Disadvantages include higher purchase costs for individual stock items, occasional supply shortages (called *back orders*), and unavailability of some pharmaceuticals.

Prime Vendor Purchasing

In some situations, pharmacies need to work with more than one vendor, getting a large amount of stock from two or more suppliers. The pharmacy may be able to set up a **prime vendor purchasing contract** with one of these vendors to secure a discount for high-volume purchasing. This is an exclusive agreement to continually purchase a specified percentage or dollar amount toward different types of ordering and delivery methods. Prime vendor purchasing offers the advantages of lower acquisition costs, competitive service fees, electronic order entry, and emergency delivery services. Prime vendor purchasing is common in both retail and hospital pharmacies.

Closed or Open Formularies

Study Idea

In community pharmacy, a therapeutic substitution cannot be made unless the prescriber authorizes the change. The third-party payer also needs to give prior approval.

Beside considering delivery times and drug costs, the selection of wholesalers for primary and prime vendor purchasing relationships may also be influenced by a drug formulary and which wholesaler can supply the drugs on the list most cost effectively. A formulary is a list of medications approved for use or coverage. With a **closed formulary**, drugs not on the list are not allowed or covered by the insurer or institution. Hospitals try to control expenses by reducing the number of pharmaceuticals of the same drug class in its formulary according to best practices established by the medical community and what is available economically in purchasing groups. For example, the hospital may purchase one proton pump inhibitor (PPI) drug and make a therapeutic substitution for any other kind of PPI ordered. If omeprazole is the least expensive, then any medication orders for lansoprazole, esomeprazole, or pantoprazole would be changed to omeprazole. Typically, any nonformulary order has to be approved by the pharmacy and therapeutics (P&T) committee, which includes members of the medical staff.

Community pharmacies have **open formularies**. They stock pharmaceuticals to serve all of the patients in their community. However, insurers sometimes have closed formularies, though most use a more open, multitiered formulary. If the pharmacy is owned by a health maintenance organization (HMO), private insurer, or the Veterans Health Administration (VHA), for example, the pharmacy may have a formulary based on the larger organization's accepted standard of care.

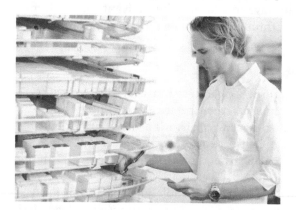

Technicians need to keep close track of the inventory, especially the most frequently purchased pharmaceuticals, to assist in deciding what needs to be purchased and how quickly.

Handling Orders

Study Idea

OOS items must be ordered in a quantity sufficient to fill waiting orders and any new orders expected.

The technician reviews and verifies each of the drugs listed on the end-of-the-day reorder list and orders to process them, alerting the pharmacist to any schedule II controlled substances. If the pharmacy is on a strict daily drug budget, you need to exercise good judgment and prioritize which drugs will be ordered for the next business day and which can wait. It is not uncommon for an independent pharmacy to wait to order an expensive drug until it is needed, rather than keep it in stock on the shelf.

When ordering next-day inventory, the technician assesses the predicted new prescriptions or refills for (1) **out-of-stock (OOS)** items, (2) partial fills, and (3) stock replenishment. Special orders for seldom stocked high-cost injectable products often require additional delivery time directly from the manufacturer if they are not in the wholesaler's on-site inventory.

For *fast movers*, the purchase decision is often based on the most economical order quantity or best value (such as ordering capsules in a 1,000 count size rather than 100 count size, or buying a case of liquid antacid rather than one or two bottles). Before purchasing a large quantity of a product on sale, the technician must estimate the additional time it will take to sell the larger quantity at a profit using the following formulas (see Example 8.9):

$$\text{time until all stock is sold} = \frac{\text{quantity to sell}}{\text{sales history}}$$

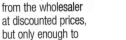

Pharm Fact

Pharmacies may buy seasonal products from the wholesaler at discounted prices, but only enough to sell in that season.

Example 8.9

The supplier offers a sale on calamine lotion: buy six cases, get the seventh case free. Each case sells for $6.00 and contains 12 bottles. All invoices must be paid in 30 days, or the pharmacy will be charged interest. Last year, the pharmacy sold 60 bottles of calamine lotion. If sales remain the same, how long will it take until all of the stock is sold?

Step 1 Determine the quantity to sell:

$$\frac{12 \text{ bottles}}{1 \text{ case}} \times 7 \text{ cases} = 84 \text{ bottles}$$

Step 2 Determine the sales history in bottles per month:

$$\frac{60 \text{ bottles}}{12 \text{ months}} = \frac{5 \text{ bottles}}{1 \text{ month}}$$

Step 3 Determine the time until all stock is sold in months:

$$\text{time until all stock is sold} = \frac{\text{quantity to sell}}{\text{sales history}}$$

$$y \text{ months} = 84 \text{ bottles} \times \frac{1 \text{ month}}{5 \text{ bottles}} = 16.8 \text{ months}$$

$$y \text{ months} = 16.8 \text{ months}$$

Answer: If sales remain the same, it will take 16.8 months until all the stock of Calamine lotion is sold

If it takes more than 16 months for the pharmacy to realize its return, is it a good idea to buy the product even if it is on sale? Probably not, because the storage space it will take up will take up space that could be given to a faster-moving product. The gross profit from the discounted price will be absorbed into the overhead costs, leaving little net profit. Calamine lotion is a low-dollar inventory item. What if this exact scenario applied to an expensive pharmaceutical like Vytorin, which is used for treating hyperlipidemia? The pharmacy pays $100.00 or more for a bottle of Vytorin. In that case, the pharmacy would not want to wait almost 17 months to see a return on its investment.

Processing Order Deliveries

Once an order is delivered from a wholesaler, warehouse, or other pharmacy, the technician must go through a number of key processes that require documentation.

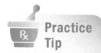
Receiving

When the wholesale delivery arrives, the process of **receiving** begins, which is a set of procedures to legally check in and accept the order. The pharmacist or technician first must sign an invoice from the wholesale representative, verifying the receipt of the correct number and type of totes or boxes. **Totes** are plastic containers for specialized medications, including those for refrigerated items (in cold packs) and for controlled substances, which all come sealed. A separate invoice and receipt are required for controlled substances. The pharmacist should check for and document intact seals and the content of these totes.

To check a delivery, you must carefully match the pharmaceutical products received against the purchase invoice for the correct products—matching the names, National Drug Code (NDC) numbers, barcodes, manufacturers, quantities, product strengths, and package sizes. You must also check for their delivery condition. In the case of a missing item or an incorrect, damaged, or improperly shipped product (not stored properly), notify the wholesaler and pharmacist immediately. Return the defective shipment and replace the ordered items as soon as possible.

Occasionally, a pharmaceutical product is temporarily or permanently unavailable from a wholesaler. First determine the reason for the unavailability—for example, the drug is (1) on back order, (2) being recalled by the manufacturer, or (3) being discontinued. If the product is not expected to be received the next day, the pharmacist should then identify a therapeutically equivalent product with permission from the prescriber. Alternatively, the pharmacy could consider borrowing the drug from another local pharmacy or one in the corporate chain if the drug is available.

Posting

As the inventory order is checked and approved, it is important that the order is accurately posted. **Posting** is the process of updating inventory in the pharmacy software database and reconciling any differences between the new and current stock. This process includes checking the newly received drug inventory for NDC numbers, expiration dates, and drug cost updates.

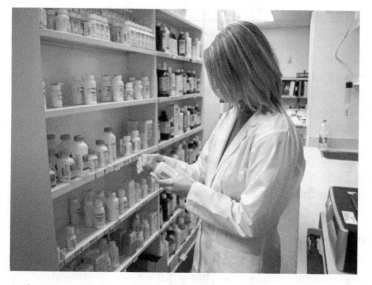

A pharmacy technician checks the label to insure proper storage.

Once the posting of the invoices is complete, a copy should go to accounts receivable for payment and the original should be filed in the pharmacy. (Controlled substance invoices should be filed separately for auditing convenience.)

The technician must also handle Drug Quality and Security Act (DQSA) documentation. This documentation includes noting the delivery transaction information and the full history or statements of the compounder/manufacturer on the lot number of the delivered medication. DSQA documentation must be kept on file for six years. Many wholesalers do not send a written copy of these reports but have them available online.

Storage

After medications are received, they must be stocked or shelved according to their proper labeling and storage requirements. Instructions for special storage and handling requirements for the pharmaceuticals are included on their product package inserts. These requirements are in line with the US Pharmacopeia–National Formulary (USP-NF) reference standards.

For instance, nitroglycerin has strict storage requirements. The sublingual tablets are unstable in the presence of air, moisture, and light, and must be stored in their original brown glass container from the manufacturer or a in specially designed airtight container. Nitroglycerin should be kept at temperatures below 77° F, or 25° C. Even body temperature will decrease its potency. To ensure potency, patients should purchase a new bottle of 25 tablets every three months. Intravenous nitroglycerin must be protected from light by covering the solution during administration.

Refrigerated and frozen pharmaceuticals are delivered in specially marked storage totes packed with ice or dry ice. These drugs should be posted and stored as soon as possible. Do not touch the dry ice. Place dry ice in a well-ventilated area until it completely dissolves.

Vaccines come in a tote with a color-coded tracking device that indicates whether the vaccine has been exposed to temperatures outside the proper storage range. If the temperature fluctuated out of the proper range in transport, the vaccine must be discarded, and the supplier should be contacted for credit or replacement. Zostavax and other vaccines and intravenous pharmaceuticals that need to be kept frozen should be stored at 5° F, or –15° C. Zostavax must be used within 30 minutes after it is reconstituted with a diluent.

Remember to check and log the freezer and refrigerator temperatures daily. Pharmacy refrigerator temperatures are kept in the range of 36° F to 46° F, or 2° C to 8° C. Refrigerated drugs include insulins, suppositories, some eye drops and soft gels, many vials, and injectable drugs. Chemotherapy agents that require refrigeration should be stored either in a separate refrigerator or isolated to prevent contamination if a leak or spill occurs. Any open refrigerated drug must be dated with its beyond-use date (BUD) to ensure it is discarded at the appropriate time.

Medications and items stored at room temperature should have a designated space and shelf label organized to minimize dispensing errors. Some pharmacies have stock alphabetized by brand name with the generic stock next to each item. Others have different systems or exceptions for look-alike or sound-alike drugs. For example, metformin 500 mg (a common diabetes drug) should not be placed on the shelf next to metformin ER 500 mg.

In a hospital pharmacy, the technician is often responsible for restocking the floor stock medications stored in automated dispensing units, such as the Pyxis or Omnicell. The automated units include a perpetual inventory system and electronically charge the appropriate patient account at the point of administration.

Patients should be informed about how to properly store medications at home. For example, a reconstituted antibiotic suspension is stable for a limited time, about 10 days, and should be discarded once the treatment is complete. Penicillin-based solutions need to be stored in the refrigerator after they have been reconstituted. Other antibiotics such as azithromycin, clarithromycin, and cefdinir are stored at room temperature, which is generally considered to be below 86° F, or 30° C. Some temperature variation may occur during a short-term power outage, but any long-term storage above room temperature can affect refrigerated medications. Patients whose medication has experienced dramatic temperature variation should contact the pharmacy or manufacturer of the product for more information.

Patients need to be made aware that if an insulin vial or syringe is frozen or left in the heat of a car or in light, the medication should not be used and should be discarded. In warm climates or in summer, patients may be advised to transport their insulin home from the pharmacy in a cooler, especially if they are not returning home immediately.

Once opened, most insulins have a BUD of 28 days, though newer agents may be good for up to 60 days. Check the package insert for the manufacturer-recommended BUD. Patients need to be instructed that insulin should be stored in the refrigerator until first use, and then discarded after the BUD. Patients do not need to refrigerate a vial or insulin pen after first use.

Handling Out-of-Stock and Medications

After receiving, posting, and shelving/storing inventory is complete, it is important to initiate the prescription filling process for any OOS or partial-fill prescriptions from the day before. The OOS prescription orders are processed, verified, and filled first, so they can be available for the patients to pick up later that same day, as promised. If possible, you should notify the patients when the prescription is ready for pickup. The completion of partial-fill orders takes priority next. These patients have commonly received three to five days worth of medication to hold them over until the order is received. Notify these patients that their medication is ready as soon as the remainder can be filled.

Handling Controlled Substances

Controlled substances require special purchasing, receiving, and record keeping of inventory, according to the Controlled Substances Act (CSA). Each pharmacy must register with the US Drug Enforcement Agency (DEA) to purchase and dispense controlled substances, and the US Food and Drug Administration (FDA) requires that all controlled-substance containers be clearly marked with their schedule designation on the product label.

Schedule III, IV, and V Drugs

In most pharmacies, the technician can order Schedule III–V (C-III–C-V) medications. However, per store policy, the pharmacist may have to verify and sign for their receipt at delivery. After comparing the invoice with the ordered drug name, dosage, and quantity, the technician can often sign the receipt and ask the pharmacist to verify it. Next, the technician can store these drugs among the rest of the drug stock, usually alphabetically by generic drug name. All C-III, C-IV, and C-V prescriptions and records, including purchasing invoices, are commonly kept separate from other records and must also be kept in a readily retrievable form.

C-II Purchasing

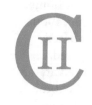

C-II controlled substances follow stricter protocols per federal and state law and regulations. Similar to other medications, PAR levels for most C-II drugs generate automated inventory alerts in the pharmacy software for reorders or for OOS or partial-fill orders. However, purchase of C-II controlled substances must be specifically initiated and authorized by a pharmacist and executed on a DEA Form 222, either online or on paper.

C-II Receiving and Documentation When receiving the C-II tote, the technician should check that the seal is not broken, then break the seal and verify the contents with the invoice. After verification, the pharmacist must document the following information on the DEA Form 222 delivery receipt section: the date, the name and amount of C-II drugs received, and the corresponding NDC numbers. The technician can then post the C-II drug inventory to the inventory database, including the NDC numbers, prices, and expiration dates.

Controlled Substance Disposal As C-II controlled substances in the inventory expire or are defective (such as a case of broken tablets), they must be disposed of properly. Any controlled drug disposal must be itemized, recorded, witnessed, and signed by a second pharmacist on the DEA Form 41. In most cases, C-II drugs are delivered or sent to an authorized destruction depot after the proper documentation of DEA Form 41 has been completed with a copy to accompany the drugs, a copy mailed to the DEA, and a copy kept on file.

C-II Perpetual Inventory Record Community pharmacies use automated or manual perpetual inventory to maintain inventory counts and close control of all C-II drug stock. A pharmacy must keep perpetual inventory record for all C-II medications on a tablet-by-tablet (or other dosage form) basis that includes product, dosage, quantity, date received or dispensed, prescription number, remaining inventory, and signature or initials of the pharmacist.

Biennial Inventory Count According to DEA regulations, a biennial (every two years) inventory of controlled substances must be taken. Some states (and pharmacies) have even more stringent requirements, such as a yearly inventory. These inventories should closely approximate the perpetual inventory record. For C-III, C-IV, and C-V substances, an estimated count and/or measure of units remaining in stock containers is permitted, unless a container holds more than 1,000 capsules or tablets. Then an exact count is required. For C-II drugs, each unit must be accounted for. The C-II inventory count should not vary by more than four days from the calendar month and date of the last biennial inventory. The pharmacy must file an original hard copy of the biennial inventory, send another to the DEA, and may also fill one out online for the DEA. Major deviations in actual counts and numbers listed in the C-II drugs must be investigated and reported if not resolved.

Additional tracking mechanisms exist by state and federal authorities to monitor the distribution of C-II drugs. If there is evidence of overprescribing by a physician, overdispensing by a pharmacy, or overselling of C-II drugs by a wholesaler, the DEA—after a thorough investigation—has the authority to temporarily or permanently revoke the DEA license of that physician, pharmacy, or wholesaler. A wholesaler can limit the monthly amount of controlled substances distributed to a community pharmacy if it deems that there has been excessive use.

Drug Returns and Credits

Sometimes, drugs must be returned to the wholesaler for credit in their original stock bottles or unit-of-use packaging and in their original condition. Pharmacy overstocks, patient declining medications at pickup or neglecting to pick them up, soon-to-be-expired drugs, manufacturer or FDA recalls, reformulated drugs, or drugs in out-of-date packaging are all reasons for a drug return. The different reasons for returns result in slightly different ways to handle them.

Study Idea

Review the FDA recall classifications in Chapter 2.

Return of Recalled Drugs

When an official drug recall alert occurs, the wholesaler will typically email or mail the drug recall information to the pharmacy drug name, strength, dose, NDC, lot number, and expiration date as well as the date and type of recall (voluntary, mandatory). This form is then returned to the wholesaler with the stock pulled from the shelves and the pharmacy is usually given a credit to their account or reimbursed for the stock that is lost.

Practice Tip

When filling prescriptions for specially ordered, high-cost drugs, do not attach the patient medication label to the drug packaging. Attach it with a rubber band or place it with the packaging in a resealable plastic bag, so it can be returned to the wholesaler if not picked up.

Return of Declined Medications

At times, patients do not pick up their filled medication within seven days, even after reminder messages. Consequently, you must reverse or cancel the online insurance billing, store the prescription in the patient profile for possible future use, and return the stock to drug inventory or to the wholesaler. For example, if a patient declines to pick up the expensive diabetes drug Victoza (liraglutide), you can store it in the refrigerator and then return it to the wholesaler for credit if the box is unopened and the prescription label (perhaps attached by rubber band) can be removed without altering or damaging the manufacturer's label.

A return-for-credit form must be completed that lists the drug(s) and quantities to be returned. You and the wholesale driver must verify the contents of the return totes or boxes, and sign for the credit. Your signature guarantees under penalty of law that the product was purchased directly from the wholesaler and that the drugs have been stored and handled in accordance with manufacturers' guidelines and all federal, state, and local laws. The containers are then sealed and returned to the wholesaler for credit. The signed form is filed for future reference.

Expired Medications

As noted, pharmacy technicians must check the dating on stock and rotate the products (including OTC drugs and dietary supplements) on a monthly basis, or per store policy. All medications that are expired or nearly expired (within three to six months) are to be removed and returned to the wholesaler or manufacturer, but the pharmacy may not be issued credit for these medications. This process of returns and credits is time-consuming, and it involves a lot of paperwork. Many pharmacies now hire **reverse distributors** to handle outdated inventory. They come to the pharmacy, prepare the drugs for return, and provide the return documentation. In some cases, pharmacies will be credited a percentage of the cost of the medication. These instances depend on the contractual agreements between the pharmacy and the wholesaler, distributor or manufacturer.

Study Idea

Refrigerated drugs that need to be returned should not be packaged in a tote until the wholesale driver is on site; then the drugs are added to the tote with proper cooling packs.

Wrongly Filled Prescriptions

At times, the incorrect medication is filled for a prescription, which occasionally happens despite safety checks. If the drug did not leave the pharmacy, the prescription can be corrected, and the drug can be returned to stock. However, if the patient left the pharmacy, discovered the error, and then came back to the pharmacy later with the medication unopened, the incorrect drug must be discarded per law and pharmacy protocol. In this case, the pharmacy cannot redispense or recover the cost of the incorrect prescription.

As you can see, inventory information takes time to get to know well. Technicians need knowledge and experience working with the various aspects of inventory management before they move into positions of greater responsibility. That is why technicians taking the ExCPT need to be well versed in the basic terms and concepts of inventory management.

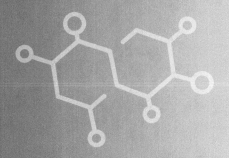

Review
and Assessment

STUDY SUMMARY

The task of inventory management in a pharmacy requires in-depth knowledge of the amount and types of drugs being prescribed and of the rate of purchases in each pharmacy. Sales reports and turnover rates are used to set up inventory PAR levels or establish maximum and minimum levels for each drug. Technicians must be aware of:

- the various wholesaler relationships and ordering procedures for prescription controlled substance and noncontrolled drugs as well as OTC products

- procedures for purchasing, receiving, and stocking of pharmaceuticals

- inventory terminology

- the importance of DQSA, FDA, and DEA rules and documentation on drug inventory

- the proper forms to order and report issues of controlled substances, and of the special storage requirements for select pharmaceuticals

- the methods to return and be reimbursed for recalled products

- the importance of monitoring, reversing claims, and returning to stock prescriptions that are filled incorrectly or not picked up by patients.

ADDITIONAL RESOURCES

For more in-depth explanations, check out *Pharmacy Practice for Technicians,* Seventh Edition from Paradigm Education Solutions. To master and extend the material presented in this chapter, take advantage of the resources available through the eBook resources links. These include digital supplements, study resources, and a practice exam generator with 1,000+ exam-style questions. End-of-chapter tests are accessible through the eBook for individuals using the self-study course and through Cirrus for individuals enrolled in the instructor-guided course.

Common Pharmacy Abbreviations and Acronyms

The abbreviations with red lines through them are ones that are still in use but are discouraged by Institute for Safe Medication Practices (ISMP). The ISMP recommends the use of the correct words instead. Many of these discouraged abbreviations are also on The Joint Commission's Official "Do Not Use" List of Abbreviations.

Abbreviation	Meaning
A-B-C	
aaa	apply to affected area
ACA	Affordable Care Act (Patient Protection and Affordable Care Act)
a̶c̶; a̶.̶c̶.̶; A̶C̶	before meals
ACE	angiotensin-converting enzyme inhibitors
a̶d̶; a̶.̶d̶.̶; A̶D̶	right ear
ADD	attention-deficit disorder
ADH	antidiuretic hormone
ADHD	attention-deficit hyperactivity disorder
ADME	absorption, distribution, metabolism, and elimination
ADR	adverse drug reaction
AIDS	acquired immune deficiency syndrome
AM; a.m.	morning
ANDA	Abbreviated New Drug Application
APAP	acetaminophen; Tylenol
AphA	American Pharmacy Association
ARBs	angiotensin receptor blockers
a̶s̶; a̶.̶s̶.̶; A̶S̶	left ear
ASA	aspirin
a̶u̶; a̶.̶u̶.̶; A̶U̶	both ears; each ear
b.i.d.; BID	twice daily
BMI	Body Mass Index
BP	blood pressure
BUD	beyond-use date
°C	degrees centigrade; temperature in degrees centigrade
Ca^{++}	calcium

Abbreviation	Meaning
Cap; cap	capsule
CDC	Centers for Disease Control and Prevention
CF	cystic fibrosis
CHF	congestive heart failure
CNS	Central Nervous System
COPD	chronic obstructive pulmonary disease
CPR	cardio pulmonary resuscitation
CSP	compounded sterile preparation
CV	cardiovascular
D-E-F	
D_5; D_5W; D5W	dextrose 5% in water
D_5 ¼; D5 1/4	dextrose 5% in ¼ normal saline; dextrose 5% in 0.225% sodium chloride
D_5 ⅓; D5 1/3	dextrose 5% in ⅓ normal saline; dextrose 5% in 0.33% sodium chloride
D_5 ½; D5 1/2	dextrose 5% in ½ normal saline; dextrose 5% in 0.45% sodium chloride
D_5LR; D5LR	dextrose 5% in lactated Ringer's solution
D_5NS; D5NS	dextrose 5% in normal saline; dextrose 5% in 0.9% sodium chloride
DAW	dispense as written
DC; d/c	discontinue
D/C	discharge
DCA	direct compounding area
Dig	digoxin
disp	dispense
EC	enteric-coated
Elix	elixir
eMAR	electronic medication administration record
EPO	epoetin alfa; erythropoietin
ER; XR; XL	extended-release
°F	degrees Fahrenheit; temperature in degrees Fahrenheit
$FeSO_4$	ferrous sulfate; iron
G-H-I	
g, G	gram
gr	grain
GI	gastrointestinal
GMP	good manufacturing practice
gtt; gtts	drop; drops
h; hr	hour
HC	hydrocortisone
HCTZ	hydrochlorothiazide
HIPAA	Health Insurance Portability and Accountability Act
HIV	human immunodeficiency virus
HMO	Health Maintenance Organization
HRT	hormone replacement therapy

Abbreviation	Meaning
~~h.s.~~; ~~HS~~	bedtime (comes from Latin *hora somni* meaning "hour of sleep"); ~~hs~~ should also not be used
IBU	ibuprofen; Motrin
ICU	intensive care unit
IM	intramuscular
IND	Investigational New Drug Application
Inj; ~~IJ~~	injection
IPA	isopropyl alcohol
ISDN	isosorbide dinitrate
ISMO	isosorbide mononitrate
ISMP	Institute for Safe Medication Practices
IV	intravenous
IVF	intravenous fluid
IVP	intravenous push
IVPB	intravenous piggyback
J-K-L	
K; K+	potassium
KCl	potassium chloride
kg	kilogram
L	liter
LAFW	laminar airflow workbench; hood
lb	pound
LD	loading dose
LVP	large-volume parenteral
JCAHO	Joint Commission on the Accreditation of Healthcare Organizations
M-N-O	
Mag; Mg; MAG	magnesium
MAR	medication administration record
mcg	microgram
MDI	metered-dose inhaler
MDV	multiple-dose vial
mEq	milliequivalent
mg	milligram
~~MgSO~~$_4$	magnesium sulfate; magnesium
mL	milliliter
mL/hr	milliliters per hour
mL/min	milliliters per minute

Abbreviation	Meaning
MMR	measles, mumps, and rubella vaccine
MRSA	methicillin-resistant S. aureus
MOM; M.O.M.	milk of magnesia
M.S.	morphine sulfate (save MS for multiple sclerosis)
MU†; mu	million units
MVI; MVI-12	multiple vitamin injection; multivitamins for parenteral administration
Na⁺	sodium
NABP	National Association of Boards of Pharmacy
NaCl	sodium chloride; salt
NDA	New Drug App
NDC	National Drug Code
NF; non-form	nonformulary
NKA	no known allergies
NKDA	no known drug allergies
NPO; npo	nothing by mouth
NR; d.n.r.	no refills; do not repeat
NS	normal saline; 0.9% sodium chloride
½ NS	one-half normal saline; 0.45% sodium chloride
¼ NS	one-quarter normal saline; 0.225% sodium chloride
NSAID	nonsteroidal anti-inflammatory drug
NTG	nitroglycerin
OC	oral contraceptive
od; o.d.; OD	right eye
ODT	orally disintegrating tablet
OPTH; OPHTH; Opth	ophthalmic
os; o.s.; OS	left eye
OTC	over the counter; no prescription required
ou; o.u.; OU	both eyes; each eye
oz	ounce
P-Q-R	
p.c.; PC	after meals
PCA	patient-controlled anesthesia
PCN	penicillin
pH	acid-base balance
PHI	protected health information
PM; p.m.	afternoon; evening
PN	paternal nutrition

Abbreviation	Meaning
PNS	peripheral nervous system
PO; po	orally; by mouth
PPE	personal protective equipment
PPI	proton pump inhibitor
PR	per rectum; rectally
PRN; p.r.n.	as needed; as occasion requires
PTSD	Post Traumatic Stress Disorder
PV	per vagina; vaginally
PVC	polyvinyl chloride
q	every
q.h.; qhour	every hour
q2h	every 2 hours
q4h	every 4 hours
q6h	every 6 hours
q8h	every 8 hours
q12h	every 12 hours
q24h	every 24 hours
q48h	every 48 hours
QA	quality assurance
QAM; qam	every morning
qDay; QD; Qd	every day
q.i.d.; QID	four times daily
QOD; Q other day; Q.O. Day	every other day
QPM; qpm	every evening
qs; qsad	quantity sufficient; a sufficient quantity to make
QTY; qty	quantity
qwk; qweek	every week
RA	rheumatoid arthritis
RDA	recommended daily allowance
Rx	prescription; pharmacy; medication; drug; recipe; take
S-T	
sig	write on label; signa; directions
SL; sub-L	sublingual
SMZ-TMP	sulfamethoxazole and trimethoprim; Bactrim
SNRI	serotonin norepinephrine reuptake inhibitor
SPF	sunburn protection factor

Abbreviation	Meaning
SR	sustained-release
SS; ss	one-half
SSRI	selective serotonin reuptake inhibitor
STAT; Stat	immediately; now
STD	sexually transmitted disease
Sub-Q; SC; SQ; sq, subcut, SUBCUT, subq	subcutaneous
SUPP; Supp	suppository
susp	suspension
SVP	small-volume parenteral
SW	sterile water
SWFI	sterile water for injection
Tab; tab	tablet
TB	tuberculosis
TBSP; tbsp	tablespoon; tablespoonful; 15 mL
TDS	transdermal delivery system
t.i.d.; TID	three times daily
t.i.w.; TIW	three times a week
TKO; TKVO; KO; KVO	to keep open; to keep vein open; keep open; keep vein open (a slow IV flow rate)
TNA	Total Nutrition Admixture
TPN	total parenteral nutrition
TSP; tsp	teaspoon; teaspoonful; 5 mL
U-V-W	
U or u	unit
u.d, UD, ut dictum	as directed
ung	ointment
USP	U.S. Pharmacopeial Convention
USP-NF	*U.S. Pharmacopoeia-National Formulary*
UTI	urinary tract infection
UV	ultraviolet light
VAG; vag	vagina; vaginally
Vanco	vancomycin
VO; V.O.; V/O	verbal order
w/o	without
X-Y-Z	
Zn	zinc, but $ZnSO_4$—should not be used for zinc sulfate
Z-Pak	azithromycin; Zithromax

Commonly Prescribed Controlled Substances

Commonly Prescribed Controlled Substances

Generic	Brand Examples	Used For
Schedule II		
amobarbital	Amytal, Tuinal	Sedative, analgesic
amphetamine/dextroamphetamine	Adderall	ADHD/narcolepsy
cocaine topical	C-Topical Solution	Nose bleed, vasoconstriction
codeine**		Analgesic
dexmethylphenidate	Focalin	ADHD
fentanyl	Duragesic, Sublimaze	Narcotic analgesic
fentanyl patch	Duragesic	Analgesic
glutethimide	Doriden, Dorimide	Hypnotic sedative
hydrocodone* (with cough/cold ingredients)	Vicotuss	Cough/cold relief
hydrocodone/APAP	Vicodin, Lortab, Norco	Analgesic
hydromorphone	Dilaudid, Exalgo, Palladone	Analgesic (for severe pain)
lisdexamfetamine	Vyvanse	ADHD
meperidine	Demerol	Narcotic analgesic
methadone	Dolophine	Analgesic
methadone	Methadose	Opioid maintenance
methamphetamine	Desoxyn	Weight reduction
methylphenidate CR	Concerta, Metadate, Ritalin LA	ADHD
methylphenidate	Ritalin	ADHD
morphine	MS Contin, Roxanol, Oramorph, RMS, MSIR	Analgesic

opium	Tincture of Opium	Antidiarrhea
oxycodone	OxyContin, Percocet	Analgesic
oxycodone/APAP	Percocet, Tylox	Analgesic
Oxycodone/ASA	Percodan	Analgesic
oxymorphone	Opana	Analgesic
pentobarbital	Nembutal	Sedative, hypnotic, anti-anxiety, anticonvulsant
tapentadol	Nucynta	Analgesic

Schedule III

anabolic steroids (such as testosterone cypionate)	Depo-Testosterone	Various indications, depends on steroid
armodafinil	Nuvigil	Stimulant
ASA/butabital/caffeine	Fiorinal	Migraine relief
ASA/butabital/caffeine/Codeine	Fiorinal with codeine	Migraine relief
ASA/codeine	Empirin with Codeine	Analgesic
benzphetamine	Didrex, Recede	Appetite suppressant
buprenorphine	Subutex, Butrans	Opioid maintenance
buprenorphine/naloxone	Suboxone, Zubsolv	Opioid maintenance
butorphanol	Stadol	Analgesic
codeine/APAP	Tylenol No. 3	Analgesic
dronabinol	Marinol	Appetite stimulant
esterified estrogen/testosterone	Estratest	Hormone replacement
hydrocodone/chlorpheniramine	Tussionex	Cough suppressant, antihistamine
ketamine	Ketaset, Ketalar, Special K	Dissociative anesthetic
phendimetrazine	Plegine, Prelu-2, Bontril, Melfiat, Statobex	Appetite suppressant
testosterone	AndroGel, Testim	Low testosterone
thiopental	Pentothal	Anesthetic

Schedule IV

alprazolam	Xanax	Anti-anxiety, benzodiazepine
APAP/dichloralphenazone/isometheptane	Midrin, Epidrin	Migraine relief
carisoprodol	Soma	Muscle relaxer
chlordiazepoxide	Librium	Anti-anxiety, benzodiazepine
clidinium/chlordiazepoxide	Librax	GI antispasmodic
clonazepam	Klonopin	Anticonvulsant. Benzodiazepine

clorazepate	Tranxene	Sedative, anti-anxiety
diazepam	Valium, Diastat	Anti-anxiety, anticonvulsant, benzodiazepine
eszopiclone	Lunesta	Hypnotic
flurazepam	Dalmane	Hypnotic
lorazepam	Ativan	Anti-anxiety, benzodiazepine
meprobamate	Miltown, Equanil	Anti-anxiety
midazolam	Versed	Sedative
modafinil	Provigil	Stimulant
Oxazepam	Serax	Anti-anxiety, benzodiazepine
phenobarbital	Luminal	Anticonvulsant
phentermine	Adipex, Fastin	Appetite suppressant
propoxyphene	Darvon	Analgesic
propoxyphene/APAP	Darvocet	Analgesic
quazepam	Doral	Anti-anxiety, benzodiazepine
sibutramine	Meridia	Weight loss
suvorexant	Belsomra	Hypnotic
temazepam	Restoril	Hypnotic
tramadol	Ultram	Analgesic
triazolam	Halcion	Sedative, hypnotic
zaleplon	Sonata	Hypnotic
zolpidem	Ambien	Hypnotic

Schedule V

atropine/diphenoxylate	Lomotil	Antidiarrheal
codeine***	Robitussin AC, Phenergan with Codeine, and others	Cough suppressant, nasal congestion, upper respiratory tract concerns
ezogabine	Potiga	Anticonvulsant
lacosamide	Vimpat	Anticonvulsant
pregabalin	Lyrica	Neuropathic pain

Note: Information updated as of August 2016. New drugs come in often. Visit http://www.deadiversion. usdoj.gov/schedules/ for the updated list.

* Combination products containing hydrocodone are Schedule II as of 2014.

** Products containing not more than 90 milligrams of codeine per dosage unit (ie tablet or capsule)are Schedule III.

*** Cough preparations with one or more non-narcotic ingredients, containing not more than 200 milligrams of codeine per 100 milliliters or per 100 grams are Schedule V.

Index

Note: Locators for figures are indicated by *f*, tables by *t*, and photos by *p* following the page number.

heparin, 70, 71*t*
herbals, 81
high blood pressure, medications for, 33–36, 34–36*t*
high-density lipoprotein (HDL), 36
high-efficiency particulate air (HEPA), 214
high-risk medications, medication guides for, 121, 121–122*t*
high-stakes exam, preparing for, 1–12
  certification, benefits of, 2
  after exam, 12
  multiple-choice test tips, 10–11, 11*t*
  right exam, choosing, 4–10
histamine-2 antagonists (H₂ blockers), 56, 57*t*
HMG-CoA redutase inhibitors, 36, 37*t*
homeopathy, 79
horizontal laminar airflow workbench (H-LAFW), 214
Humira, 72, 72*t*
Humulin R, 77*t*
hydralazine, 39*t*
hydrochlorothiazide, 64, 65*t*
hydrocodone/acetaminophen, 61*t*
hydrocortisone, 74*t*, 77*t*
Hydrodiuril, 64, 65*t*
hydromorphone, 61*t*
Hygroton, 65*t*
hyperthyroidism, 52, 52*t*
hypnotic drugs, 23
hypothyroidism, 51–52, 52*t*

I

ibandronate, 63*t*
ibuprofen, 62*t*, 76*t*
iloperidone, 28*t*
Imdur, 38, 39*t*
imipramine, 26*t*
Imitrex, 30, 32*t*
immunization, 82–83
Imodium, 56, 58*t*
Imodium AD, 77*t*
Incruse Ellipta, 54*t*
indacaterol, 53*t*
indacaterol/glycopyrrolate, 55*t*
indapamide, 65*t*
Inderal, 36*t*
Inderal LA, 36*t*
Indocin, 62*t*
indomethacin, 62*t*
inflammatory bowel disease medications, 58*t*
Inflectra, 72, 72*t*
infliximab, 72, 72*t*
informed consent form, 119
infusion rate, 222
inscription, 151
insomnia, medications to treat, 23–24, 24*t*
Inspra, 65*t*
Institute for Safe Medication Practices (ISMP), 18, 118
Institutional Review Board (IRB), 119, 155

insulins, 50–51, 50*p*, 51*t*
insurance information, 148–149
integrative medicine, 78–79
interchangeable biological drug, 144
intervention, Pulverization by, 201
intradermal (ID), 211
intramuscular (IM), 211
intravenous (IV), 211
Invanz, 44, 44*t*
Invega, 28*t*
inventory turnover, 244
inventory value, 243
Investigational New Drug (IND) Application, 119
Invokamet, 49*t*
Invokamet XR, 49*t*
Invokana, 48*t*
iPLEDGE program, 123, 123*t*
ipratropium, 53*t*
ipratropium/albuterol, 54*t*
irbesartan, 35*t*
irritable bowel syndrome (IBS), 56
  medications, 57*t*
Isordil, 38, 39*t*
isosorbide dinitrate, 38, 39*t*
isosorbide mononitrate, 38, 39*t*
Isotretinoin, 123
IV bolus injections, 211
IV push (IVP) injections, 211

J

Janumet, 50*t*
Janumet XR, 50*t*
Januvia, 48*t*
The Joint Commission (TJC), 118
  official Do Not Use list, 130, 130*t*
Jolivette, 69*t*
just-in-time (JIT) ordering, 245
juvenile diabetes. *See* type I diabetes

K

Kadian, 61*t*
Kazano, 49*t*
Keflex, 41*t*
Kenalog, 74*t*
Keppra, 32*t*
Keppra XR, 32*t*
ketoconazole, 45*t*
ketorolac, 62*t*
Klonopin, 24*t*
Kombiglyze XR, 50*t*
Kristalose, 58*t*

L

Llabetalol, 36*t*
Lactaid, 77*t*
lactase, 77*t*
Lactobacillus rhamnosus, 77*t*
lactulose, 58*t*
Lamictal, 32*t*
Lamictal CD, 32*t*
Lamictal ODT, 32*t*
Lamictal XR, 32*t*
Lamisil, 45*t*
Lamisil AT, 77*t*

lamotrigine, 32*t*
Lanoxin, 38, 39*t*
lansoprazole, 56, 57*t*, 77*t*
large-volume parenteral (LVP) solutions, 211
Larissia, 69*t*
Lasix, 64, 65*t*
Latuda, 28*t*
lead time, 248
Lescol, 37*t*
Lescol XL, 37*t*
levalbuterol, 53*t*
Levaquin, 43*t*
levetiracetam, 32*t*
levigation, 201
Levitra, 66*t*
levocetirizine, 55*t*
levodopa/carbidopa, 31*t*
levofloxacin, 43*t*
levonorgestrel, 68–69, 69*t*, 77*t*
levothyroxine, 52*t*
Levoxyl, 52*t*
Lexapro, 26*t*
licensure, 3
lidocaine, 62*t*
Lidoderm, 62*t*
linaclotide, 56, 57*t*
linagliptin, 48*t*
linezolid, 44, 44*t*
Linzess, 56, 57*t*
liothyronine, 52*t*
lipids, 36
Lipitor, 37*t*
lisdexamfetamine, 30*t*
lisinopril, 34*t*
Lists of Licensed Biological Products with Reference Product Exclusivity and Biosimilarity or Interchangeability Evaluations, 144
lithium, 30, 32*t*
Lithobid, 30, 32*t*
Livalo, 37*t*
lixisenatide semaglutide, 48*t*
Loestrin 21, 69*t*
Loestrin Fe, 69*t*
Lomotil, 56, 58*t*
Lonhala Magnair, 53*t*
loop diuretics, 65*t*
Lo/Ovral 28, 69*t*
loperamide, 56, 58*t*, 77*t*
Lopid, 38
Lopressor, 34, 36*t*
loratadine, 55*t*, 76*t*
lorazepam, 24*t*
losartan, 35*t*
loss, 242
lot number, 160
Lotensin, 34*t*
lotion, 199
Lotrimin, 45*t*
Lotrimin AF, 77*t*
lovastatin, 37*t*
Lovaza, Vascepa, 38
Lovenox, 70, 71*t*
low-density lipoprotein (LDL), 36

Photo Credits

Cover © Shutterstock/topnatthapon

Preface pg. xi © iStock/sunnyfrog; pg. xii © Paradigm Education Solutions; pg. xiv © Paradigm Education Solutions; pg. xv © Paradigm Education Solutions

Introduction pg. 2 © Shutterstock/Dmitry Kalinovsky; pg. 8 © Shutterstock/Rawpixel.com

Chapter 1 pg. 50 © Shutterstock/Ondrej83; pg. 70 © iStockphoto/Eraxion; pg. 74 © Shutterstock/Tomas Nevesely; pg. 75 © Shutterstock/Keith Homan; pg. 82 © Shutterstock/MaraZe

Chapter 2 pg. 105 © Paradigm Education Solutions; pg. 106 © Paradigm Education Solutions; pg. 113 © Shutterstock

Chapter 3 pg. 120 © iStockphoto/sjlocke; pg. 126 © Marharyta Pavliuk; pg. 132 © Paradigm Education Solutions

Chapter 4 pg. 142 © Paradigm Education Solutions; pg. 150 © Paradigm Education Solutions; pg. 160 © Medical Packaging Inc.; pg. 162 © George Brainard; pg. 166 © Shutterstock/Draw

Chapter 5 pg. 171 © iStockphoto/Murat Sen; pg. 173 © Paradigm Education Solutions

Chapter 6 pg. 195 © George Brainard; pg. 198 © Paradigm Education Solutions; pg. 200 © George Brainard

Chapter 7 pg. 210 © Paradigm Education Solutions; pg. 228 © Paradigm Education Solutions; pg. 229 © Paradigm Education Solutions; pg. 231 Image Courtesy of Tova Wiegand Green

Chapter 8 pg. 250 © Shutterstock/Tyler Olson; pg. 252 © iStock/sjlocke